More Attention, Less Deficit

Success Strategies for Adults with ADHD

Ari Tuckman, PsyD, MBA

Specialty Press, Inc.
300 N.W. 70th Ave., Suite 102
Plantation, Florida 33317

Cover Design: Michael Wall, Kall Graphics
Layout: Babs Kall, Kall Graphics

Specialty Press, Inc.
300 Northwest 70th Avenue, Suite 102
Plantation, Florida 33317
(954) 792-8100 • (800) 233-9273

Printed in the United States of America

ISBN-13: 978-1-886941-74-8

ISBN-10: 1-886941-74-2

Library of Congress Cataloging-in-Publication Data

Tuckman, Ari.
More attention, less deficit : success strategies for adults with ADHD / Ari Tuckman.
p. cm.
ISBN 978-1-886941-74-8 (alk. paper)
1. Attention-deficit-disorder in adults. 2. Attention-deficit disorder in adults–Treatment. I. Title.

RC394.A85T834 2009

616.85'89–dc22

2009005972

What the experts are saying about this book!

More Attention, Less Deficit is outstanding. Written in a clear and easy-to-understand style, the book brings together a vast amount of information, ideas, suggestions, and research. Dr. Tuckman's energy and empathy sustain the book throughout. All adults with ADHD can benefit from this book, as well as all people who care about them. Superb!

Edward Hallowell, MD, author of various books
and founder of The Hallowell Centers in New York and Massachusetts

Dr. Tuckman has provided us with a richly detailed discussion of ADHD in adults and especially how it should be managed, directly written for the adult with ADHD in mind. Wonderfully supportive and informative, this book provides countless recommendations for addressing the myriad symptoms of poor self-control and time management, inattention and disorganization, and impulsive and careless behavior that afflicts nearly every major domain of life activities for adults. The book should prove enormously instructive for both adults with ADHD and for clinicians who specialize in its diagnosis and management.

Russell A. Barkley, PhD, Clinical Professor of Psychiatry
Medical University of South Carolina (Charleston)
And Research Professor of Psychiatry, SUNY Upstate Medical University (Syracuse)

More Attention, Less Deficit is a great "life manual" on how to live successfully with any, and all ADHD challenges. It is full of great strategies and helps the reader to understand the underlying issues so the strategies can truly stick. Dr. Tuckman's book is comprehensive, practical and easy to read—just what the adult with ADHD needs and wants!

Nancy A. Ratey, EdM, MCC, SCAC
Strategic Life Coach, Author, The Disorganized Mind

Dr. Tuckman has done a fantastic job at providing a virtual smorgasbord of information for adults with ADHD. By using the menu provided at the beginning of each chapter, the reader can select articles specific to their situation resulting in greater reader interest and satisfaction. I wholeheartedly recommend this book for all adults with ADHD. It's like getting an individualized consult with Dr. Tuckman!!

Patricia O. Quinn, MD
Director, The Center for Girls and Women with ADHD, Washington, DC
www.addvance.com

More Attention, Less Deficit is the new "Bible" of ADHD. Dr. Tuckman brilliantly maps out strategies and tips while peppering it with facts in a way that makes it interesting and easy for the adult with ADHD to devour in bite-sized pieces. A must-read for all who are touched by ADHD.

Terry Matlen, ACSW
Author of Survival Tips for Women with ADHD, *Director, www.addconsults.com*

Dr. Tuckman has given us a thorough compilation of science-based information on Adult ADHD that is down to earth, easy to understand, practical, and highly useful. This book provides the essential ingredients of hope, guidance, and knowledge for anyone who wants to understand and gain better control of this complex disorder.

Kevin Murphy, Ph.D. President, Adult ADHD Clinic of Central MA

This valuable book will help adults with AD/HD and those who care about them, have a greater understanding of the disorder—and more importantly—learn what to do about it. Written in a very user-friendly manner, the book can be read in any order the reader finds useful. Packed with strategies for successfully managing symptoms, adults with AD/HD will also find ways to come to terms with all that the disorder adds and subtracts in their lives. This is no small feat, believe me! An excellent resource from an author who really "gets" what it is like to have AD/HD.

Marie Paxson, President, CHADD (Children and Adults with Attention Deficit/ Hyperactivity Disorder);
Personal opinion as CHADD does not endorse publications.

This is the first book I have read where a healthcare professional has conveyed an accurate overview of the coaching process and how it fits into the whole, comprehensive picture of successful ADHD management. Dr. Tuckman's book represents an excellent educational resource, for not only understanding ADHD, but as a strong starting point to identify potential strategies which can powerfully enhance the treatment of ADHD.

David Giwerc, MCC, Founder & President, ADD Coach Academy
Former President of the Attention Deficit Disorder Association

As a follow up to his highly respected book for professionals, *Integrative Treatment for Adult ADHD,* Dr. Ari Tuckman has done a masterful job culling the scientific literature to design a user-friendly, comprehensive blueprint for living well with adult ADHD. *More Attention, Less Deficit* will be an invaluable resource for adults living with ADHD, their loved ones seeking to understand the disorder, and clinicians looking for tried and true coping strategies that will help their patients.

J. Russell Ramsay, Ph.D., Co-Director, Adult ADHD Treatment & Research Program,
University of Pennsylvania School of Medicine
Author of Cognitive Behavioral Therapy for Adult ADHD:
An Integrative Psychosocial and Medical Approach

Ari Tuckman offers an insightful, practical and most important user friendly guide for adults with ADHD. This book is chock full of great ideas and exceptional strategies. Most importantly, Tuckman provides a reasoned and reasonable appreciation of ADHD, an essential foundation to help those with the condition find the strength and motivation to take charge of their condition.

Sam Goldstein, Ph.D., Co-Author Clinician's Guide to Adult ADHD

Dedication

For Bailey, my little love.
Somehow I managed to write this book
despite the sleep deprivation.
Hopefully we'll sell enough copies
to pay for all the coffee.

Table of Contents

Acknowledgments

would like to acknowledge a number of people who contributed to making this the best book it could be. First, I'd like to thank Jenneane Jansen, Sandy Wolofsky, and Hernan Visani for pushing me to come up with a great title (and rejecting my crummy ones). Jenneane also helped me polish up the article on the Americans with Disabilities Act. I'd also like to thank Barbara Luther, David Giwerc, and Rory Stern for helping me refine my thoughts on the difference between coaching and therapy. Roberto Olivardia provided information for the article on the connection between ADHD and eating disorders. It's nice to have friends and colleagues to lean on!

I would like to thank the researchers who get into the nitty-gritties of ADHD and give the rest of us the solid information that we need to improve the lives of our clients, patients, students, loved ones, and ourselves. I would also like to thank all my clients, support group attendees, and audience members at presentations who've shared their experiences and taught me so much.

Finally, I'd like to thank my wife, Heather, for putting up with all the time that I spent writing. I swear I don't have ideas for any other books. Well, maybe just one...

Other Books by Ari Tuckman

Integrative Treatment for Adult ADHD: A Practical, Easy-to-Use Guide for Clinicians (2007). New Harbinger Publications.

How to Read This Book

Any way you want, that's how! It's yours; you can do whatever you want with it. Mark it up. Highlight stuff. Scribble in the margins. Dog-ear the pages. Yell at it. Stick it under someone else's nose to prove a point or help her understand you better. Books are meant to be actively used, not worshiped.

When I was thinking about writing this book, I kept coming back to one question:

Why are none of the books about adults with ADHD written for readers with ADHD?

It's kind of a strange question to ask, but it really seems to be true. Whenever I ask a new adult ADHD client whether he has read any of the available books, I almost always get something along the lines of "Well, I started a couple, but I didn't finish any of them."

Since most readers will read only parts of this book, I designed it in such a way that it's easy to find what you want and jump around. You can flip to any page and read just a few pages that will make sense all by themselves. Here's the structure:

4 Sections General groupings of material.

17 Chapters More specific groupings of material.

189 Articles 1 to 5 pages on a particular topic.

Each article can easily stand alone, so you don't need to read everything (or anything) that came before in order to get something out of it. If you're only up for reading for a few minutes, you can read an article or two and not feel like you're leaving in the middle of something. And definitely don't feel guilty about it!

To make it easier to keep track of which articles you have already read, you can tear off the bottom corner of the page so you don't waste your time rereading when you don't want to.

You may also find it helpful to subscribe to the podcast version of this book, to reinforce what you're reading. You can find more information at www.adultADHDbook.com.

What Makes This Book Different?

There are quite a few books out there about ADHD in adults. Why should you spend your precious dollars and time on this one? In my obviously biased opinion, this book is better in a number of important ways:

- *An ADHD-friendly structure.* This book is a collection of articles, each on a particular topic. It's organized in a way to make it easy to find exactly what you want. Most adults with ADHD do not read books straight through, so I purposely wrote this book to cater to that tendency to jump around and not make it to the end. So jump around!
- *Reader-friendly article summaries.* Each chapter begins with an introduction and the main points contained in each article to help you decide which articles are most relevant to your situation and thereby worth reading. These summaries can also help you remember better by cueing you what to focus on.
- *A unique feature.* The lower corner of each page is perforated to make it easy to tear off the corner to indicate that you have already read a particular article. This is helpful if you want to read the book out of order (and you probably will).
- *Rock solid information.* Although my goal is to make this book highly useful, I base most of it on what research has found. The rest of it comes from my decade of treating ADHD adults, running a support group, and hundred-and-something presentations. Information that is factually accurate tends to be most useful.
- *Accompanying podcast.* I will be doing a free weekly podcast where I read portions of the book, so you can learn in more than one way. You can find more information at: www.adultADHDbook.com

Introduction: A Million Things to Make Your Life Better

Whenever I meet a new client with ADHD, I always feel compelled to tell her a million things that can help her understand her ADHD and enjoy life more. This book is those million things. It's everything I want to tell new clients and audiences at presentations. It's incredibly interesting and extremely important. This is the kind of information that can change your life. Yes, I will be that bold to say that it can change your life. It won't change everything, but it can change a lot. You will do some things differently, and you will feel different about some of the things that stay the same. Knowledge has that kind of power.

As I was writing this book, I kept coming back to the idea that life is different after being diagnosed with ADHD. ADHD can make your life really difficult—before you know what's tripping you up. Once you know it's ADHD, life gets much easier. Then you know what you're wrestling with and can start to get a hold of it. Then it becomes a fair fight.

The goal here is merely to tilt the odds of success, to make you more likely to do the right thing at the right time. Not all the time, but most of the time. Not perfect, but better. ADHD takes away your ability to be consistent, so the information and strategies in this book are here to give you back some of that consistency.

It's odd that ADHD is still more thought of as a childhood disorder, since there are actually more adults with ADHD than children. This is mostly a quirk of the math, because there are approximately three times as many adults as there are children in the United States (U.S. Census, 2000). But the fact remains that current estimates suggest that there are eight million adults with ADHD in the United States and only two to three million children (Ramsay and Rostain, 2007). Besides, where do you think all those ADHD kids came from?

Unfortunately, only a few of these adults have been diagnosed and are receiving appropriate treatment. The National Comorbidity Study found that only 10 percent of adults with ADHD had received treatment within the prior twelve months (Biederman, Spencer, Wilens, Prince, and Faraone, 2006). Even if that estimate is pretty far off, it still makes for a lot of people working harder than they should have to. I hope that this book will help you work a little less but have more to show for it.

What We Cover—and How We Cover It

I've broken the chapters in this book into four sections:

I. Understanding ADHD in Adults

II. Start with Effective Treatment

III. Build the Necessary Skills

IV. Improve Specific Areas of Your Life

The material progresses step by step from basic information about ADHD to practical day-to-day strategies. Section I lays the foundation, section II tells you about the professionals who could be helpful to you, and sections III and IV give you a ton of strategies you can use.

I'm a psychologist in private practice. People come to me for information about ADHD, so I need to know my stuff. But my clients don't want grad school lectures—they want strategies to make their lives better. Balancing these two needs has given me the two guiding principles for writing this book:

1. *Scientifically accurate.* The information I present comes from research and clinical experience. Accurate information is more helpful.
2. *Totally practical.* You're not reading this book because you think ADHD is interesting. You want practical strategies to make your life better.

I found that there weren't enough books that struck the right balance between these two goals. Some of them contained too much information that I was skeptical about, whereas the academic books don't explain to readers how to apply the information in daily life. So this is the book that Goldilocks would pick—not too fluffy, not too dense, but just right.

Section I

UNDERSTANDING ADHD IN ADULTS

Introduction: Knowledge Is Power

The more you know about ADHD, the better off you will be—not just knowing the obvious stuff, but really understanding why your brain does what it does (and sometimes doesn't do). This will set you up for success in a way that you just can't achieve without fully understanding your ADHD. Before you learned about your ADHD, you pretty much had to figure out the hard way what worked best for you. This also meant finding lots of jobs, relationships, and strategies that *didn't* work for you. Instead, by looking at your life through the lens of ADHD, you can explain all sorts of things that happened in your past, as well as create new approaches to make a better future. This is big.

It's easy to explain away ADHD-based behaviors as something that people should be able to control. If so, then they should feel badly about themselves if they don't control it. Of course, this raises the obvious question: *Why in the world would someone bring himself so much trouble if he could possibly avoid it?* It just doesn't make any sense. Unfortunately, if you buy into the idea that you should be able to control these behaviors simply through desire and willpower, you won't get very far—you probably bought this book because you've figured that out the hard way. Desire and willpower aren't enough if you don't have a solid understanding of ADHD—how it affects you and what you can do about it. Let's talk about both of these, because they're equally important.

Learning that you have ADHD gives you a better explanation for why you do what you do (or don't do). It gives you an explanation that you don't have to feel bad about. This may be a trivial example, but it works: I have bad eyes, so I have to wear glasses. It's a hassle, but I do it because it's better than driving into other cars. But I don't feel bad about myself for having bad eyes, and I certainly don't blame myself for it. No one asks me to try harder to see well. So how are bad eyes any different from ADHD brain wiring? Both are caused by factors beyond one's control. Both require adjustments in how one does things. Obviously, ADHD's impacts are far greater than just having to wear glasses, but as for how it should affect how you feel about yourself, it should be no different. It's a lot easier to feel good about yourself if you know that it's a brain wiring issue that causes your difficulties, rather than a moral failing. This also sets you up to be more likely to make the necessary adjustments to improve your life.

In addition to these self-esteem gains from explaining your difficulties as being brain based, it also helps you predict which strategies are going to be most effective. This is crucial. Rather than having to haphazardly try every suggestion someone gives you or that you read in a magazine, you can pick from a short list of strategies that are likely to work for someone with ADHD. You don't need to reinvent the wheel, because others have already figured lots of these things out. With this understanding and these strategies, all sorts of options open up that weren't present before. Now you can get traction from that effort and really get somewhere.

Of course, since ADHD tends to not be invisible, your family and friends may have noticed some of these things about you, too. You will probably want some better explanations for them as well, even if you don't tell them that you have ADHD. The more you know about ADHD in general and your own strengths and weaknesses in particular, the better you can explain some of these things to them. That may take some of the heat out of your arguments and enable you all to work better together.

This book isn't a bunch of empty claims about being able to do anything you put your mind to or a collection of inspirational sayings that raise you up, only to fall flat. This is scientific research and clinical experience applied to your daily life. The more you learn about ADHD, the more you will realize that it fits for you. It will explain a lot. The more you use these solid, ADHD-based strategies, the more successful you will be. No one can take those successes away from you. It's not just pretty words, it's actual successes. *That* is why knowledge is power.

What This Section Covers

To give you that foundation of knowledge, this section includes the following chapters:

1. *Executive Functions: It All Flows from Here* (p. 5) We use executive functions to stay on top of the various demands in our complicated lives. Research is finding that people with ADHD have certain information-processing weaknesses that interfere with their ability to perform at their best. Understanding how this works will explain a lot of the difficulties you've had, as well as offer suggestions for ways to do better.

2. *Diagnosing ADHD: Accurate Diagnosis Guides Effective Treatment* (p. 21) There are several ways to diagnose ADHD, some of which are more reliable than others. It's important to get the diagnosis right, though, if you want to have the best chance of improvement. We will cover all the various diagnostic issues, from who can do it to what other conditions can cloud the picture.

3. *The ADHD Brain: Wired a Little Differently* (p. 58) ADHD is absolutely a brain-based disorder. Although it can lead to psychological effects, it is neurologically based. We will cover the basics of the brain areas involved as well as the causes.

4. *ADHD Affects Everything: No Wonder My Life Was So Hard!* (p. 65) Research clearly shows what adults with ADHD already know—life is harder with undiagnosed and untreated ADHD. We will cover all the various ways that ADHD can affect someone's life.

This may be more information than you need, at least right now, but you may find that you come back to it later. I would rather give you extra than have you wish for more. If you can absorb these chapters, or even most of them, you will be in great shape to really understand what comes in the rest of the book.

CHAPTER 1

EXECUTIVE FUNCTIONS: IT ALL FLOWS FROM HERE

ADHD involves far more than merely not enough attention or too much hyperactivity. It affects many aspects of how you process information and manage the demands in your life. This chapter covers *executive functions*, our highest-level brain processes that enable us to make good decisions in a complex world. Research is increasingly finding that people with ADHD display specific weaknesses in certain executive functions. This explains why people with ADHD tend to have the particular struggles that they do—and also why they don't have other struggles.

This is why I chose to start the book with a chapter on executive functions, rather than the obvious choice of beginning with getting diagnosed (that comes second). If you understand how executive functions operate, everything else in this book and about ADHD makes perfect sense. It explains

- all the difficulties that people with ADHD face in various parts of their lives, as well as the areas where they don't have trouble;
- why certain time-management and organizational strategies tend to work well for people with ADHD, whereas others don't; and
- why some treatments are effective for ADHD, whereas others aren't.

This unifying framework not only explains why your past looks the way it does but also offers some promise for making the future look better. This foundation means that you don't need to reinvent the wheel every time you're faced with a new challenge, since you already know how your brain tends to operate. This makes life much easier.

This chapter includes a series of related articles on the topic of executive functions. Since most adults with ADHD struggle with reading books cover to cover, I've included summaries here so that you can choose the articles that are most helpful to you or most relevant right now.

Executive Functioning: Who's Calling the Shots Around Here, Anyway? (p. 7) The executive functions are our highest-level brain processes. They enable us to make good decisions in a complex world. Research is increasingly explaining ADHD struggles as deriving from executive-functioning weaknesses.

Response Inhibition: It Starts with Stopping (p. 8) The key to successful decision making is that tiny little pause where we think through our options and make a good choice. People with ADHD have difficulty creating this pause and therefore get distracted, forget things, and leap without looking.

Working Memory: The Brain's RAM (p. 9) We use working memory constantly to hold information in mind as we remember what just happened, relate it to long-term memories, and think ahead into the future. People with ADHD tend to have blinky working memories, which leads to a variety of problems in their daily lives.

Sense of Time: It Can't Be 5:00 Already! (p. 11) People with ADHD have difficulty monitoring the passage of time and planning accordingly, a skill that's really important in today's busy world. As a result, they tend to spend too long on some activities and not plan enough time for others. This contributes to their well-known time-management problems.

Remembering to Remember: It's All About Timing (p. 12) In our busy lives, we all have dozens of little (and not so little) things to remember to do over the course of a day, such as phone calls and appointments. People with ADHD have great difficulty reminding themselves of these tasks at the right time, often forgetting completely or remembering only when it's too late.

Emotional Self-Control: Having Feelings Without Acting on Them (p. 13) People with ADHD tend to express their feelings more strongly than others do and are more influenced by their feelings than other people are. This also affects their ability to see beyond their emotions and to take others' perspectives into account.

Self-Activation: Getting That Heavy Ball Rolling (p. 14) Everybody has to use a certain amount of force of will to get going on boring tasks, but people with ADHD have a much steeper hill to climb. As a result, they tend to procrastinate until the pressure of a looming deadline pushes them into action.

Persistence of Effort: The Little Engine That Sometimes Could (p. 16) Once someone with ADHD gets going on something, there's the second challenge of sticking with it all the way through. Unfortunately, most of our daily obligations don't give partial credit for tasks that are mostly done.

Hindsight and Forethought: Using the Past and Future to Guide the Present (p. 17) We use the lessons from past experiences to make better choices the next time around. People with ADHD have a hard time stopping long enough to remember those lessons and apply them forward, so they're more likely to make the same mistakes.

Executive Functioning: Who's Calling the Shots Around Here, Anyway?

There is growing consensus among researchers that ADHD involves weaknesses in *executive functions*, a broad range of high-level information-processing functions that are crucial to success in life, especially as an adult. Rather than respond automatically and thoughtlessly to whatever the environment throws at us (like amoebas do), we use executive functions to modify our behavior for a better outcome, to maximize future gains, even at the price of losing out in the short term. This can mean forgoing something enjoyable in the moment (like a fat piece of chocolate cake) or pushing ourselves to endure something boring but important (like studying for a test). We could almost say that the executive functions enable us to see beyond the current moment by bringing back the lessons from the past and bringing forward the goals of the future to better guide our behavior. Executive functions enable us to resist distractions and temptations to go for the greater gain.

Although we can intentionally choose to approach situations in certain ways, many of the executive functions operate without conscious awareness, like breathing. If you watch little kids talking themselves through a difficult task, they are sort of verbalizing their executive functions—for example, "one step at a time," "slow down," "don't look over there." Eventually it becomes automatic and we don't have to think about it as much, but we may still find that we talk ourselves through challenges sometimes.

Different researchers have created somewhat different lists of executive functions. I've found that Russell Barkley's *response inhibition theory* is the most thorough and useful of these, so most of what I talk about in this chapter is an outgrowth of his work. His theory is incredibly detailed and impressive but contains far more information than most nonclinicians need to know. So I've pulled out the aspects that are most useful for your daily life—the parts that not only explain why some things are so hard for you but also set the stage for the rest of the book to offer helpful strategies. Even though I talk about specific executive functions, keep in mind that they interact constantly and the lines between them can be pretty blurry.

In case you're interested in the details, Barkley breaks the executive functions into four connected types: nonverbal working memory; verbal working memory; self-regulation of affect, motivation, and arousal; and reconstitution (planning). There's a lot to the executive functions, but the details are less important in terms of your day-to-day life.

As you will see in the rest of this chapter, the executive functions give rise to all sorts of important abilities, some of which I'll talk about in detail. And as you probably know far too well, a significant price is paid by people who are weak in these various skills. Life as an adult in this society is complicated, so those who have weak executive functions will struggle and stand out. They will have trouble managing all the details of life and making "responsible" choices (i.e., ones that benefit the future more than the present). As a result, many adults with untreated ADHD are seen as irresponsible or immature because they tend to react too much in the moment and lose sight of the bigger picture. Society expects and forgives this of children, but not of adults. As a result of these difficulties with managing the thousand and one details of daily life, people with ADHD spend a lot of time scrambling to hold it all together and prevent disaster. It takes a lot more energy to put out fires than to prevent them. This reactive lifestyle is much more stressful than the one led by adults without ADHD.

We expect adults to be able to show self-control and not need as much direction from others. Because people with ADHD struggle with making themselves do the right thing at the right time, parents and romantic partners often step in to provide these executive functions to keep their loved one from going too far off the rails—for example, by reminding her about upcoming appointments, organizing her stuff, or stopping impulsive purchases. Alternatively, she may find tools that can do the job for her—for example, setting up automatic debits to eliminate having to remember to send out the bills or using a PDA to remind her of upcoming meetings.

Spend some time on this chapter and maybe even come back to it later. I think you will find that it explains a lot.

Response Inhibition: It Starts with Stopping

What makes ADHD *ADHD* rather than Asperger's syndrome or whatever? Russell Barkley, Ph.D., indisputably the top ADHD expert in the world, has created the *response inhibition theory* to explain why ADHD people have certain typical weaknesses, yet don't have other weaknesses. This sophisticated theory places primary emphasis on response inhibition—that is, the ability to hold back a response.

Barkley proposes that our executive functions can work only when they have a space to work in. Unlike simpler life forms that respond automatically to stimuli from the environment, humans are able to pause and think through the various response options and then choose the best one. This may ultimately lead to choosing a larger payoff in the future instead of a smaller payoff in the moment (also known as *delay of gratification*). But what we're talking about here is much more fundamental than consciously deciding to resist impulse buys. It's an almost invisible information processing that happens in a split second. An example is almost subconsciously deciding to ignore the sound of someone dropping a pen while you're working at your computer (i.e., not getting distracted), or holding your thought to what someone is saying until she finishes talking (i.e., not impulsively interrupting).

This explains why people with ADHD don't always do what they know they should—they have trouble filtering out external and internal stimuli, so they react to the "wrong" thing. An example is getting lost in a magazine rather than paying the bills sitting next to it. This can look like bad judgment, but what really happens is that these other stimuli have too big an impact on the ADHD person's decision making, so a less-than-optimal choice is made. It isn't bad judgment because he didn't stop long enough to judge. This is why those dreaded questions of "why did/didn't you..." lead to such unconvincing answers along the lines of "I don't know. I just didn't think of it," which is actually pretty accurate. Their brains didn't stop long enough to get a chance to think about it.

Because people with ADHD tend to be so vulnerable to external and internal stimuli, many of the strategies to help them be more effective focus on increasing the strength of the desired stimuli or decreasing the strength of less desired stimuli so that they do the right thing in that moment. For example, a beeping PDA that tells the person to leave for a meeting overrides the focus on what else he was doing. Medications (and possibly neurofeedback) work directly by increasing the brain's ability to create that delay, thereby reversing the fallout that comes from an insufficient delay. This is also why admonitions to "just try harder" don't work—they ignore the fundamental problem that people with ADHD have trouble creating that moment of pause to try harder in. It's like telling someone who needs glasses that she just needs to try harder to see.

As you read about the rest of the executive functions in this chapter, remember this delay, because this is the tripping point for many executive functioning malfunctions.

Working Memory: The Brain's RAM

Even though we often talk of memory as if there were only one kind, we actually have many kinds of memory. People with ADHD sometimes complain that they don't remember well. (And their family members probably complain more!) This is somewhat true, but not completely. Their *long-term memory* is fine—for example, Columbus discovered America in 1492 or my third-grade teacher was Mrs. Phillips. Although ADHD folks may get distracted at times when trying to remember this information, their memories actually work well. (For more on long-term memory, see *The Fundamentals of Memory* on p. 237.)

Where they run into trouble is in getting information into that long-term memory—if something never gets into long-term memory, then there is nothing there to remember, so it isn't really a memory problem at that point. Where things break down is in the *working memory*, which is the part of memory that holds information in the moment as it is being processed. We use working memory whenever we do anything that involves integrating two or more pieces of information. Here are examples:

- Integrating two or more things that happen close together in time, such as tracking the things that are said in a conversation or following events in an article or book
- Connecting a new piece of information with something from long-term memory, such as considering how a new task will fit into an existing schedule
- Holding some pieces of information while simultaneously paying attention to others, like keeping in mind that you need to change the laundry while you stop to answer a child's question

We use working memory constantly and in almost every aspect of daily life. If a person's working memory tends to blink and drop pieces of information, all sorts of problems occur, as you may know far too well. So, even if the rest of your brain works great and you are absolutely brilliant, a weak working memory will limit your ability to perform to your potential (something else you may know too well).

To use a computer analogy, long-term memory is like the hard drive and working memory is like the RAM. So ADHD folks' hard drives work well, but their RAM is kind of glitchy. Just as when you try to do too many things at once on your computer and a program crashes, ADHD people are prone to working-memory dumps where something important gets pushed out by something new. For example, while walking back to your desk to get some information for your boss, your cell phone rings and your attention goes to that, so your boss's request gets pushed out the back. If you're lucky, some bits and pieces got recorded into your long-term memory, so you may remember it later, especially if reminded by something else. So you get back to your desk and see the paperwork that your boss wanted and suddenly remember her request. Other times the memory is completely gone, so even a lie detector wouldn't pick anything up when your boss asks why you didn't get her the information. (What information? You didn't ask for any information.) It's easy to get the feeling that other people enjoy making things up if you have no memory of things that others swear happened. This also makes for all sorts of fun arguments.

Another example of a working-memory blank is forgetting where you put your keys down the instant that they leave your fingers, making it impossible to remember when looking for them the next day.

One outgrowth of a blinky working memory is that many people with ADHD learn better by doing something than by reading or hearing about it. This is because actively engaging in a task requires less working memory than remembering what one was told, picturing oneself doing the task, and then applying it later.

An unreliable working memory explains some of the distractibility, impulsive decision making, not listening, and poor use of time that plague many with ADHD—and frustrate their family members. But since so much of our thinking is based on our working memories, other more complicated problems can develop. For example, someone with ADHD may know that he should live within some budget constraints, but when faced with a tempting purchase, he may not be able to call to mind his entire weekly or monthly budget to see how this purchase fits into the bigger picture. So he spends the money, only to realize later that he forgot about some upcoming expenses and won't have enough money. Many of these processing problems look like bad judgment or foolhardiness, but it's really that the person has lost some of the relevant information from his mental calculations and therefore makes a flawed decision based on partial information.

Because these problems are based in working-memory glitches, judgmental lectures won't help the person make a different decision next time (but *will* help the person feel bad about himself and/or resent the lecturer). The second half of this book is packed with techniques that take these processing problems into account and are therefore more likely to help you be successful. So stay tuned; it does get better.

Sense of Time: It Can't Be 5:00 Already!

We all have an internal clock that tells us how much time has passed. For some people, this clock ticks loudly and consistently, and they're pretty good at judging the passage of time and knowing when to go on to something else, like going to a work meeting or getting into bed. They have a loose schedule in mind and they know where they are in relation to that schedule—what they have left to do and how much time they have to do it. For ADHD folks, the clock ticks too softly, so it doesn't guide their behavior reliably enough. As a result, they may stay absorbed in fun activities when they should really transition to more obligatory, less fun activities. This can even spill over into obligations, like picking up the kids at school, a situation that causes great anguish for all involved.

Besides the fact that their internal alarm clocks don't go off, they aren't good at predicting how long things will take. When planning ahead, they may use "best-case-scenario planning," basing predictions on everything falling into place perfectly without unexpected detours or delays. Of course, rarely does it work out this well, so they tend to run over their deadlines or show up late. (Some of this is also based in difficulties with getting going on things until the pressure of the last minute drives them into action, which is covered further in *Self-Activation* on p. 14.)

Once people with ADHD start something, time can still be really flexible. When doing something boring, like vacuuming or paperwork, time slows to a crawl and what feels like an hour may be as little as ten minutes (which is a horrible realization). So it takes a real force of will to spend as much time on that boring activity as they had hoped to. On the other hand, when doing something fun, an hour can feel like ten minutes, so they may spend too much time on it. In both cases, they may not get as much done as they had planned.

This sense of time is extremely important in today's society, not just at work but also with family and friends. Almost all parts of life require planning, forethought, and otherwise remembering what needs doing and, just as important, *when* it needs to be done. ADHD adults usually know what they need to do but have trouble doing it at the best times. Probably one of the most common and problematic examples of this is getting into bed on time each night. Assuming you have a specific bedtime, it takes a fair bit of planning, monitoring the passage of time, and making adjustments to climb into bed at the designated time and with everything done. Most ADHD adults fall victim to at least one of the many landmines as they make their way through the night's various activities. In fact, getting into bed on time requires that a lot of things go right, so we can almost say that being able to consistently hit your bedtime is a good sign that you're doing well overall. For more information on this specific topic, see *Actually Get a Good Night's Sleep* on p. 300.

Remembering to Remember: It's All About Timing

Related to the prior article, *Sense of Time*, another ability that is crucial these days is *prospective memory*, which is the ability to remember to remember. It's the capacity to remind yourself to do the right thing at the right time. Not an hour before or an hour after (those don't usually count for much, unfortunately), but right on time. Examples are "I need to call that guy after I check my email," and "I have a report due at work at the end of the week." It could even be something like remembering to bring an umbrella with you when you leave the house—remembering before you pass the umbrella doesn't help much, and remembering after you left really doesn't help much. It all comes down to remembering at exactly the right moment as you get ready to leave. We all have dozens of these sorts of tasks to keep track of every day. I would go so far as to say that one reason electronic organizers are so popular is that our brains can't handle all the information we're trying to store, so we use electronic brains to do some of that work for us.

For many people with ADHD, this is where good intentions come to die—they have trouble holding the thought from the moment that they think of it until the moment when it's the time to act. They have trouble bridging that gap in time, of carrying that thought reliably into the future.

Let's be clear, though, about a really important distinction. This forgetfulness is fundamentally different from situations in which someone consciously decides that she won't do something. When the situation is due to a failure to remember, the task doesn't even enter consciousness for a decision to be made—and that's the key difference. On these occasions, the ADHD person may be as surprised and disappointed as everyone else that the task wasn't completed.

Of course, most people expect our words and actions to line up, so they eventually run out of patience and stop believing that the ADHD person simply forgot to do what he said he would. This is especially true when the promised task is boring or difficult. Instead, they may peg the person as irresponsible or selfish—and a liar, to boot. For the ADHD person, this can add insult to injury, because he is forced to deal with both the practical consequences of the forgetfulness, such as a late fee on the electric bill, and the social fallout, such as his girlfriend becoming upset with him (again). Unfortunately, even the most trusting people eventually stop believing the promises. Most people use their own experience to understand why other people do what they do, so someone who has a pretty decent memory will assume that the ADHD person purposely chose to not do something, since that would be the reason that the non-ADHD person didn't do something. Of course, in this case that reasoning may be wrong.

In fact, when doing an ADHD evaluation, I ask about times when the person forgets and pays a price for it. This is fundamentally different from the times that he might have something to gain from supposedly forgetting. He should have no incentive to forget something that then comes back to bite him.

Emotional Self-Control: Having Feelings Without Acting on Them

Although it isn't part of the official diagnostic system, people with ADHD are often known for their strong reactions. And not just anger—every feeling may be more intense. It's sometimes said that people with ADHD are more spontaneous than others. I think what this is referring to is that people with ADHD are more likely to be guided by their strong feelings, whereas others may stop and think for a moment before acting. (By the way, it's labeled "spontaneous" if it works out well, and "impulsive" or "irresponsible" or worse if it doesn't.) For example, I had a client who would get excited about things, like taking a trip, and start talking about the trip as if it were a done deal. His kids would of course get excited about it, only to be disappointed later when it turned out that they couldn't take the trip. He would get excited about things and let that show, without stopping to think about the effect that it would have on others who got caught up in his excitement. They would be equally surprised when that excitement would quickly fade and he would forget about the potential trip that they were still fantasizing about.

By contrast, adults without ADHD are more likely to display a diluted version of their initial feelings. They're more likely to hold back that initial response and temper what they express rather than show their feelings at full strength. They may have strong feelings, but they tend to consider the larger situation before expressing them—they still have them but don't act on them as much.

The ability to create this pause is important because it gives us objectivity when we can see beyond our own initial reaction and change how much the feeling colors our thoughts and affects our actions. For example, we may get angry at our boss but remember that we need a steady paycheck, so we don't tell him how we really feel, even if he deserves it. Adults are expected to be able to pause long enough to talk themselves down from their initial feeling and talk themselves out of acting rashly. By contrast, adults with ADHD are more prone to letting their initial feelings guide their behavior without considering this bigger context.

In addition, being able to view our feelings with objectivity gives us the ability to see someone else's perspective even when it differs from our own. We're able to set our feelings aside and see that someone else may feel differently about the same situation. As with anyone who gets caught up in the moment, adults with ADHD will have trouble with this, at least in the heat of the moment. They may see it more clearly afterward when things have cooled off, but it may be too late by then. This is one of the reasons that adults with ADHD are sometimes perceived as self-centered. It isn't really that they think only of themselves; it's just that they sometimes have a hard time seeing beyond their feelings in the moment to be able to appreciate another person's needs. Unfortunately, apologies afterward aren't always enough to mend fences.

Finally, being able to exert at least some control over our feelings leads to motivation to start and stick with tasks and get things done. By focusing on the rewards for a job well done or some enjoyable aspect of the task, we create the appropriate feelings within ourselves when the task itself doesn't motivate us. This is discussed further in the next two articles, *Self-Activation* and *Persistence of Effort*.

Self-Activation: Getting That Heavy Ball Rolling

When we're kids, the various adults in our lives help us get going on tasks such as doing homework, getting dressed, and doing chores. You know, all the boring stuff that we don't really want to do. As adults, we're expected to get ourselves going—and people assume all sorts of negative character traits for those who can't get themselves going reliably—lazy, self-indulgent, or irresponsible. (Any of these sound familiar?) Unfortunately, ADHD folks have two strikes against them on these matters. The first, as described in the article *Remembering to Remember*, is the not-so-simple act of remembering what needs to be done. But assuming that the person is aware of the task, she needs to make a choice to do it.

Two things determine whether someone will get going on something—external pressure and internal pressure. *External pressure* comes from the world around us. A report that is due tomorrow has much more external pressure than one that is due in a month. A boss who is breathing down your neck creates greater external pressure than a boss who says nothing. Everyone is more likely to start tasks with high external pressure.

Internal pressure is motivation that comes from within us. It's easy to get going on things that we enjoy. The trick is firing up that internal pressure for things that aren't fun. Some people have lots of internal pressure and get going on things long before they're due. This is mostly a good thing but can be problematic if someone takes it too far, for example by stressing out and slaving away on that report for the entire month, even past the point of diminishing returns. So, more isn't always better. Especially for boring tasks, people with ADHD have a hard time mustering up that internal pressure. They may think about it occasionally, but they just won't hit that magic threshold where they can get themselves going.

Since people with ADHD aren't as good at generating that internal pressure, they are more dependent on external pressure. This is why they procrastinate. That last-minute pressure gets them going and provides the focus that their weak internal pressure just can't. Of course, as you probably know well, this procrastination tends to drive non-ADHD people crazy because they can't understand it. Their internal pressure builds as the deadline approaches and nothing is being done, so to make themselves feel less anxious, they begin applying external pressure upon the ADHD person, even though it's probably not appreciated. Not that it makes it any less annoying at the time, but try to remember that the person isn't trying to control you, he's just trying to make himself feel less anxious. At its worst, the non-ADHD person just does the task himself, resenting that the responsibility fell to him, even if he took it upon himself.

To make matters worse, the non-ADHD person sees the ADHD person self-activate pretty easily for enjoyable things but not for boring things. The non-ADHD person therefore might see it as a matter of choice and become resentful about having to pick up the slack on the boring jobs. This is where those negative assumptions about character traits come in. The thing is, for people with ADHD, this is usually more about brain-based low internal pressure than it is about character. We'll talk more about how to prevent and clean up some of these messy assumptions in chapter 15, *Relationships and Friendships: Strive for Balance*. Someone with

ADHD may also avoid dealing with a situation that she feels pessimistic about. As a result, there is a feedback loop where past failures fuel current doubts and reduced effort. So ADHD struggles in the past also contribute to current avoidance.

Persistence of Effort: The Little Engine That Sometimes Could

As discussed in the previous article, *Self-Activation*, getting going can be hard enough, but keeping going can be just as hard. There are two possible reasons for this difficulty with *persistence of effort*, depending on the situation:

- *Distractibility.* Sometimes it's a simple matter of getting interrupted or distracted by something else, so the person never returns to finish the first activity, even if she intends to.
- *Boredom.* Whereas some people take great pleasure in completing something, this doesn't do much for many ADHD people. They get something mostly finished, then lose interest. They've figured it out, the challenge is gone, and it no longer lights their fire, so it falls by the wayside. Even if they know they should just go through the motions to finish something, it can feel almost impossible to force themselves to bring something to completion. Repetition can be deadly.

Of course, this mostly applies to boring activities, because fun things are easy. It's kind of like riding a bike downhill—it doesn't take much effort. But it takes effort to force yourself to do something you find uninteresting, just as it takes effort to ride a bike uphill. Of course, this is true for everyone. It's just that for people with ADHD, that hill is much steeper on the boring stuff, so it takes a much greater force of will to stick to it all the way through. This means that ADHD folks get more mentally tired from doing boring jobs and are therefore more likely to take a break sooner. Meanwhile, those fun distractions have much steeper downhills, so it's easy to take a detour rather than trudge ahead.

For people with ADHD, the difference between the downhills and the uphills is much greater than it is for people without ADHD. Unfortunately, a lot of the family members, friends, and coworkers of people with ADHD often don't understand this and take the attitude that the ADHD person should "just bite the bullet and get it done," not realizing that it isn't that easy. If it was, they would just do it. As discussed in the previous article, *Self-Activation*, since their ability to self-generate motivation is weak, external pressure helps those with ADHD not only start something but also push themselves through to the end. By analogy, you'll probably pedal harder up the hill if a big dog is chasing you.

Success in life often requires the ability to complete all sorts of uninteresting tasks on a pretty regular basis. If this is hard for you, it can affect every area of your life: school, work, finances, family, and friends. Unfortunately, life rarely gives partial credit for things that are only partially done.

The irony, of course, is that most of these activities aren't really that hard, in and of themselves. It's not like people with ADHD don't have the skills to handle these tasks. For example, doing laundry, paying bills, and filing papers aren't inherently difficult—fighting the boredom is the hard part. Before a diagnosis, though, it can lead to accusations from oneself or others that these activities are easy, so the person should just do it. I had a client who had a really hard time getting all the groceries put away. After probably spending too long at the store and getting behind schedule on other things, it was all she could do to get the groceries into the kitchen and throw the perishables into the fridge. It would make her husband nuts to find the counters piled high with full bags. He would get on her about it, wondering why she couldn't just spend a final five minutes and get them all put away, since it's not like she didn't know where everything went. Unfortunately, it's more complicated than that.

Hindsight and Forethought: Using the Past and Future to Guide the Present

With age comes wisdom (usually). After going through an experience once or twice, ideally we learn something that will make the next time better. The struggle for most people with ADHD is to apply that wisdom in the heat of the moment. If you were to ask them beforehand how to best handle a particular situation, they could tell you. If you were to ask them afterward, they can tell you how they could have handled it better. Unfortunately, this knowledge doesn't translate reliably enough into doing the right thing at the right time.

The snag occurs when they aren't able to use their hindsight (a.k.a. wisdom) to guide their actions in the moment. The reason is that we need to stop for a moment to think before acting in order to have time to bring back the lessons of those past experiences. This is that crucial pause I was talking about in *Response Inhibition* on p. 8. For too many people with ADHD, they've already leaped before looking and only afterward realize that they're in trouble. As a result, they're often in a position of having to explain why they did something that even they know wasn't such a good idea—why they bought something from the telemarketer without getting all the details, and why they used a butter knife to pry the lid off the paint can. The problem is that there are no good explanations, since they know they made a bad decision. This leaves them with "I don't know. I just didn't think about it," which is actually pretty accurate. Maybe not satisfying, but accurate.

One of the reasons they make these less-than-ideal choices is that adult life involves lots of situations where we're faced with a choice that offers an immediate small reward but a larger punishment later. For example, staying up too late watching a movie is fun in the moment but painful the next day. Impulse buying is exciting at the time but problematic when the credit card bill arrives. As kids, we have adults around us who know these things and prevent us from making these kinds of choices. As adults, though, we're expected to be able to do this for ourselves, which is easier said than done for those with ADHD.

Another reason people with ADHD make these problematic choices is that they may not do enough planning ahead, so they have to figure things out on the spot. We use forethought to look ahead to see likely challenges and think about what kinds of responses will probably work best. To predict the future accurately, we have to be able to stop and think about how similar situations worked out in the past, evaluate current circumstances, mentally sort through our options, and choose the best one. So there's a lot going on here, even if it occurs in an instant. Without this ability, people with ADHD are forced to constantly reinvent the wheel and make things up on the spot, often with predictable results.

Of course, for this forethought to work well, we have to have a pretty good idea of what's going on so that we can prepare for the right situation. This involves both self-awareness as well as awareness of other people and outside events. Therefore, we have to monitor all of these internal and external events as they unfold so that we can plan and respond accordingly. To work well, this monitoring requires a gap between stimulus and response—we have to be able to take it all in and think about it before doing anything. This means not just reacting to the most obvious aspects of the situation, but also considering the more subtle parts.

Unfortunately, people with ADHD tend to react too quickly and without looking at the full picture of what's going on. When they do stop and take stock, they drop bits and pieces out of their working memory when mentally manipulating all the various details of the current situation and comparing their options of what to do next. As a result, they may respond in a way that fits only part of the situation but looks like bad judgment when you consider the forgotten pieces. For example, during a meeting with her boss, a person may go into a long story about an interaction with a customer without noticing that her boss is looking at his watch and giving signs of needing to stop. If she had noticed that, she could have cut her story short and gotten to the important question that she needed to ask but ran out of time for.

Or if they need to create a multistep plan, they may have trouble putting all those steps into the optimal order (known as *sequencing*). As a result, they lose efficiency when they need to go back to a step they didn't plan for or forgot. Perhaps the classic example of this is the child who tells his parents at dinner that he has a science project due the next day, not figuring into his planning that he should have gotten supplies from the store earlier in the day or week. Parents love these moments.

This brings up the idea of being able to sense when events are slipping away from us and changing course to get things back on track. In addition to drifting off onto the "wrong" activities, people with ADHD may not notice when it's time to change gears to do something else. In both cases, whether it's doing something they shouldn't or not doing something they should, it's a matter of being out of sync with the current situation.

The ultimate goal of hindsight and forethought is to create the best possible future by managing the interactions in the present most effectively. People with ADHD often have trouble following through with these plans, even if they know how to create them. For example, they can tell others how to handle situations but then can't follow their own advice. This is frustrating for family members and others who don't understand why the person with ADHD doesn't plan ahead more or follow the plans that he does create. It's not that he can't ever create these plans; it's just that he doesn't do it often enough, so he winds up flying by the seat of his pants.

This is where the indignant lectures often occur, even though they don't address the real problem. I can appreciate the frustration, but lectures aren't part of the solution. Rather, the solution lies in setting things up to make it more likely that the person with ADHD will stop long enough to consider these lessons from the past before jumping into action. That's what most of the rest of this book is about.

CHAPTER 2

DIAGNOSING ADHD: ACCURATE DIAGNOSIS GUIDES EFFECTIVE TREATMENT

Most of the people reading this book have been officially diagnosed by a competent clinician. There will also undoubtedly be some readers who bought this book to learn more about ADHD to see if it's worth seeing a clinician for a diagnosis. There are also some people who bought the book to see if *someone else* has ADHD! This is all good, as far as I'm concerned, since more information is usually better. Nevertheless, it's easy to misdiagnose yourself if all you do is read about a condition in a book, so don't let this chapter substitute for seeing a well-informed clinician.

This chapter covers the various ways that adults can be diagnosed with ADHD, from brief discussions with one's family doctor to full-day neuropsychological evaluations. If you haven't yet been diagnosed, this will help you decide which approach to take. If you've already been diagnosed, this may help you better understand the process by which the clinician came to a decision. I also cover why you probably struggled through most of your life before finally being diagnosed.

Although ADHD can be relatively easy to diagnose by a knowledgeable clinician, the situation can sometimes be less than straightforward since many adults with ADHD also have symptoms of anxiety and depression. This makes for a fuzzier picture and therefore requires more finesse from the clinician to tease it all apart.

This chapter is fairly long. I did that on purpose. A wrong diagnosis tends to waste a lot of time and money (and optimism). So take the time to get it right.

This chapter contains the following articles:

long time, still most adults haven't been diagnosed. Of those who have been, it's been mostly in the last decade or less. The slow evolution of ADHD as a diagnosis may explain why it took so long for you to be diagnosed.

Say Good-bye to ADD (and Hello to ADHD) (p. 27) Although many people still use *attention deficit disorder* and *ADD*, that term was officially replaced by *attention-deficit hyperactivity disorder* and *ADHD* in 1987. Some of this confusion comes from the fact that some people with ADHD have trouble with attention but aren't hyperactive.

What's in a Name: Attention-Deficit or Deficit in Attention Regulation? (p. 28) "Attention-deficit" implies that people with ADHD don't have enough attention, but the real problem is that they don't control their attention effectively. Mostly, they get distracted and shift their attention when they should have stayed on the original task. Sometimes, though, they stay glued on something when they should really shift.

Official Diagnostic Criteria: You Should Recognize These (p. 29) *The Diagnostic and Statistical Manual-IV* sets the official criteria that someone needs to meet in order to qualify for a diagnosis. The criteria for ADHD aren't great for adults, but they're what we have for now.

Unofficial but Common Symptoms: You'll Probably Recognize These (p. 30) In addition to the official criteria, people with ADHD often have other symptoms or difficulties. You may find that many of these look familiar, too.

How Distracted Is Distracted Enough? (p. 32) Although everyone gets distracted sometimes, those with ADHD have paid a price for their symptoms. In fact, this suffering is required in order to qualify for the diagnosis.

New Diagnostic Criteria Are Coming (Finally) (p. 33) The official diagnostic manual is going to be revised in 2012. Hopefully the authors will expand the criteria, since ADHD looks different in adults than it does in kids. I've listed here the criteria that research has found to be the most reliable.

Including Other Sources of Information (p. 34) When diagnosing ADHD, it can be helpful to include information from other sources, such as report cards, parents, or romantic partners. They can validate the information you provide as well as offer an additional perspective. All of this gives the clinician a fuller picture of your functioning and greater faith in the outcome of the evaluation.

Assessment Instruments: Not Necessarily the Best Tool for This Job (p. 37) Psychological tests are sometimes used when diagnosing ADHD and other conditions. Although testing can be very helpful in some situations, it isn't required in order to make an accurate diagnosis of ADHD.

Brain Scans: Not Enough Science, Too Much Fiction (p. 40) Although a small number of clinicians use brain scans to diagnose ADHD, there just isn't enough research available on this technique for it to be considered reliable. Therefore, I advise people to save their money.

Getting Diagnosed: How Do You Know It's ADHD? (p. 41) There are several ways to get diagnosed with ADHD. Which one is best for you depends on several factors, including how complicated your situation is.

Comorbid Conditions: Other Conditions Often Come Along for the Ride (p. 43) People with ADHD are more likely to have another condition, such as anxiety, depression, bipolar disorder, or substance abuse. These overlapping symptoms can make it more difficult to get the diagnosis right, but a skilled clinician can tease them apart.

Missed Diagnoses: Why Did It Take Me So Long to Be Correctly Diagnosed? (p. 48) Most adults with ADHD have been diagnosed only recently. There are many reasons why these people were missed for so many years, even when it was painfully obvious that there was something going on.

The Good News and Bad News of Greater Public Awareness (p. 52) The increase in awareness about ADHD in adults cuts both ways. It's good that more people are being correctly diagnosed and treated. However, the adults who are incorrectly diagnosed with ADHD aren't better off for it.

ADHD Changes with Age: Less Hyper, More Distracted (p. 55) If you were hyperactive as a child, you probably found that it quieted down as you entered adulthood. ADHD may also be less obvious later in life because we have more options as adults than we do as children, so we can choose situations where our weaknesses aren't as obvious.

Is ADHD the Same in Men and Women? (Short Answer: Yes) (p. 56) ADHD is still more likely to be diagnosed in males than in females, even though the condition creates the same information-processing weaknesses in both sexes. However, society places different expectations on men than on women, so because their demands are different, their struggles are, too.

The Relief of Being Diagnosed: Wow, That Explains a Lot! (p. 57) After years of falling short, it can be a relief to have an explanation for those difficulties that isn't a character indictment. This is equally true for the person with ADHD as it is for his family members.

ADHD Is Real

I wish I didn't have to actually type the words "ADHD is real," but unfortunately, I still do. This is especially true when it comes to ADHD in adults. There are some great organizations, like ADDA and CHADD (see the appendix, page 368) and individuals working hard to increase awareness of ADHD and to build credibility for the condition. For all their success, we still have a lot of work to do.

Myths abound regarding ADHD: people call it everything from excuse making for poor parenting to a creation of the pharmaceutical industry in order to sell pills. Research, however, consistently shows that those with ADHD are more likely to run into trouble at school, at home, with friends, on the job, with money, and in managing the mundane tasks of daily life. For these people and their families, ADHD is very real. They live it every day, struggling more than it seems they should have to—and why would they let themselves struggle if they didn't have to?

Critics use the fact that everyone has an "ADHD moment" every now and then to claim that ADHD is bogus. But a diagnosis of ADHD isn't made based on someone losing his keys every now and then (whoops, silly me!). Diagnoses are made based on a clear and consistent pattern of behavior that persists across time and circumstances and causes significant impairment. If the person isn't suffering for it, then it isn't ADHD. This quickly thins the crowd of people who qualify for the diagnosis.

If the critics want to argue based on what the research says, I'm happy to debate them. That will be an easy argument to win. If you or someone you care about has ADHD, then you also have plenty of data to contribute to that discussion.

Effective Treatment Starts with Accurate Diagnosis

The key to any effective treatment program is an accurate diagnosis. This is as true for mental health and medical care as it is for car repair. For example, if you bring in your car with noise from one of the wheels and the mechanic replaces the brake pads, but the problem is really in the bearings, you will still have the same squeak. Same story if you have ADHD but are diagnosed with something else. An accurate diagnosis allows you and your treatment providers to choose interventions that are most likely to be helpful. It's much easier to hit the bull's-eye if you're shooting at the right target.

The alternatives are to shoot blindly or to pursue a path that is unlikely to help you. As you may already know, this is especially true of adult ADHD since it's a condition that's often missed, so using an inappropriate treatment doesn't work that well. One reason for the diagnostic difficulties is that adults with ADHD often *also* have at least some symptoms of anxiety and depression, so it takes finesse to tease apart what exactly is going on—and then address it most effectively.

I talk in *Getting Diagnosed* on p. 41 about how to get diagnosed accurately. However, I will make the point here that I am often concerned about primary care physicians diagnosing ADHD. First, they rarely have enough time to really find out what is going on, including looking at other possible explanations. Second, they often don't know enough about ADHD and the other conditions that can be confused for it. This is no criticism—they have to know about all sorts of other things and no one can be an expert in everything. (I'm a psychologist, so don't ask me to diagnose a rash or stomachache.) I know they mean well, but the problem here is not just that a misdiagnosis leads to ineffective treatment and wasted time; in some cases it can make things much worse. When used alone, the main medications used to treat ADHD can exacerbate anxiety and send those with a bipolar tendency into a manic episode, which really makes a mess of things. Some primary care physicians do a really good job with diagnosing ADHD, so exceptions definitely exist. You may want to ask about your physician's experience and comfort with diagnosing and treating ADHD.

To prevent these potential problems, a comprehensive ADHD evaluation will look for anxiety, bipolar disorder, and other conditions. I have seen many clients who superficially seem to have ADHD, and would have been diagnosed with it if I had spent less time with them, but as we took a deeper look, they did not actually have ADHD. For these reasons, a number of local primary care physicians send me their patients to be evaluated for ADHD. Once I make the diagnosis, they feel comfortable prescribing, but they know their limits with diagnosing it.

Although a quickie evaluation may hit the bull's-eye, there are some potential problems, so I strongly encourage you to find someone who really knows ADHD in adults and can spend the necessary time to see if there is anything else going on. You will save more time in the long run if you start off right.

A Century of ADHD: We're Finally Getting It Right

As much as ADHD may seem like a new diagnosis, it has actually been part of the official diagnostic classification system for more than a hundred years. The evolution of the diagnosis shows an increasing understanding of the myriad effects of the disorder that go beyond the obvious behaviors.

Unfortunately, until the last couple decades, ADHD was thought of exclusively as a disorder of childhood that disappeared in late adolescence. This has had important implications for the majority who continue to struggle with the symptoms as adults. As you know, it's not that the symptoms of ADHD change that much over time so much as the demands placed on us do. I talk more about this in *ADHD Changes with Age* on p. 55.

Unfortunately for students with ADHD, the classroom is an excellent screening tool for difficulties with inattention, hyperactivity, and impulsivity, so the problems are obvious there. When we enter the world of work and have more options to choose from, we all tend to choose situations that favor our strengths and minimize the impact of our weaknesses. So, the child who could not sit still becomes a deliveryman who doesn't have to. This doesn't mean that all of his ADHD difficulties have disappeared but rather that, at least in this aspect of his life, his ADHD difficulties may be less apparent. What this all means is that it is easy to understand why ADHD was thought to disappear in adulthood.

One of the first official references to what we now call ADHD was made by G.F. Still in 1902 when he dubbed it "moral deficit disorder." This rather judgmental interpretation of ADHD behavior will be familiar to anyone who has been on the receiving end of these sorts of assumptions. This may even have come from well-meaning family members and teachers looking for an explanation for the ADHD person's seemingly self-destructive actions. In the 1930s, ADHD was renamed "minimal brain damage" and later "minimal brain dysfunction." (Not really getting any better, huh?) It wasn't until 1968 that the official diagnostic bible, the *Diagnostic and Statistical Manual-II*, called it "hyperkinetic reaction of childhood," highlighting the hyperactivity and missing the entire group of people with only inattentive symptoms.

The first studies demonstrating that ADHD persists into adulthood began to come out in the late 1960s, followed by the first published empirical studies on the diagnosis and treatment of ADHD in adults in the late 1970s. In 1980, the *Diagnostic and Statistical Manual-III* called it "attention deficit disorder" and included two subtypes: "with hyperactivity" and "without hyperactivity."

The *Diagnostic and Statistical Manual-III-R* was published in 1987 and changed the name to "attention-deficit hyperactivity disorder," making the hyperactivity a key feature. Three years later, the first newsletters targeted specifically at ADHD adults *(ADDendum* and *ADDult News)* began publishing, followed shortly thereafter by the first book for the public, Lynn Weiss's *Attention Deficit Disorder in Adults: Practical Help for Sufferers and Their Spouses* (1992).

The first journal article focusing on psychotherapy for adults with ADHD was published in 1994. This goes a long way toward explaining why ADHD adults (probably undiagnosed) often had such a hard time finding therapists who could go beyond traditional psychotherapeutic techniques and give them the kind of help they really needed. There just wasn't much information out there. It wasn't that long ago that I finished graduate school (1997) and I barely heard anything about ADHD in adults.

The *Diagnostic and Statistical Manual-IV (DSM-IV)* was published in 1994 and made an easily missed grammatical change with significant implications. The

DSM-IV renamed the condition "attention-deficit/hyperactivity disorder." It added the slash between attention-deficit and hyperactivity to signify that the disorder may include one or both symptom types. This was formalized by the inclusion of three subtypes: the predominantly inattentive type, the predominantly hyperactive-impulsive type, and the combined type who have both. The seemingly minor addition of the slash is important, since those people with only the inattentive symptoms still technically have ADHD (even though they don't have any H).

Although the *DSM-IV* criteria have a lot of solid research behind them, they are focused primarily on what ADHD looks like in children rather than in adults. What this means is that, if a clinician is strictly following the official guidelines, many adults who truly do have ADHD will technically not have enough of the symptoms to qualify for the diagnosis. It's likely that the next version of the diagnostic manual will contain separate criteria for adults, but until then, we are stuck with these second-best criteria. For those practicing in Europe and/or in some hospital settings, the *International Classification of Diseases-10* diagnostic coding system contains criteria that are very similar but not identical to DSM-IV's for ADHD.

The first medication approved by the Food and Drug Administration for adults with ADHD was Strattera in 2003. Of course, the medications used for kids are also used for adults (sometimes called "off-label use"), but it is still significant that it has been only a handful of years since adult ADHD was officially recognized in this sense. Since then, most of the other major medications have been approved for use in adults.

If you look at the history here, ADHD in adults is still very much a new discovery. If you struggled for years and wondered why nobody ever figured it out, this is probably why. Unfortunately, you're in very good company.

Say Good-bye to ADD (and Hello to ADHD)

Lots of people still use the terms *ADD* and *attention deficit disorder*, often to refer to those people who are inattentive but not hyperactive. They may use *ADHD* for those who do have hyperactivity and impulsivity. Although this makes sense, it's technically incorrect. The term *ADD* was retired in 1987 with the publication of the *Diagnostic and Statistical Manual-III-R* and replaced by *ADHD*. As I explained in the last article, *A Century of ADHD*, ADHD contains three subtypes, one of which is for people who have only the inattentive symptoms. So these people have ADHD, even though they have no H. I know, it's confusing.

Actually, it gets worse. If we're *really* going to be technical here, we would call it *AD/HD* (with the slash) since the most recent term is *attention-deficit/hyperactivity disorder*. But the slash is kind of awkward, so I'll stick with plain ol' *ADHD*.

The new version of the diagnostic manual (due out in 2012 or so) may change the names and make some of this easier. Meanwhile, we're stuck with a name that can be misleading.

What's in a Name: Attention-Deficit or Deficit in Attention Regulation?

It's unfortunate, but the term *attention-deficit* is actually kind of inaccurate and misleading. It implies that people with ADHD have a deficit in attention—that is, they don't have enough attention. Believe it or not, this actually isn't quite right. What ADHD folks have is a deficit in attention *regulation*—that is, keeping their attention on what is most important at that moment. An error in attention regulation can occur in two ways.

- *Shifting too soon.* This occurs when someone shifts her attention when she shouldn't have, such as by looking up to see who is walking by her office rather than staying focused on her email and ignoring the passersby.
- *Sticking too long.* This occurs when she keeps her attention focused on something when she should have shifted. For example, she should have noticed those people going by and joined them on their way to a meeting rather than continuing to read her email.

Both are failures in attention regulation. Effective attention regulation means shifting when it's best to shift and sticking when it's best to stick. This decision process happens many times per second.

At its extreme, this locking-in of attention is called *hyperfocus,* wherein the person becomes completely absorbed in an activity to the exclusion of awareness of the rest of his environment. For me, the classic example of hyperfocus is the kid who becomes so intent on a video game that he doesn't even hear his name being called. Another example is the adult surfing the Internet who doesn't notice that several hours have gone by. Recognizing how easy this was for her husband, the wife of a member of my adult ADHD support group suggested that he install a timer on the light switch in the study so that he couldn't help but notice when it was time to stop. Unfortunately, he got used to working in the dark! Obviously, that solution didn't really work, but then it was no longer a matter of hyperfocus. When the lights went out, he was making a conscious choice. I don't know that this made his wife any happier.

Unfortunately, hyperfocus is often used as an example of someone having good attention skills, at least when he wants to. Therefore, as the reasoning goes, this means that his attention is voluntarily controllable and he is merely choosing not to pay good attention at other times. For people without ADHD, this reasoning may be more accurate, but for folks with ADHD, hyperfocus actually shows poor attention regulation in that this obliviousness to everything else is actually a problem.

People with ADHD have the greatest difficulty keeping their attention on tasks that are boring and don't have an immediate reward or punishment—like paperwork, cleaning, and organizing. In contrast, exciting, novel, or personally meaningful activities are easy for people with ADHD to focus on (as they are for everyone). A frustrated spouse will point out this discrepancy, angry that he has to handle most of these less interesting tasks. It looks like a conscious and selfish choice rather than a problem with attention regulation. What separates those with ADHD from those without it is the degree of difference between their performance on boring activities and their performance on enjoyable activities. Everyone does worse on less interesting activities—but folks with ADHD do much worse. I discuss this difference further in *Persistence of Effort* on p. 16.

It's also worth noting that distractions can be external (e.g., noise from outside the conference room makes it hard to concentrate on what the presenter is saying) as well as internal (e.g., you suddenly remember that you need to send off an email, and start thinking about that rather than listening to the presenter). A client of mine is notorious among his friends for drifting off into thought in mid-conversation—both in response to what someone else said and because of his own private thoughts. Fortunately, they know him well enough not to take it personally.

Official Diagnostic Criteria: You Should Recognize These

The fourth edition of the *Diagnostic and Statistical Manual* (DSM-IV) is the official source that defines which symptoms make up each psychiatric diagnosis. I've shortened the official criteria for ADHD and listed them below. I go into more detail in *New Diagnostic Criteria Are Coming (Finally)* on p. 33, but some have criticized that these symptoms more accurately describe ADHD in children than in adults. So you may need to translate them a little into your adult life.

Note that reading this list isn't a substitute for a thorough evaluation with a professional who really understands ADHD in adults.

Six or more of the following symptoms of inattention have persisted for at least six months:

- Poor attention to details or makes careless mistakes
- Often has difficulty sustaining attention
- Doesn't listen well

- Trouble following through on commitments
- Disorganized
- Dislikes activities that require sustained mental effort
- Tends to lose things
- Easily distracted
- Forgetful

Six or more of the following symptoms of *hyperactivity-impulsivity* have persisted for at least six months:

Hyperactivity:

- Fidgety
- Has trouble sitting still
- Feels restless
- Has difficulty engaging in leisure activities quietly
- Always on the go
- Overly talkative

Impulsivity:

- Blurts out answers before questions have been completed
- Has difficulty waiting turn
- Interrupts

Adapted with permission from the Diagnostic and Statistical Manual of Mental Disorders, *Text Revision, Fourth Edition, (Copyright 2000). American Psychiatric Association.*

Unofficial but Common Symptoms: You'll Probably Recognize These

In addition to the official symptoms, adults with ADHD tend to display a wide range of other symptoms. Many of these are caused by or develop out of the official symptoms. These lists are certainly not exhaustive, but they do illustrate the pervasive effects that ADHD can have.

Inattention Difficulties

- Some ADHD adults work hard at being organized but have little to show in terms of results. Although they move things around, the objects don't wind up in better places because the person doesn't have a good organizational system into which to put things. This can lead to feelings of hopelessness and avoidance of organizing.
- They don't live up to potential. Others may assume that they could do better if only they cared more or tried harder.
- They frequently miss turns and exits when driving, especially when going down familiar roads.
- They have poor time management and/or procrastination, which causes big problems at work and at home.
- They hyperfocus on an enjoyable activity to the point where other activities are forgotten or ignored for longer stretches of time than planned.
- They have a tendency to miss pieces of conversation or be briefly tuned out. This may or may not be visible to others.

Hyperactivity/Impulsivity Difficulties

- They have a tendency to leave too many projects unfinished, both at home and at work. They get bored once they have the project figured out or it becomes routine. The project will be finished only because of external pressure from an impending deadline or someone else pushing on them.
- They have trouble sitting and reading. If they do read books, they may read several simultaneously and probably not finish most of them (which is why this book is written the way it is!).
- They have a tendency to blurt things out, based on a fear that otherwise they will forget their thought.
- They have a higher-than-average number of traffic citations for speeding or reckless driving.
- Money burns a hole in their pocket, so they tend to buy things they don't really need. They have trouble sticking to a budget or mentally figuring how individual purchases fit into the bigger picture.
- They engage in thrill-seeking behavior. This may be most obvious in physical tasks, such as motorcycle riding. However, it may also

be seen in relationships, such as by creating dramatic situations or breaking up when the relationship becomes familiar and routine.

Other Difficulties

- They have a high intake of caffeine, perhaps because it's the only thing that helps them to focus.
- They are pessimistic about their ability to make a better life. This is based on a long history of struggle and too much failure. They may minimize their strengths, always feeling that they could have done better. New failures and mistakes bring back to mind a laundry list of past blunders.
- Family or coworkers may feel more of the pain of the ADHD symptoms as a result of covering for the ADHD person's limitations.
- Related to the previous items, they may show a tendency to be with caretaker types in relationships who are then seen as too controlling.
- They may compensate for inefficiencies at work by putting in extra hours just to finish the normal workload. In addition, they may find that it's helpful to come in early or stay late because they are less distracted when the workplace is quieter.
- They have great difficulty with the overly loose structure of college, leading to dropping out or needing extra semesters to graduate. They have hodgepodge transcripts with a broad array of courses, wide range of grades (A to F), and many dropped classes.
- They have school difficulties such as inconsistent grades, behavioral problems, horrible homework performance, and generally performing below their potential.
- There is a family history—at least one parent, sibling, or child has ADHD.
- They are prone to strong emotional reactions that come on quickly and then dissipate almost as quickly.

How Distracted Is Distracted Enough?

Since everyone has moments of poor concentration, how do we tell the difference between ADHD and other mental health conditions or just the stress of normal life? Obviously we can't diagnose the entire world with ADHD, so we have to draw a cutoff line somewhere. The official diagnostic manual requires that, for a symptom to count, it has to cause some significant impairment. So, for example, someone who once in a blue moon loses her keys and needs to spend a few minutes looking for them doesn't suffer much from it. However, the person who routinely loses his keys and is getting written up at work for repeated lateness is suffering. The keys are probably only the tip of the iceberg. Without this impairment and suffering, something is merely a personality quirk that makes the person interesting or is kind of annoying. ADHD struggles, by contrast, are far more than annoying.

In addition, the symptoms need to have been present for most of the person's life and in multiple settings—not just at school but also at home, at work, and with friends. If the symptoms occur in only one or two settings, then I would look for aspects of those situations that are triggering the symptoms.

Those who truly have ADHD will have no shortage of examples of times when they paid a price for their ADHD weaknesses. If you've lived it, you know it.

New Diagnostic Criteria Are Coming (Finally)

It will be interesting to see what the upcoming version of the diagnostic manual does with ADHD, especially in relation to adults. There is talk of possibly changing the three subtypes (i.e., inattentive, hyperactive/impulsive, and combined). The inattentive subtype might even become a different diagnosis altogether. More subtypes might also be added, such as something that has been called *slow cognitive tempo*, which is for people with ADHD who tend to be more passive, have low energy, and are given to daydreaming.

Most important, it will be interesting to see if separate criteria are given for adults, since the current criteria are more relevant for children. This improvement would make it easier for adults who still have ADHD to qualify for the diagnosis. Psychologists and researchers Russell Barkley, Kevin Murphy, and Mariellen Fischer did a thorough analysis to determine which symptoms best describe ADHD in adults. These are the nine symptoms they found to work best:

- Is often easily distracted by extraneous stimuli or irrelevant thoughts.
- Often makes decisions impulsively.
- Often has difficulty stopping his or her activities or behavior when he or she should do so.
- Often starts a project or task without reading or listening to directions carefully.
- Often shows poor follow-through on promises or commitments he or she may make to others.

- Often has trouble doing things in their proper order or sequence.
- Often more likely to drive a motor vehicle much faster than others (excessive speeding). (Substitute item for adults without driving experience: Often has difficulty engaging in leisure activities or doing fun things quietly.)
- Often has difficulty sustaining attention in tasks or play activities.
- Often has difficulty organizing tasks and activities.

Reprinted by permission from ADHD in Adults: What the Science Says *by Russell Barkley, Kevin Murphy, and Mariellen Fischer. © 2007 Russell A. Barkley.*

You may see more of yourself in this list than in the current criteria.

Including Other Sources of Information

As with many diagnostic processes, it can be helpful to include information from additional sources, if possible. The most obvious additional source is a romantic partner or a parent. Sometimes these other people notice different things that complement the information you provided. Of course, many symptoms of ADHD are internal experiences that may not be directly visible by others—for example, others may not realize that you feel restless while sitting through a lengthy dinner. Regardless, assuming the information is generally pretty accurate, more tends to be better. It helps the clinician get a fuller picture of your strengths and weaknesses and what your life looks like. I prefer to have the other person present during the diagnostic interview, but this information can also be collected over the phone or by mail through rating scales, questionnaires, or written descriptions.

Information About Your Past

A diagnosis of ADHD requires that you have had these symptoms since childhood, so a clinician needs to find a way to look back in time and make sure that you actually had those symptoms. Obviously, you can tell the clinician about your childhood and teen years, providing specific examples of times when ADHD symptoms caused difficulties for you. Although you may be completely truthful, some clinicians worry about how accurate anyone can be when talking about old behaviors. (To be honest, I don't know how accurate or complete I would be in describing my childhood in detail.) Some people will tend to minimize their difficulties, whereas others will exaggerate them, so it's hard to know what to do with that information.

One solution is to bring a parent to the meeting with the clinician. Parents can often provide more accurate and detailed information about how someone performed in childhood, since adults tend to remember things better than children do. Of course, given the strong genetics of ADHD, there's a decent chance that one or both of your parents also have ADHD. If so, they may not see your symptoms as noteworthy or may minimize the degree of those symptoms. Nonetheless, it's usually helpful to bring a parent, if possible.

The one saving grace here is that report cards can provide a snapshot of past performance. Of course, this assumes that you can locate those report cards. Given that those with ADHD tend to have parents with ADHD, and organizing is not a strength of those with ADHD, this may be a bit of a stretch unless you are still a fairly young adult. If those report cards aren't available, I ask clients before our meeting to ask their parents what they remember about their report cards. It isn't as good as the real thing, but I'll take what I can get. Generally speaking, I'm less interested in the specific grades that someone received and more interested in the comments that teachers made, if any. However, keep in mind that report cards tend to be more sensitive to hyperactive and impulsive symptoms than to inattentive ones, particularly if the student is a nice kid who seems to be trying. Besides grades that seem noticeably below the student's abilities, I look for comments like these to suggest that the person has ADHD:

- Needs to try harder
- Doesn't work to potential
- Needs to pay attention better
- Doesn't hand in assignments
- Is disruptive in class
- Work is sloppy or rushed
- Talks too much
- Doesn't follow directions

Probably the single best indicator of ADHD symptoms in childhood is unreliable and incomplete homework performance. Those with ADHD really struggle with homework. The work itself isn't necessarily difficult, but rather the kids struggle with keeping track of the assignments, bringing home all the relevant books and papers, and then remembering to bring everything back to school. Even assuming all of these things happen, there is still the challenge of actually doing all the work without getting sidetracked into other, more interesting activities. This may be especially true of bright students who get the concepts pretty quickly but still have to slog through the boring and pointless repetition of a dozen more problems to complete the assignment. It's not that ADHD students are unable to complete any homework, but rather that they have difficulty keeping up with the constant flood of new assignments, especially once they hit high school.

So I always ask about homework performance. For me, the biggest single indicator is that the person would complete homework but then not hand it in—this just doesn't make sense in any case except for those with ADHD. In addition, those with ADHD will often say things like this:

- "I never did homework."
- "If I did it at all, it was always like five minutes before class."
- "I could never sit still long enough to do it."
- "I could never keep track of all the books and papers."
- "Even if I did it, I would lose it or forget to hand it in."
- "My parents were always on my case about doing it. Otherwise it didn't get done."

Of course, there can be other reasons why someone didn't do homework consistently, such as overly permissive parenting, a chaotic home life, or caregivers who didn't value academics. The difference is that these other people could have done more of their homework if they had chosen to, whereas those with ADHD had great difficulty maintaining their concentration and effort long enough to get it done consistently, despite their best intentions. Over time, of course, those who find homework difficult or painful may begin to avoid doing it, especially when they start to fall behind in the class. This makes sense, even if it only makes things worse. What started as a matter of ability becomes a matter of choice. So the ADHD student gives up on homework or just does the bare minimum. However, beneath that seeming apathy is a thick layer of frustration, embarrassment, and even shame.

By contrast, some students may have done all right on their homework simply because a parent sat with them the entire time, ensured that it all got done, and even contacted the teacher or other students to track down what the assignment was. In this case, it's diagnostic that it took so much effort for the parent to assist with something that other students did mostly by themselves. Predictably, these students' performance plummeted when this support was removed, either just for a few days or when they went away to college.

Information About Your Present

Just as it can be helpful to get a parent's perspective on past functioning, it can be helpful to get a romantic partner's input on more recent functioning. Your romantic partner's opinion might not be more right than yours, but she may notice some interesting things about your way of doing things. This may be especially true if you had a parent with ADHD, so those difficulties may feel normal to you. For example, I had a client who didn't think that his running out of gas on a semiregular basis was noteworthy—but his wife sure did!

Of course, some romantic partners may have an agenda to make the other's ADHD symptoms seem either worse or better than they actually are. Some partners may want to see the other person as the troubled one in the relationship in order to take the spotlight off her own difficulties, or even to play the role of the long-suffering martyr. Other partners may resist the idea of ADHD, instead explaining the difficulties as a lack of effort or other shortcomings, such as selfishness or irresponsibility. (For more on this, see *Relationship Patterns to Avoid* on p. 323.) As I said before, more information is generally helpful, but only if it is generally accurate. A skilled clinician should be able to read between the lines on these sorts of matters and get a clear picture, even from fuzzy data.

Assessment Instruments: Not Necessarily the Best Tool for This Job

Some people feel uncomfortable with the idea of just talking to a clinician and relying on her judgment about whether they have ADHD. *Isn't there a more objective way of determining the diagnosis?* they wonder. Well, there is, but it isn't really that great, at least not for this diagnosis. Yes, a formal battery of psychological or neuropsychological tests can provide a tremendous amount of potentially useful information, but the tests that we currently have aren't really that great for ADHD. By analogy, an X-ray is just the thing to diagnose a broken bone, but it doesn't tell you much about a strained muscle. Of course, an X-ray can be a good way to ensure that the problem isn't a broken bone and, similarly, a battery of tests can be used to rule out other possible reasons for trouble with concentration and restlessness.

Before we go into the pros and cons of testing, let's talk about what it is. Probably the best-known example of psychological testing is IQ tests, but there are all sorts of tests available, depending on what questions the evaluator wants to answer. For example, one would use a different set of tests to determine whether a student qualifies for extra time on the SAT than to determine whether Grandma is still capable of managing her own finances. The tests are specifically designed to discern and measure a person's various abilities—for example, short-term versus long-term memory, or verbal skills versus spatial skills. By having the person do all sorts of tasks, the evaluator can isolate these distinct abilities and get separate measures of each. After spending anywhere from an hour to a full day with the person, the evaluator scores all the tests, puts all the data together, analyzes the results, and writes up a report. The rough rule is that the evaluator spends an hour by herself for every hour spent with a client, so it's a pretty big endeavor in both time and money.

The Good News About Assessment Instruments

Assessment instruments can be efficient ways to gather a standardized and presumably accurate sampling of a person's abilities. For example, compared to others his age, what are this person's strengths and weaknesses, and does this pattern tell us anything about a potential diagnosis? A skilled evaluator can also use the testing data in offering suggestions for strategies to help her clients use strengths to compensate for weaknesses. This can be really helpful, especially when other interventions haven't been as successful as everyone would have hoped. So, if you have tried all sorts of interventions to little or no avail, testing may reveal something that you and your treatment providers haven't yet taken into account. Identifying this missing piece may help you overcome the barriers to progress or help you adjust your expectations.

Testing can also be useful if something other than just ADHD is suspected—for example, learning disability, brain injury, compromised intelligence, or personality disorder. Testing can reveal whether someone has something in addition to or instead of ADHD that is contributing to his difficulties.

Another advantage of testing is that it can be harder to fake than an interview. For example, if someone is trying to look as though he has ADHD or a learning disability in order to get medication or accommodations (known as *malingering*), the testing will probably pick that up. Here's a little insider information from my wife, who does a lot of testing: Some people with legitimate disabilities intentionally perform worse just to make sure that it shows up in the results. Unfortunately, this blows the entire thing, because the tests pick up that the person is intentionally making mistakes, so it casts a shadow of doubt on everything. So try your best and have faith in the assessment instruments—if you have a disability, the instruments will pick it up!

Speaking of accommodations, there will be times when someone needs to have a formal battery of testing in order to justify accommodations, such as on tests like the SAT or MCAT, for college, or for a job. The people setting these requirements assume that testing is more objective and thereby more accurate than the results from a diagnostic interview. This is not necessarily true, but if that is the requirement, then we have no choice but to comply when seeking accommodations.

The Bad News About Assessment Instruments

Probably the biggest negative aspect related to using testing for diagnosing ADHD is that the tests we have today just aren't that great at picking it up. This is partly because folks with ADHD shine when being tested in a quiet room, without interruptions, with an evaluator who keeps them on task and provides a new activity every few minutes. So, lots of folks with ADHD look pretty good on these tests (this is called a *false negative*), whereas they have much more trouble managing the chaos, distractions, multitasking, prioritizing, and interruptions of real life.

Although these tests may not pick up an individual's ADHD, they do find differences at the group level. That is, a group of people with ADHD tend to score lower than a group of people without ADHD. While this is useful for researchers to know, it is less useful for a clinician who is trying to diagnose one person. By analogy, we can definitively prove that men tend to be taller than women, but there is some overlap in the middle, so you have some men who are shorter than some women. So there is a difference in the group averages, but we can't necessarily predict someone's sex based on height (most people would probably get huffy if you got that one wrong).

Nonetheless, some people think that testing is better because it is more objective. They like the fact that it produces scores, percentiles, and graphs, under the idea that these data make the test more accurate or reliable. This kind of makes sense, except that in this case it isn't really true. Fuzzy and subjective as it may seem, still the best tool for diagnosing ADHD is a thorough diagnostic interview performed by a skilled clinician who really knows what to look for. In my practice, I do a two-hour interview, reviewing how the person is doing now, as well as how the person did at other times of life. I also look for other explanations for the person's difficulties, since other things can look like ADHD.

Although assessment instruments can yield a tremendous amount of information, that information doesn't come cheap. As mentioned previously, it takes a lot of time from a trained clinician who needs to be compensated for all that time. A typical evaluation will run from $1,500 to $3,000, depending on how many tests are administered. Unfortunately, insurance reimbursement for these services tends to be rather limited. So the question then becomes one of value—if you want that extra information and are willing to pay for it, then it is a good deal. As with any other service, if you would like to be tested, find someone who has significant experience with ADHD in adults or whatever condition you think you might have. Administering the tests is easy; it's the interpretation that takes real skill, so find a professional who can really do a good job and provide targeted, detailed recommendations—that's the *real* point of going through the whole process.

Some Specific Tests

Let's talk about a couple of the assessment instruments that are most specific to the diagnosis of ADHD.

Rating Scales

There are many rating scales available to assist in the diagnosis of ADHD and other conditions. Some of them were heavily researched and are sold only to healthcare professionals, whereas others are available to anyone and may be less research based. They can be good ways of gathering information from other people about how they see your functioning. They also make it easy to add up those answers and obtain a score that shows how mild or severe your functioning is in various areas, at least according to this scale. This can boil down a lot of information and make it easier to see patterns across the answers that you or others gave.

However, the results should not be considered as written in stone or definitively accurate. For example, a client of mine was diagnosed by his family physician as having ADHD, partly based on the results of a rating scale. When we really talked about what was going on, it was anxiety that was driving his difficulties, even though superficially they seemed like typical ADHD symptoms. To his credit, this physician had referred this young man to me for a second opinion. So rating scales can be helpful, as long as you don't overread the results.

Continuous Performance Tests (CPTs)

CPTs are computer-based tests that assess attention by giving subjects a boring, repetitive task that requires accurate responding over time—in other words, something that will separate those who have attentional issues from those who don't. These tests usually involve responding to some stimuli, either visual or auditory, but inhibiting responses to other stimuli. They compare the subject's results to the pattern of results from various groups—ADHD, depression, anxiety, brain injury, those without any diagnosis—in order to determine which group this one person belongs in.

Unfortunately, since many conditions can affect attention and this kind of performance, CPTs don't necessarily distinguish ADHD from these other conditions, so they can't be used alone. This may change with time as further research improves their accuracy. But they are a great way to tell if someone is fraudulently trying to look like he has ADHD, since it's virtually impossible to intentionally respond in a consistent pattern that looks like ADHD.

Brain Scans: Not Enough Science, Too Much Fiction

Some interesting work has been done on the use of brain scans to better understand the role of various brain areas in different conditions, including ADHD. Various scans are available, although the best known is probably *single photon emission computerized tomography (SPECT)*. SPECT works by measuring where injected radioactive glucose is metabolized in the brain. Areas of the brain that are more active metabolize more glucose, and thereby show up brighter on the SPECT scan. *Functional magnetic resonance imaging* (or *fMRI*) is a newer technology that also measures brain activity, although in a somewhat different way.

Regardless of how it's measured, the clinician then matches up the subject's brain activity pattern to those of groups of people who have been diagnosed with various conditions. So the clinician makes a diagnosis based on which group an individual seems to most closely resemble.

Research has found that there are indeed differences between groups of people with various psychiatric diagnoses on these brain scans. Unfortunately, as discussed in *Assessment Instruments* on p. 37, the fact that researchers can find differences between groups does not mean that we can use these techniques to diagnose individuals. Put simply, these brain scans are too often wrong when you try to diagnose an individual. Yes, they are super cool and totally sci-fi, but that doesn't make them accurate (i.e., helpful). There are simply too many errors, where a person's brain scan says one thing but her behavior and symptoms say another. It may be interesting to know how your brain looks, but your symptoms and functioning in your life are the things that really matter.

Despite the sometimes grand promises of these practitioners, it's hard to justify using brain scans diagnostically. Considering how much they cost (about $2,000), they just don't add anything to the diagnostic process that a skilled clinician can't figure out in other, less expensive ways. Perhaps further research will change that but, at this time, save your money. Low-tech procedures are still the best way to go.

Getting Diagnosed: How Do You Know It's ADHD?

It can be confusing to figure out how best to get an official diagnosis of ADHD. The possibilities range from quickie online surveys to full-day batteries of neuropsychological tests. Which one is best? Well, it depends on several factors:

- *How complicated is your situation?* Some people have relatively clear-cut cases of ADHD without any other obvious explanations for their difficulties. Others also have anxiety, depression, addiction, learning disabilities, or complicated histories of abuse, and the ADHD may be only one small piece of the puzzle. Generally speaking, the more complicated your situation, the more in-depth an evaluation you should seek.
- *Why are you being diagnosed?* Some people are looking for a diagnosis so they can pursue the treatments that will be most effective. If so, a thorough interview will probably be sufficient. Others are looking to receive accommodations at college or at work, which often require formal testing and a more involved process.
- *How much additional information do you want besides a yes or no about ADHD?* The more involved the evaluation, generally the more information you gain from it about how you process information, what your strengths and weaknesses are, and how you relate to other people. This information can be useful but will

generally cost you more in time and money since it involves more time from the clinician.

- *Are you feeling lucky?* This is kind of a silly question, but it's worth asking. After all, we could use a coin toss to determine if someone has ADHD—and sometimes we'll actually be right. Of course, sometimes we will also be wrong, so I don't think that I would want to stake my own treatment on whether it comes up heads. Related to this, some people go to their primary care physician, do a brief interview, maybe fill out a rating form, and voilà!, they've been diagnosed with ADHD. This is fine if your physician knows his stuff and you actually do have ADHD, but isn't so helpful if your physician doesn't know his stuff or you don't have the condition.

In my own practice, I do a two-hour interview for diagnosing ADHD. I ask about the person's current functioning and then ask about how she functioned at other times in her life, as far back as elementary school. I'm looking not only for symptoms of ADHD but also for other difficulties, weaknesses, and strengths that the person may have. If the person reports that she has a particular symptom, I need to answer several important questions in order for it to count toward a diagnosis of ADHD:

- *How long has the symptom been present?* If someone has ADHD, the symptoms have been present for pretty much the person's entire life. Someone who just began having trouble over the last few years, or less, probably has something other than ADHD.
- *How frequently does the person display the symptom?* Someone who only occasionally spaces out in conversation is less likely to have ADHD than someone who does it frequently.
- *Does the person display the symptom in more than one setting?* If the symptom is present in only one or two parts of the person's life, but everywhere else is fine, then it probably doesn't count. If it's ADHD, it shows up in most parts of the person's life. Of course, how noticeable or problematic the symptom is may depend on the circumstances—forgetfulness may be less obvious at work if a PDA gives constant reminders.
- *How much impairment does the symptom cause?* Is it kind of annoying, or has it cost this person jobs and relationships? The more severe, the more likely it is to be ADHD.

At the end of it all, once we've talked about all the areas where the person is struggling and the places where she is doing well, I sort through it all to see if

ADHD is the best explanation. In other words, does the pattern of strengths and weaknesses suggest ADHD, or does the pattern look like something else instead, or is it both? There are four possibilities:

- *The person has ADHD but nothing else.* The person has the required number of symptoms, without a lot of symptoms of other conditions. This also requires that the person doesn't have strengths that contradict a diagnosis of ADHD. For example, someone who had minimal trouble managing all his homework, without help from parents, is unlikely to have ADHD.

- *The person doesn't have ADHD but does have some other condition.* The person is indeed having difficulties, but they seem to be better explained by something else, like anxiety, depression, bipolar disorder, or stress. For most of these people, the symptoms haven't been lifelong, as they would be for ADHD.

- *The person has both ADHD and another condition.* Many adults with ADHD have at least some symptoms of anxiety, depression, or sleep problems, which can make it harder to determine which condition is driving a particular symptom.

- *The person has neither ADHD nor another condition.* This is pretty rare, since if someone isn't having some significant difficulties, he probably won't seek out a diagnosis. So the person may have a touch of something, but not enough to cross the threshold to a formal diagnosis. However, there are some people who try to get diagnosed so that they can fraudulently gain accommodations at school or work. Of course, this may indicate a condition of another sort...

Once in a blue moon, I have clients who are disappointed or upset by the outcome of our evaluation. Some thought they did have ADHD, and some didn't. Regardless, I'm not doing them any favors if I tell them they have a condition that they don't have or withhold a condition that they do have. The truth may not always be pretty, but it is helpful if it enables you to pick the most effective strategies.

Comorbid Conditions: Other Conditions Often Come Along for the Ride

After a lifetime of struggle, it shouldn't be surprising that most adults with ADHD also suffer from some other condition, such as anxiety, depression, or substance use. Unfortunately, this can make it harder to get an accurate diagnosis since some of the symptoms can look the same, at least superficially. ADHD is only one of many conditions that can affect concentration and make someone distractible and forgetful. In a way, poor concentration is kind of like a fever in physical health—a fever can come from a cold, malaria, cancer, or all sorts of other conditions, so knowing that someone has a fever doesn't help that much in making a diagnosis. In the same way, trouble concentrating just tells us that *something* is going on, but it doesn't tell us *what*.

There are three important differences that tend to distinguish ADHD from every other mental health condition:

- The symptoms of ADHD have been present in one form or another from childhood or at least the early teen years.
- The symptoms don't change that much over time (except for the hyperactivity, which tends to settle down).
- The symptoms are present in most settings and parts of the person's life.

Let's talk more specifically about the other mental health conditions that most commonly come along for the ride with ADHD or are mistaken for it, since you may need or want to seek treatment for these other conditions as well.

Depression

One study found that up to one out of three adults with ADHD experience major depression or *dysthymia* (a longstanding but milder depression) at some point in their lives (Barkley and Gordon, 2002). These are pretty big numbers and not surprising given the additional struggles that people with ADHD face. Because both disorders can affect concentration and the ability to get things done, a clinician who doesn't know ADHD well enough or doesn't spend enough time getting the details may assume that the only diagnosis is depression and miss the ADHD that is driving it. Women and girls are probably more likely to be misdiagnosed in this way.

Both ADHD and depression can cause people to be down on themselves. Whereas depressed people tend to focus on or exaggerate their perceived shortcomings, ADHD adults will often have a larger kernel of truth in their feelings of worthlessness after years of underachievement. Unfortunately, they have better reasons for being hard on themselves, at least until treatment enables them to do better in their lives.

Anxiety

ADHD can give you a lot to worry about. Sometimes they're things that you know you should worry about ("I really didn't spend enough time on that report for work—my boss won't be happy," or "I forgot to pay that bill!"). The things that you don't yet know about but fear are out there somewhere are often worse. These ticking time bombs can be things like appointments that you scheduled and forgot about, only to find out after you've already missed them. Or the school function that you agreed to help out with but forgot immediately. So even if there isn't anything that you know you should be worried about, there is always the possibility of something else coming up to bite you. Not a fun way to go through life...

There is also the constant grind of daily stress that comes from not making efficient use of time because of distractibility, avoidance, and procrastination. Life keeps moving, so tasks pile up and the stress builds until it finally explodes in a mad dash of activity.

Additionally, some ADHD adults are at greater risk for developing social anxiety as the result of a lifetime of embarrassment and social fallout from not waiting their turn, putting their foot in their mouth, forgetting, and interrupting or intruding. They come to learn that they do inappropriate things but can't stop it, so they may simply avoid some social situations or be anxious when they are in them. I had one client who would, in an effort to make sure he didn't say the wrong thing, overthink things so much that he wound up saying very little at all. He felt bad about it afterward but became so overloaded with checking himself that he couldn't just be himself.

Over time, ADHD adults learn that life is unpredictable and that bad things can happen suddenly and without warning. Obviously, having a layer of anxiety on top of ADHD doesn't make anything any better. It affects how you feel about yourself, how clearly you think, and what kind of odds you place on being successful. Add it all together and you will be less willing to take a chance on new strategies that might make your life better and reverse some of those other negatives.

In the diagnostic process, it's important to keep in mind that inattention can be caused by both anxiety and ADHD, so it's important to figure out if the inattentiveness is coming from both conditions or just one. One way to tell the difference is to look at the timing—if you have trouble concentrating only when you feel nervous, then it probably isn't ADHD. On the other hand, if your concentration is always bad but gets noticeably worse when you're nervous, then you probably have both.

Bipolar Disorder

The symptoms of bipolar disorder can look somewhat like those of ADHD. In ADHD, the symptoms are less extreme but more common; in bipolar disorder, they are more pronounced when they occur but will also wax and wane more significantly and even disappear completely for stretches. We also look at the age of onset—often in childhood with ADHD, later for bipolar. Although folks with ADHD can be prone to sudden bursts of emotion, those bursts tend to come and go much more quickly, whereas they last much longer and can be much more intense in those with bipolar disorder.

Some people with ADHD will be misdiagnosed with bipolar disorder, and vice versa, in childhood, only to have it later become clear in early adulthood that they really have the other condition. More so than with most other conditions, it's important to be sure that someone diagnosed with ADHD doesn't also or instead have bipolar disorder, since the medications used to treat ADHD can exacerbate untreated bipolar symptoms and send someone into a manic episode, which can lead to extremely reckless and dangerous behavior.

Learning Disabilities

People with ADHD may be more likely to have learning disabilities. (Some researchers think that it just *seems* like folks with ADHD have more learning disabilities because ADHD folks are more likely to be evaluated, so their learning disabilities are more likely to be found.) If you do have a learning disability, this added wrinkle can have a significant impact on your functioning and ability to be successful. How much impact it has depends on the nature and severity of the learning disability, how it interacts with your ADHD symptoms, and what skills are required of you in your life. A psychoeducational evaluation may be necessary to identify and better understand the precise learning disability that you have. Although it's overkill to put every adult through a full battery of tests, it may be helpful for those who seem to have more processing problems than just ADHD or don't respond well to typical treatments.

Substance Abuse and Other Addictions

For several reasons, people with ADHD are more likely to abuse alcohol or drugs or engage in other addictive behaviors like gambling, pornography, or overspending. It may not be full addiction, but it is still enough that it creates problems for them. Some people use these problematic behaviors to self-medicate the frustration, anger, disappointment, sadness, shame, and guilt that can come from a lifetime of undiagnosed and untreated ADHD.

Even for those who don't approach the level of addiction, they may impulsively drink too much at the wrong times and then regret their behavior afterward. Or it may ruin what they had hoped would be a productive day. I had a client who had a tendency of going along with his roommate's offers to grab a couple beers—even though he knew it rarely stopped at a couple beers and even when he had planned to take care of some important things later that night. That foresight and those plans went out the window as soon as his roommate made the offer. Another client would lose himself in the moment and wind up spending far more time and money on Internet pornography than he had planned.

It's interesting that, contrary to what we might expect, those with ADHD are not more likely to abuse cocaine or stimulants. Rather, as with the general population who uses drugs, marijuana is the most second popular, behind alcohol.

If someone has a strong history of substance abuse, it can be difficult to know which symptoms come from the effects of that abuse rather than from ADHD. Of course, someone with ADHD will have had those symptoms before he started abusing substances, but if the person has been engaging in substance use since the middle-teen years, there may not be that much history that is untouched. Assuming one has the time, it can help to stay clean for several months, perhaps with the help of a treatment program, and then see if any of the ADHD symptoms remain. This may be easier said than done, though, in that it may be necessary to address the ADHD in order to improve the likelihood of the person staying clean. This is the unfortunate irony of those with the double whammy of ADHD and substance abuse—it can become a real dilemma about which to address first. The unfortunate irony is that the stimulants, which are the most commonly prescribed medication class for treating ADHD, also have a potential for abuse, making most clinicians hesitant to prescribe them for those with a history of substance abuse.

Antisocial Personality Disorder

Children with ADHD, especially those with hyperactive and impulsive symptoms, are more likely to evoke negative reactions from their caregivers, especially if they also have untreated ADHD. A self-reinforcing process can be created wherein the child is labeled a bad kid because of his ADHD-based unruly behavior. As a result, he gets more negative reactions from adults, which causes him to act out even more, so the situation gets worse. In extreme cases, this can evolve into oppositional defiant disorder (ODD) and conduct disorder (CD), the childhood precursors to antisocial personality disorder in adulthood, for some people. People with antisocial personality disorder have little regard for the rules and frequently run into trouble with authority figures and the law.

As you probably know far too well, people often assume that ADHD-based behaviors are intentional or reflect irresponsibility and selfishness. Although ADHD people may do some of the same bad things as those with ODD, CD, and antisocial personality disorder, it's less intentional with ADHD—they may be just as surprised and disappointed as everyone else about their mistakes. For example, I had a client who was a lawyer and got arrested for shoplifting when he accidentally walked out of the store with a CD he hadn't paid for yet. This was completely unintentional. By contrast, those with ODD, CD, and antisocial personality disorder know they are stealing but don't really care—or get a thrill from breaking rules. The ADHD adult's mistakes come more from a neurologically based lack of awareness or spillover from poor planning that make negative outcomes more likely.

Head Injury and Medical Conditions

Injury to the frontal lobes of the brain can cause symptoms that can look very similar to those of ADHD. This shouldn't be surprising given that the frontal lobes are affected in those with ADHD. The difference for those with brain injury is that they won't have had any of these symptoms before the injury. They may also have a different set of symptoms (some extra deficits, perhaps), but also may not have some that are typically associated with ADHD. I evaluated a man who had been in a car accident as a teenager, leading to a mild brain injury. He had struggled ever since at work and managing his life. In this case, his troubles mostly came from the accident, since he didn't really have them before, but he definitely resembled someone with ADHD.

As for other medical conditions, it's generally not necessary to get a medical workup, such as a physical or neurological evaluation, unless you have other symptoms that go beyond the usual for ADHD that are worth getting checked out. Of course, we should all get good physical exams regularly, just to make sure there isn't anything sneaking up on us. However, there is currently no medical test for ADHD.

Missed Diagnoses: Why Did It Take Me So Long to Be Correctly Diagnosed?

Although things are getting better, the sad reality is that most adults with ADHD haven't been diagnosed or treated for it. So if you're someone who suffered for a long time before finally being diagnosed, you're in very good company. The main problem is that ADHD in adults is a relatively new concept, as these things go, so it's just making its way into most therapists' and physicians' knowledge bases. The good news is that we're learning a lot more about ADHD, but the bad news (for adults with ADHD) is that we're learning a lot more about everything else, too, so it's impossible to keep up with it all.

Let's talk about some of the reasons why so many of these adults are being diagnosed so late.

"ADHD Is for Kids"

Probably the biggest reason is that many healthcare professionals don't look for ADHD once someone reaches adulthood. As a result, other diagnoses or explanations are given instead, such as anxiety, depression, fear of success, passive-aggressive behavior, or self-destructive tendencies. (Any of those sound familiar?) Although the person may in fact be anxious, or whatever, that's not the full picture, so an important piece is missed if the ADHD is ignored.

In many cases, these other conditions come out of a lifetime of ADHD struggles, meaning that treatment of the effects will be of limited benefit. Unfortunately, because it works a little, everyone assumes that that must be the real problem and then settles for some partial treatment response. I've seen many clients who, even after seeing multiple therapists or psychiatrists over the years, were never diagnosed with ADHD or treated effectively.

Another Condition Masks the ADHD

Some people may also have another condition that hides the ADHD symptoms. Adults with ADHD are more likely than folks without ADHD to also have some other condition, mostly anxiety and depression. Some people have enough anxiety or depression that they officially qualify for the diagnosis, whereas others have some of these symptoms but not enough to cross the threshold. Of course, given the troubles that undiagnosed ADHD brings, it shouldn't be surprising that someone would be anxious or depressed. Unfortunately, having more than one condition can create a tangled web of symptoms that can be difficult to tease apart—for example, is the person distractible because she is anxious or because she has ADHD? So what this means is that a healthcare professional may see the other condition instead of the ADHD and therefore treat only that other condition. This treatment probably won't do anything for the ADHD but may have some benefit for the other condition. Ironically, this partial progress may convince the professional that the problem here is indeed anxiety or depression, so he doesn't look further, even though the person doesn't make the full progress one might expect.

It's human nature that we tend to find what we're looking for, so if someone tends to look for anxiety and depression and doesn't think about ADHD, then probably only the most severe cases of ADHD will stand out. Increasing awareness of ADHD in adults has the effect, then, of making professionals more likely to consider this condition, even when clients or patients also have symptoms of something else.

Clinicians Don't Know Adult ADHD

Another possibility is that many healthcare professionals are unfamiliar with how ADHD looks in adults. If someone uses the wrong characteristics to make a diagnosis, that person will obviously be less likely to pick up on it if someone has a particular condition. For example, if clinicians assume that everyone with ADHD has obvious hyperactivity (as the stereotypical ADHD boy does), then they will miss all the people who have only the inattentive symptoms or the adults who have grown out of the obvious restlessness. As another example, a member of the adult ADHD support group I ran was told by her psychiatrist that she couldn't have ADHD because she had managed to get a Ph.D., so therefore she must have been able to concentrate. What he didn't take into account was the fact that this very bright woman had had to work twice as hard as her classmates just to keep up, leaving her constantly exhausted and stressed out. She was successful, but she suffered for it.

As this woman illustrates, some people manage to achieve significant success despite their ADHD, so success should not necessarily rule out an ADHD diagnosis. There are many ways to compensate for sometimes significant weaknesses in certain skills and still achieve greatness. For example, high intelligence, a strong work ethic, charisma, or a supportive social network will help anyone be more successful. In addition, some people may do very well in one part of life but really struggle in other parts. For example, someone with untreated ADHD may do very well at work if she has an attentive and organized assistant, but her house and personal life may be disasters.

Success Despite ADHD—Until Something Changes

Some people do OK or even become quite successful until their circumstances change and their ADHD weaknesses become more obvious, resulting in "sudden" difficulties. Here are examples:

- Promotion or transfer to a less structured or more demanding job
- Leaving the workforce to stay home with children
- Divorce from a well-organized spouse
- Retirement from the structured life of the military
- Reduced involvement by parents who keep the young adult on track

This last one is especially common among new college students who drown in the sudden lack of structure of campus life. This is a big transition for any student, but those who have difficulty organizing their time and assignments and resisting temptation will very quickly run into trouble. In later life, this organizing may be provided by roommates, romantic partners, and assistants. In other cases, the ADHD person may have to work much harder or longer for the same successes. For example, he may need to come in early or stay late to get the same amount of work done, which works fine until he has kids and can't spend the extra time at work.

The official diagnostic manual requires that someone has to have had ADHD symptoms since childhood. If the symptoms weren't present from early life, then some other diagnosis needs to be made. Unfortunately, not all ADHD adults will have shown obvious symptoms in early life. This does not mean that the symptoms weren't present, but rather that they may not have been as obvious. Individuals with high intelligence who weren't hyperactive may have done OK in school, even if teachers thought they could have done better. This is because the inattentive symptoms are quiet relative to the "noisy" symptoms of hyperactivity. The inattentive kid may not be paying attention, but he's not disrupting the class, so the teacher may not realize when he's daydreaming. As Tom Brown, Ph.D., joked at the 1999 CHADD conference, the hyperactive kids are so obviously different from classmates that even the school janitor can diagnose them.

For the hyperactive and impulsive students, high intelligence isn't much of a protector in the areas of self-control, organization, time management, or good judgment. The problem is that the hyperactive or impulsive kids know what they're supposed to do, but they can't make themselves do it reliably enough. However, even these difficulties may not be as obvious if the person attended an extremely structured school where teachers and aides kept him in line. Alternatively, if someone attended an unstructured school, his impulsive misbehavior may not have stood out as much. For example, I once evaluated a college freshman who went to a private high school with small, supportive classes and had a mother who supervised his homework very closely. As a result, despite the fact that he could be the poster child for ADHD, his grades were generally quite good because others kept him from going off the rails. If he did go off, he could charm his way out of it and get extra time for the missing assignment. Not surprisingly, he wound up on academic probation his first year in college when all that structure and support were left behind because he didn't have the skills within himself to do well.

Other Explanations Are Used

Even if someone's struggles were obvious, explanations other than ADHD may have been used, such as "She just needs a better attitude," "He'll grow out of it," or "Her parents just need to crack down more." Of course, most adults were children during a time when ADHD was not frequently diagnosed, even in children. For people who were born before 1980, unless they were really hyperactive, it's unlikely that they would have been diagnosed as children. So other reasons were used in explaining the troublesome behavior.

This may be especially likely if a parent also has ADHD (probably undiagnosed), something that's pretty likely given ADHD's strong genetics. As a result, the child's struggles may be normalized under the logic of "I was the same way but I turned out fine. We don't need to do anything about this." Ironically, some of these ADHD adults are even less tolerant of excuses by their ADHD children, perhaps because it brings up their own painful pasts, so they hold fast to a boot-strap mentality even if it isn't working.

Everyone Supposedly Has ADHD These Days

Some people dismiss the diagnosis of ADHD with the simple explanation that everyone has a bit of ADHD these days, so we don't really need to concern ourselves with it. I had a client tell me that her doctor completely discounted ADHD in general, as well as her suffering and need for medication. What's happening is that people without ADHD superimpose their own experiences onto those of people with ADHD. For example, the person who sometimes forgets things won't realize how often someone with ADHD forgets things. Or they will assume that stories of trouble managing finances means that the person with ADHD occasionally puts too much on the credit card rather than that bills are lost completely and that the person receives phone calls about late payments.

The Good News and Bad News of Greater Public Awareness

ADHD has become a much better recognized condition. This is both good and bad, depending on whether someone actually has it or just thinks he does. There are various reasons why more people are being diagnosed with ADHD. Some of these reasons are legitimate and helpful, whereas others are not. Let's start with the good reasons first.

The Good News: We're Better at Diagnosing Adults with ADHD

There are two main reasons why more adults with ADHD are being successfully diagnosed.

First, there has been increased awareness over the last decade that ADHD doesn't end in adolescence. This is probably the biggest reason. It has been barely three decades since the first studies on ADHD in adults were published. As with any condition, greater awareness means that more people are diagnosed. This is the whole point behind public awareness campaigns and advocacy organizations, such as ADDA and CHADD (see the list of resources in the appendix). The adults who are now being diagnosed have always struggled with distractibility, disorganization, and poor time management before educational campaigns put the term *ADHD* into the public awareness. Because they didn't have ADHD as an explanation for their difficulties, they came up with other explanations. Labels don't change the facts, but they can change our understanding of those facts (and, hopefully, suggest likely solutions).

Second, ADHD struggles are more obvious in our fast-paced world. Our lives have become much more complicated and harder to manage over the last several decades, compared to simpler times of the past. We are all dealing with a constant flood of information, demands, and stuff. Those who have a harder time handling this deluge will be more obvious—so the ADHD folks stand out more.

Of course, I am by no means suggesting that the increased complexity of modern life causes ADHD; it just makes it easier to *see* who has ADHD and who doesn't. It's kind of like how exposure to milk makes it more obvious who has lactose intolerance. ADHD has been found to be pretty much as common in every country where it has been studied, making it difficult to claim that there is anything about Western society that causes it.

With cell phones and email, we're expected to be instantly available and respond immediately, so there is less wiggle room than there was when we could buy ourselves some extra time by claiming that something was "in the mail." In addition, the workplace has become leaner and meaner in that the secretaries, clerks, and assistants who would have covered some of an ADHD employee's shortcomings have been trimmed away. Finally, we're all working more hours and spending more time commuting, and we have larger houses to take care of, meaning that there is more to do and less time to do it. So anyone who is less efficient, for whatever reason, will struggle more—and stand out more.

But the majority of adults with ADHD (perhaps as much as 90 percent) have not been diagnosed and are not being treated for it (Biederman, Spencer, Wilens, Prince, and Faraone, 2006). So for all the good work that has been done, there is still more to do. If you're reading this book, it means that you (or someone you care about) are part of a far too exclusive club.

The Bad News: Some Diagnosed People Don't Actually Have ADHD

Advocates have worked long and hard to increase awareness of ADHD. Although this is a good thing for those people who truly do have ADHD, it can be a bad thing when people who don't have it are being diagnosed with it. Giving someone a diagnosis that he doesn't have is not actually helpful, since some of the treatments used for that condition will not be of much benefit and may even be problematic. So let's talk about some of the reasons why people without ADHD are being incorrectly diagnosed with it.

First, ADHD can be easy to overdiagnose, especially in self-diagnosis. Because everyone has times when they are distractible or make impulsive decisions, it's easy to say that it's ADHD, especially if the person doesn't really understand the multifaceted ways in which ADHD affects functioning. So, if someone is a little overenthusiastic when taking a brief questionnaire in a magazine, it's easy to self-diagnose as having ADHD.

There are many reasons why people do not achieve as much as they would like, but ADHD can be a one-size-fits-all diagnosis for some people seeking an explanation for their difficulties. Most people who seek a diagnosis of ADHD are truly experiencing problems of one sort or another and are looking for ways to feel better. That makes sense to me. But ADHD is only one possible reason for those problems. For example, people with anxiety, depression, personality disorders, poor social skills, addiction, bipolar disorder, or unrealistic expectations may also seize the label because it seems to explain their difficulties. These people aren't necessarily actively lying about it; it's just that they've chosen the wrong explanation. As I sometimes joke, even the common cold has inattention and poor concentration among its symptoms, but we would never say, "I had a really bad case of ADHD last week, but I'm feeling better now."

The big difference between ADHD and most of the other causes of trouble concentrating is that people with ADHD will have had those troubles for their entire life. For people without ADHD, the troubles will have begun over the last months or maybe years or will come and go over time. ADHD difficulties will always be there.

I once evaluated a woman in her midforties for ADHD. She did have many of the expected symptoms, but they had started only over the last couple of years, a period of time when she began menopause, became depressed, and began drinking heavily. For her, these other reasons were a better explanation for her difficulties.

Second, some healthcare professionals don't know enough about ADHD in adults but are diagnosing it anyway. Just as with self-diagnosis, this can happen when a professional is involved. Most of these professionals mean well and are trying to help a patient or client who is suffering, but a misdiagnosis isn't helpful. Some professionals feel more comfortable than others in admitting that they don't know something or are unsure and would prefer a second opinion. Of course, this assumes that there are some better-informed local professionals to get that second opinion from, but that isn't always the case.

Third, some people may be seeking special accommodations at school or work or on tests. Although this is legitimate for those who truly have ADHD or another disability, for others it may be seen as a way to get an edge in a competitive world. Often these accommodations aren't really all that helpful if the person doesn't have a true disability. See chapter 17, *Work: Hopefully More Than Just a Paycheck*, for more information about accommodations.

Finally, some people mistakenly diagnose themselves with ADHD after getting some benefit from someone else's medication. (Doctors get nervous if you tell them you did this.) Unfortunately, feeling more focused and productive after taking stimulant medication doesn't mean anything—most people do better on a stimulant. That's why everyone loves caffeine so much! Most of these people genuinely believe they have ADHD, but some of them will deceptively seek a diagnosis of ADHD to gain access to prescription stimulants, believing medication will give them an edge at school or work, or they enjoy the buzz. The difference between people with ADHD and those without it is that those with ADHD (hopefully) show a much greater improvement on the stimulant than non-ADHD people will. Of course, the converse here is not true—failure to show an improvement on a stimulant does not necessarily mean that someone doesn't have ADHD.

ADHD Changes with Age: Less Hyper, More Distracted

ADHD looks different in children than it does in adults. There are two unrelated reasons for this.

Hyperactivity Settles Down in Adulthood

Outright hyperactivity tends to quiet down into fidgetiness, internal feelings of restlessness, and difficulty with or aversion to sitting still. So the kid who couldn't sit still for more than a few minutes becomes an adult who can force himself when he has to. He may not enjoy sitting through a long meeting, for example, but he can make himself do it when necessary. Of course, he will try to avoid those situations when he can. Many adults with some remaining hyperactivity avoid going to the movies because they get restless if the movie doesn't totally grab them. I actually ask new clients whether they go to the movies when I do an ADHD evaluation, since an answer of no and the reasons can be pretty informative. .

Adults may also find better ways of coping with their restless energy, like working long hours, working in very active jobs, working two jobs, constantly puttering around the house on various projects, or having active hobbies. Whereas kids tend to be aimless in their restlessness, adults with ADHD may be more productive and put that energy to better use.

It's probably this reduction in hyperactivity that led clinicians to assume that most kids grow out of ADHD, since it is the most obvious symptom. Ironically, though, in adulthood the consequences tend to be more severe, even if the symptoms themselves are somewhat less. This is partly because adults have a greater ability to cause big changes in their lives. For example, impulsively calling out in class may get a student a detention, but impulsively confronting a boss (even if the person is correct about what she is saying) may get an employee fired. Overspending as a child may lead to an inability to join friends who are going out, but it can lead to crippling credit card debt as an adult. Or the impulsive choice to not use birth control may lead to an unplanned pregnancy—something that is quite well documented in the research.

Adults Have More Options Than Kids

Adults tend to choose situations where their difficulties are less obvious. Of course, we all tend to choose situations that favor our strengths and minimize the effect of our weaknesses. We have more options as adults, where there are many ways to live life and to earn an income. But as kids, we all have to go to school, which isn't a very ADHD-friendly place. Paying attention to long lectures that aren't always thrilling requires more force of will than most ADHD students can muster. Same for keeping track of multiple homework assignments, completing all those assignments, and actually remembering to turn them in. An adult who finds it difficult to stay interested in reading books just doesn't read books—and he doesn't have to. If an adult hates cleaning, she can hire someone to come in and do it, or she can do just the minimum.

Granted, this second reason for why ADHD looks different in adults than kids is actually more reflective of the choices that adults make than it is of the ADHD itself changing. As with many other conditions, these symptoms can be more or less obvious, depending on the situation that the person is in. Someone who tends to be forgetful may not have problems with that if she works in a very structured job where there are many built-in reminders. I evaluated a young man who had a job with lots of meetings but could count on several email reminders before each meeting, so he didn't need to work that hard to keep track of them all.

Although adults with ADHD may be able to make some tactical decisions about certain parts of their lives, even the most creative problem solving will not eliminate all the difficulties. Whereas the problems that result from hyperactivity and impulsivity tend to be more dramatic, such as car accidents, large purchases, or quitting jobs, it is the slow erosion of inattention-based difficulties that can cause some of the biggest problems for adults. For example, ordinary tasks like grocery shopping, paying bills, and staying organized prove to be a constant challenge for ADHD adults, especially if they don't have an organized and supportive romantic partner. As a person's life becomes more complex, as she is promoted to more demanding jobs and children arrive, these difficulties with inattention become more disabling. The symptoms that remain become more problematic since we expect adults to function more independently, consistently, and accurately than kids.

There are advantages and disadvantages to having ADHD as an adult compared to as a child. The good news for adults is that they have a greater ability to choose their situations, so they can set themselves up for success. The bad news is that adults are expected to function at a higher level and with less assistance from others, so there are more opportunities for the ADHD to trip them up. If you're reading this book, you're probably tired of being tripped up and are looking for something better.

Is ADHD the Same in Men and Women? (Short Answer: Yes)

Most people still tend to think that ADHD is more common in boys and men than in girls and women. This is partly true, but it may also be wrong. It is definitely true that more males are *diagnosed* with ADHD, but this doesn't necessarily prove that the condition is actually more common. Some researchers argue that because clinicians are more likely to look for ADHD in males, they are more likely to give the diagnosis to males than to females, even if they have the same symptoms. In other words, we tend to find what we look for (and not find what we aren't). It becomes a self-fulfilling prophecy.

Whereas males are more likely to be diagnosed with ADHD, females are more likely to be diagnosed with depression or anxiety. A woman may actually be depressed or anxious, but that is only part of the picture, and the important ADHD part is left out. It may be that males are more likely to have the hyperactive and impulsive symptoms or at least be more obvious about them, which makes it easy for a clinician to see their ADHD. By contrast, females may have more of the inattentive symptoms, which can look like depression and anxiety if one doesn't look closely enough.

So males are more likely to be diagnosed with ADHD, but is the disorder any different between the two sexes? Some research has found that the outcomes of a life of ADHD are the same for men as for women (Barkley, Murphy, and Fischer, 2007). Some new research is also finding that symptoms of inattention are affected by women's hormone levels as they go through their monthly menstrual cycles and menopause, so there may be some benefit to increasing medication doses for particular days of the month (Brown, 2005).

Probably the biggest difference, though, is based more in societal expectations than in ADHD itself. That is, although gender roles in Western society are less rigid than they used to be, men and women still tend to live different lives and have different demands. Women are still more likely to have greater responsibility for raising children and managing the household, which presents different challenges than focusing primarily on earning an income—and doing both is even more complicated. Also, because female friendships tend to be deeper than male friendships (speaking stereotypically, of course), they may be more sensitive to disruption by untreated ADHD. When it comes to unproductive ways of coping with adversity, men with ADHD are more likely than other men to abuse alcohol and marijuana, and there is mounting evidence that women with ADHD are more likely than other women to have trouble with overeating and obesity. So, even if ADHD is exactly the same in men as in women, men and women aren't the same.

The Relief of Being Diagnosed: Wow, That Explains a Lot!

As you may know yourself, many adults feel a tremendous sense of relief once they are finally diagnosed with ADHD. After years of struggle, they finally have a better explanation than having a bad attitude, being selfish, or needing to try harder. Even if they didn't know about ADHD, they certainly knew about the problems it caused and how it made them feel different from everyone else. After years of not knowing why they were having so much trouble and why the strategies that seemed to work for others didn't work for them, it can feel as though a giant weight is lifted to finally have a good explanation.

Romantic partners and family members may also feel better for knowing, since by the time someone shows up in my office, they have usually tried all sorts of other solutions, with not enough to show for it. There are times when having an answer, any answer, is better than not knowing. At least if you have an answer, you can begin to do something about the situation.

This relief may be mixed with overwhelming feelings of sadness or anger for the time lost and the struggles and failures that could have been prevented. I ran into a former client at a presentation. As we caught up, he told me about his experience at a recent conference, about listening to the presenters talk about the struggles of ADHD and how he felt furious at the world for the injustice of it all. Sitting in that crowded room, with so many others affected by ADHD, evoked a lifetime of frustration that he could barely contain. It brought back memories of his punitive father who never understood why he did the things that he did. Although he found some perspective with time, the visceral reaction in the moment was overwhelming.

This process of adjustment is addressed further in *The Four Stages of Adjustment to a New Diagnosis* on p. 195.

CHAPTER 3

THE ADHD BRAIN: WIRED A LITTLE DIFFERENTLY

Research has clearly shown that ADHD is a brain-based condition. Some parts of the brain tend to work differently or are different sizes than in people who don't have ADHD. The better our science gets, the more obvious these differences become. It isn't caused by bad parenting (although that doesn't make things any better), but it is often caused by the genetics that parents pass down to their kids. This can actually be liberating for both the person with ADHD and the parents who struggled to do the best job they could.

I don't go into too much detail in this chapter about the very complicated neurology of ADHD. I provide just enough of this kind of information to help you understand it, without drowning you in details. It's important to have a foundation in it, but not a doctorate.

This chapter contains the following articles:

The Many Facets of Attention

When most people think of attention, they think that someone is either paying attention or not. In reality, attention is a very complex neurological function made up of numerous subfunctions and probably involving different parts of the brain. It may be helpful to be aware of this, since we all have different strengths and weaknesses in these areas. We can break attention into these four subfunctions:

- *Selective attention*—the ability to focus on specific things while ignoring others, such as reading while ignoring background noise (sometimes also called *freedom from distractibility*)
- *Divided attention*—the ability to simultaneously attend to two or more stimuli, such as talking while driving
- *Shifting attention*—the ability to intentionally shift attention back and forth between two or more sources of information, such as shifting between the TV and newspaper
- *Sustained attention*—the ability to maintain attention on something boring with only limited reinforcement, such as folding a giant stack of laundry

People with ADHD can have trouble in all of these areas, but you may find that you're generally stronger or weaker in some than in others. Each can have a different effect on our ability to manage our lives. However, it may be that difficulties with sustained attention cause the most problems for folks with ADHD, since we all have to handle long and boring tasks to keep our lives running smoothly.

What Causes ADHD? More Nature Than Nurture

Research has found that ADHD is primarily caused by genetics, although environment may also play some role. So it's more about who your parents are than how they raised you (although their parenting style may affect whether you develop any of the conditions that tend to come along for the ride with ADHD). About one in four first-degree relatives (parents, siblings, and children) of someone with ADHD also have ADHD. In practical terms, we can therefore assume that if someone has ADHD, there is a very good chance that at least one other person in the family has it as well. This makes ADHD one of the most heritable mental health conditions, up there with bipolar disorder and schizophrenia. Researchers are still working on identifying all of the genes that are involved, since there are likely about half a dozen, each of which contributes in its own way.

Of course, as with most conditions, there is still some room for environmental influences. Since ADHD is a brain-based disorder, anything that affects brain development in pregnancy or during early childhood could have the potential to affect whether someone develops ADHD and how severely. This can include prenatal exposure to nicotine or alcohol; early exposure to lead, stroke, brain trauma; and low birth weight. Maternal smoking has been found to be the strongest predictor of ADHD symptoms in children (Barkley, 2006a). However, this may be an indirect effect in that ADHD children are more likely to have ADHD mothers who are more likely to smoke. So the smoking itself may not cause the ADHD in the child.

Things like parenting style and socioeconomic status have very little effect on who displays ADHD symptoms.

Things That Don't Cause ADHD (But Some People Still Think They Do)

Even though solid scientific research has proven what does and doesn't cause ADHD, there is still a lot of information out there about supposed causes that either have no scientific support or have been disproved. So let's go through those, since knowing what isn't true can be as important as knowing what is.

Diet and Food Additives

Probably the best-known unsupported theory is that ADHD is caused by diet, such as refined sugar, food additives, food allergies, or vitamin or mineral deficiencies. Refined sugar and artificial food colorings, in particular, gained notoriety from supporters of the Feingold diet. Of course everybody does better with a healthy diet, but study after study has found that diet does not create ADHD. A small minority of people may have reactions to certain foods that make them feel less focused, but ADHD involves far more than that. So, to state the obvious, if you find that certain foods affect you negatively, don't eat them.

Some of the confusion related to these diet theories is that many studies have indeed found that ADHD kids tend to eat more junk food. There are two reasons for this. First, impulsive ADHD kids may not delay gratification well and therefore are more likely to eat unhealthy foods that taste good. Second, ADHD kids are more likely to have an ADHD parent who will have a harder time doing the extra work that eating healthfully entails—junk food tends to be easier. So, in both cases, having ADHD causes the eating of junk food more than junk food causes ADHD. These early researchers were right in what they measured, but they got it reversed in what caused what.

The bottom line here is that changing your diet to treat your ADHD is a waste of time. It's good for you in other ways, so there's no harm in it. But focus on proven treatments. In a way, if you're able to maintain a generally healthy diet, it probably means that overall you're doing pretty well with your ADHD, since it takes stability and consistency to eat healthfully.

Bad Parenting

Probably every parent of an ADHD child has received comments that a better parenting style would get that kid to behave. This only adds insult to injury—not only is that parent struggling with raising a more challenging child, but the comments blame the parent for those challenges! Even when said in a supportive way and with good intentions, these comments can still increase feelings of helplessness and frustration. This is especially true for kids who were born before 1970; at that time ADHD was not well known, so those parents had to figure things out on their own, just as you did. So just as you hopefully cut yourself some slack once you learned about your ADHD, cut your parents some slack too (especially if they also had undiagnosed ADHD).

Just as with the early research done on diet, the researchers were right about what they measured, but they got the causes reversed. That is, ADHD kids cause bad parenting more than bad parenting causes ADHD, so the researchers measured the result rather than the cause. Untreated ADHD children are better at pushing their parents past their limits, so those parents use fewer positive behavior-management techniques and more negative ones. As further proof, some really interesting studies have found that when ADHD kids are prescribed medication that controls their problematic behaviors, their parents wind up using more positive parenting techniques and fewer negative ones (Barkley, 2006b). Amazing—the parents perform better when their kids take medication! Of course, most of the parents of the ADHD kids in my practice could have told you this, too.

Modern Society

A third theory holds that the sometimes frenetic pace of modern life makes us all more distractible and hyperactive and even gives some people ADHD. This is used to explain why ADHD seems so much more prevalent now than it used to. As much as our electronics-driven information overload can distract even the most single-minded among us, there simply is no connection between our increased pace of life and the development of ADHD. If this theory were true, we would find that slower-paced societies have fewer cases of ADHD—but they don't.

At most, we can say that ADHD symptoms are more obvious and debilitating in our fast-paced and complicated world. This is similar to saying that a white shirt is more obvious against a black background than it is against a white one, but we would never say that the black background caused the white shirt.

Natural Selection for a Different Time

Some people claim that those with ADHD are the descendants of hunters from our distant past, in contrast to the majority, who were farmers. The theory is that the quick reaction times and distractibility characteristic of ADHD actually were evolutionarily adaptive at one time. By contrast, the farmers were better at routine and repetition. Unfortunately for these hunters, modern society no longer values those traits, so the hunters are forced to live in a farmer's world.

These romanticized notions may make some people feel better about themselves in the moment ("Wow, I'm just a misunderstood hunter!"), but it doesn't change the reality that people with ADHD need to function now in our current society, not in some inaccurate vision of life many thousands of years ago. As I will repeat countless times in this book, I prefer to build people's self-esteem by helping them change what they can, then accept the rest. This is easier if you start out with rock-solid information, because then no one can take that away from you by disproving your beliefs.

Neurology of ADHD

ADHD is a brain-based disorder. The brains of those with ADHD have been found to be different than the brains of those without ADHD in several ways. Most functions involve the interaction of more than one brain area, but the primary area affected by those with ADHD is the frontal lobes. This is the area right behind the forehead. It is involved in some of the highest-level information processing, including the executive functions, which are discussed in other parts of the book.

Research has found that the affected areas are less active in those with ADHD compared with those without ADHD, at least when you take groups of people. (However, this doesn't mean that brain scans can be used to diagnose individuals—see *Brain Scans* on page 40.) So because these parts of the brain don't operate as effectively, folks with ADHD don't process information as well in certain ways.

Our brains use dozens of different compounds as neurotransmitters, which serve as the signal between nerve cells and allow them to communicate. In ADHD, the affected areas use mostly dopamine, although some use norepinephrine. The medications used to treat ADHD increase the amount of these neurotransmitters and thereby correct the shortfall. This also explains why the antidepressants, which mostly affect serotonin, have no direct benefit for ADHD, whereas the couple antidepressants that also affect norepinephrine have some potential benefit for ADHD. Unfortunately, at this time, there is no way to reliably predict which medication will work best for which person without using trial and error. Interestingly, medication tends to make the brain scans of people with ADHD look more like those of people without ADHD, which makes sense, since it does the same to their performance.

Promoting Brain Health

Anything that is generally good for our brains is probably good for people with ADHD. I'm referring to the obvious things like eating a fully balanced diet, getting enough sleep, and exercising regularly. The opposite can be said for the things that are generally bad for our brains and are best avoided, like cigarettes, alcohol, drugs, sedentary lifestyles, unhealthy foods, various toxins, and excessive stress.

However, the fact that these things affect our brains doesn't mean that we consider them as part of the cause of ADHD—or use them as a central part of the treatment. Adding in more of the positives and minimizing the negatives will allow someone with ADHD to perform at her best but won't change the fact that she still has ADHD. By contrast, not doing enough of the good things and doing lots of the bad will only make the ADHD person perform worse. This is true for everyone, so it isn't really an ADHD-specific intervention. So those New Year's resolutions are good for all of us. Of course, sticking with them is easier said than done...

CHAPTER 4

ADHD AFFECTS EVERYTHING: NO WONDER MY LIFE WAS SO HARD!

Hi Dr. Tuckman,

I was diagnosed with ADD last year. I have suffered from various symptoms since childhood. I often find myself not being able to handle the pressure of life. Just getting simple things done, and I am single with no kids. ADHD has long affected my relationships, my work habits, my finances, etc. I am now at the point where I really can't deal with it any longer. Last year after my diagnosis, I refused to take my meds. And this just perpetuates the problems. My anxiety level is extremely high. And I get to the point where I want to shut myself off from society…which is where I am now. My doctor retired last winter, and I am looking for someone new. Please let me know if you are accepting new patients.

This email from a prospective client neatly captures all of the struggles faced by adults with ADHD. If you are an adult with ADHD, none of this should be surprising or unfamiliar. In one short paragraph, this woman summarized what a life with untreated ADHD is like. She is generally overwhelmed yet is ambivalent about treatment. She's feeling anxious and depressed, which is hardly surprising, given the difficulties she's having. As you probably also know well, it can be a real challenge to find treatment providers who really understand the many complicated and subtle effects of ADHD in adults. The bottom line here is that this woman is going under.

I wish that I could say that this email is a fluke, one in a thousand. But I get a fair number of them. And it's not just locals who send me these—I get them from people all around the country, hoping that I might know of someone near them.

What all these emails tell us is that life is much harder with untreated ADHD. If you didn't know this already, you wouldn't be reading this book, whether you're the person with ADHD or you're reading it for someone else. In this chapter, I review and summarize the abundant research that shows the pervasive effects that untreated ADHD can have on someone's life. This goes far beyond the well-publicized effects on academic performance and covers pretty much every other area of an adult's life.

This chapter discusses the various ways that ADHD affects people's lives, including both the direct and indirect effects of a lifetime of undiagnosed and untreated ADHD (you could call this the downer chapter). Of course, sweeping generalizations don't accurately tell everyone's story, but most readers should find a fair bit they can relate to in this chapter. Some readers may find great relief in having their experiences validated and may even suspect that I spied on them to write this chapter (no comment). Others may feel kind of depressed to see a long list of problems, some of which they hadn't even realized they have. Hang in there—it does get better. I strongly believe that you need to know what you're dealing with before you can do anything about it, but if you need some more immediate solutions before you can stomach looking at problems, then no biggie. Come back around to this chapter later, if you feel like it. Or not.

This chapter contains the following articles:

Risk Factors, Protective Factors (p. 68) Research has found that certain factors tend to contribute to worse outcomes and others to better. Although you can't change your past, it may help explain why certain things worked out for you the way that they did. It may also be helpful to keep in mind if you have a child with ADHD.

Consistently Inconsistent: I Can Do Anything Once! (p. 69) Most successes in life require consistency. Unfortunately, one of the most confusing aspects of ADHD is that most people with it have the ability to do what they need to, but somehow they can't do it reliably enough.

Knowing Is Easy; Doing Is Hard (p. 70) Most people with ADHD tend to know what they're supposed to do and how to do it but have a tough time making it happen.

ADHD and the Evolving Personality (p. 71) As with many things, growing up with ADHD can influence how your personality develops because it tends to make some situations more likely and other situations less likely. This is also affected by when you were diagnosed and whether you were treated.

Living Without a Diagnosis: Living the Hard Way (p. 73) It's easy to get down on yourself if you have ADHD but don't know it. Without this possible explanation, you're left with a bunch of other explanations like laziness or bad attitude, none of which anyone would feel good about.

ADHD at School: Sometimes Intelligence Isn't Enough (p. 74) One of the reasons why so many more kids than adults are diagnosed with ADHD is that school tends to reveal ADHD weaknesses. The older a student gets, the more he is expected to manage increasingly complex assignments and the more that difficulties with concentration, time management, and organization reveal themselves.

ADHD at Work: More Options Than in School (p. 77) The work world offers many more options than school does, which can be great news. It makes it easier for all of us to find a situation that is a good fit for our strengths and weaknesses.

However, ADHD difficulties may be more problematic when an adult is expected to function at a higher level than children and teens are.

Daily Life Functioning: Doing Everyday Stuff Every Day (p. 79) For most people, daily life involves a thousand little things that need to be done, pretty much every day. Juggling all these unrelated tasks can be a real challenge for adults with ADHD, causing too many things to slip through the cracks.

Money Management: Where Does All My Money Go? (p. 81) Research has found that adults with ADHD have more money troubles than those without. There are several reasons for this, including impulsive spending, late fees from forgetting to pay bills, and general disorganization.

Social Skills and Friendships (p. 83) Social interactions are pretty complex and easily affected by ADHD symptoms, from blurting things out to forgetting what someone told you.

Romantic Relationships: Where's Cupid Now? (p. 85) A good romantic relationship requires the best that each person can give. Unfortunately, untreated ADHD symptoms tend to undermine your ability to consistently give your best. (They also may bring out some of the worst in your partner.)

Parenting: Hard Enough Under the Best of Circumstances (p. 87) Having children adds stress to any relationship. If one of the parents has ADHD, it can really exacerbate the couple's ability to work cooperatively to handle the million daily demands, especially if one of the children also has ADHD.

Self-Image and Sense of Effectiveness: A Little Bit Dented (p. 90) We come to understand ourselves through the various successes and failures that we have as well as other people's reactions to them. Someone growing up with untreated ADHD will tend to find herself in certain kinds of situations and evoke certain kinds of reactions that can affect how she later sees herself.

Unhelpful Coping Strategies: Common Habits and Defense Mechanisms (p. 91) People with ADHD tend to use certain coping strategies to deal with the difficult situations that they find themselves in. Although these coping strategies reduce the discomfort in the moment, they tend to bring more troubles later. It can be helpful to identify which ones you tend to use so that you can perhaps choose a different approach.

Substance Use and Addiction: When the Solution Becomes a Problem (p. 101) Teens and adults with ADHD are more likely to engage in addictive behaviors than other people are. There are several understandable reasons for this, but it tends to make things worse.

Driving: No Big Deal, Until It Is (p. 102) Driving is a very attention-intensive task, especially because we need to maintain our attention even when not much is actually happening. Most of the time, brief lapses in attention or impulsive choices don't cause any problems, but the consequences can be extremely serious.

Crime and Punishment: ADHD and the Legal System (p. 103) People with untreated ADHD are more likely to run into trouble with the law—yet another reason why early treatment is important.

Risk Factors, Protective Factors

In the most general sense, we can say that the more ADHD symptoms someone has and the more severe they are, the more parts of his life will be affected. This probably isn't surprising. However, an interesting shift takes place as a person enters adulthood. The hyperactivity and impulsivity (if you had them) that created so many problems in childhood tend to settle down, but the inattention symptoms remain. What's worse, the demands for careful attention greatly increase as a person leaves the family nest. So the inattention symptoms become more problematic as one enters adulthood.

Researchers like to figure out which factors predict positive or negative outcomes for those affected by various conditions. We can then use this information to select the interventions that are most likely to have a beneficial effect. Keep in mind, though, that we're complicated creatures, so no single factor is as predictive as a combination would be. Also remember that researchers deal with groups, whereas you as an individual may have had different factors affect you. For example, you may have had pretty bad ADHD, but you were a real charmer and were able to get teachers to work with you, so you managed to do OK in school.

If you are already an adult, these two lists may help you understand why certain things worked out the way that they did. If you are the parent of a child, teen, or young adult with ADHD, this list may help you choose what to focus most on. Most of these shouldn't be surprising

Negative Outcomes

The following factors have been correlated with negative outcomes for those with ADHD:

- More severe ADHD symptoms and/or other conditions, such as anxiety, depression, or substance abuse
- The presence of impulsivity or aggressiveness, since then the child is far more likely to also have oppositional defiant disorder or conduct disorder, which leads to other difficulties
- Poor social skills or self-care abilities

- Traumatic experiences
- Lower socioeconomic status, if it creates additional psychological and emotional strain on the family
- Family instability, such as divorce or job loss
- Parental depression, law breaking, and/or substance abuse

Positive Outcomes

By contrast, these factors have been correlated with positive outcomes for those with ADHD:

- A protective effect of treatment (earlier and more intense treatment probably leads to better outcomes)
- Lack of hyperactivity or impulsivity (i.e., only the inattentive symptoms)
- Greater intelligence, in that more raw intellectual power partially compensates for some of the lost efficiencies resulting from the ADHD
- Special talents, interests, and experiences that build self-esteem
- An environment that promotes structure and predictability so one can perform at one's best
- A school or work environment that does not overly punish ADHD traits
- Social support from family and friends who accept the negative and appreciate the positive in the person

Conclusion

You can't change your past, but there is value in understanding how the past has shaped the present. Life isn't fair, so some of us have had to work much harder to find success and happiness. If you were born at a time when ADHD was still relatively unknown, you have had a harder road than those who are being born today. You may have some catching up to do to get to where you feel you should have been, but better late than never! I've done ADHD evaluations on clients in their sixties and have colleagues who have clients in their seventies, so it's never too late.

Consistently Inconsistent: I Can Do Anything Once!

People with ADHD can do anything once. The problem is, most things in life need to be done repeatedly—especially the boring things. The electric company isn't much impressed if you get one payment in on time. Unfortunately, they're really good at noticing if your payment arrives late.

People with ADHD perform some tasks quite well but not others, or they can't maintain a consistent performance for the same task over time. This means that sometimes they do great on mundane activities, like doing all the laundry in a flurry of activity, but most of the time it looks like a mountain of dirty clothes is trying to eat the hamper. Or they may do well on a new activity but then lose momentum over time as the novelty wears off.

For example, I had a client who was the top salesman for his company when he started. Within a few months, when the job had lost its spark, he became one of the lowest producers, much to his supervisor's confusion and chagrin. Unfortunately, this occasional good performance can be the most damning evidence against ADHD folks because it's seen as proof of their abilities. When they perform badly, people assume it's more about attitude than ability. What they don't realize is that the ability to be consistent over time and across situations is a skill in itself. For example, filling out checks and licking envelopes aren't really that hard, but remembering to do it (every month!) is.

In fact, when I am doing an ADHD evaluation, I look for these kinds of inconsistent performance. If someone has no problem being consistent on these sorts of maintenance activities, then she probably doesn't have ADHD. On the flip side, though, if the person almost never does these things well, then I wonder if the problem is actually some other learning disability or lack of ability.

Success in life is built not on doing a few things really well but on doing lots of things at least reasonably well. Or just doing them. It's built on doing a thousand little things a day for a thousand days in a row. ADHD folks run into trouble on the stuff that's really pretty easy—as long as they remember to do it when it's time to do it, have all the necessary stuff on hand, and take it all the way to completion. Life rarely gives partial credit. The reasons for this inconsistency are covered in more detail in chapter 1, which discusses executive functions, so you may want to review that if you haven't read it already.

Knowing Is Easy; Doing Is Hard

Most people with ADHD generally know what they're supposed to do, how to do it, why it's a good idea to do it, and probably when it would be ideal to get it done. That's the easy part. The hard part is actually doing it. That's kind of a contradiction—the task isn't hard, but it's hard to do it. For example, filing papers isn't inherently difficult, but sitting down and following through with it is. Going to the grocery store is easy, but actually getting there *before* the fridge is empty is hard.

This is why it's easy to tell other people what to do, but it's harder to follow that advice ourselves. All the complexities of daily life get in the way of following the plans and priorities that we set for ourselves, whereas those don't exist when we're sitting around offering advice. Also, when we're giving advice to others, we're able to hone in on just the relevant matters and screen out other factors, something that's harder to do when we're emotionally involved in our own lives.

As a result, a lot of ADHD folks get down on themselves for having such a hard time on such easy tasks. They may knock on themselves for being stupid or self-destructive for not doing these simple tasks (and others may happily chime in on the criticism). Sometimes the challenge is the task itself, but sometimes the challenge is managing the rest of their lives so that the task actually gets done.

Sometimes the Hard Part Is Boredom

Many tasks in life are pretty easy but really boring: filing papers, paying bills, mowing the lawn, and loading the dishwasher. These tasks aren't hard, but adults with ADHD often have a hard time doing them. The challenge is to fight the boredom and actually start and then stick with these brain-numbing activities. So it's really more about boredom management than anything else.

Sometimes the Hard Part Is Juggling

Other tasks may not be that boring, so it's more a matter of remembering and planning ahead to be in a good position to do them at the right time. It's kind of like how throwing a ball a few feet up in the air and catching it is easy. No problem. But catching that ball when you're also juggling five other balls, that's much harder. For many ADHD folks, life feels like they're forced to keep ten balls in the air when they can really manage only four. Or three. So they wind up flailing around, dropping some and flinging others, randomly jumping from one task to the next without any real plan. Important tasks are forgotten while trivial ones are completed. It's not that they aren't good at catching one ball; it's that they aren't good at catching ten.

ADHD and the Evolving Personality

Even if you're not big on Freud, we can all agree that what happens in childhood has some effect on who we become as adults. This can be both good and bad, depending on the temperament we're born with and how well our environment fits with and caters to those innate tendencies. We've all had experiences that have positively shaped the people we've become, and we've also all had negative experiences that we found a way to overcome. If you have ADHD, especially if you were born before ADHD was well understood, you probably had more than your fair share of negative experiences. It's hard to not bear some scars from that.

You don't want to live in the past or allow old bad stuff to get in the way of enjoying new good stuff, but it helps to understand how those old experiences shaped who you are now. With knowledge comes the power to do things differently, to make the future better than the past.

ADHD can have both direct and indirect effects on someone's life. An example of a direct effect is the undiagnosed student who did poorly in school and now doesn't have the necessary degrees to get the jobs that are at her level of ability. Even if this is ancient history by now, it will obviously carry forward and continue to affect her life. An indirect effect is a situation where someone's ADHD caused problems with maintaining friendships because of forgetfulness and interrupting. Even if many of his ADHD symptoms have subsided or medication mostly cleans them up, he may still hold himself back socially because of an expectation that he doesn't do well socially. Although it is easy to understand this pessimism, things might be different now as an adult, but he will never discover that if he doesn't try again and push himself beyond his comfort zone. So the past lives on in the present.

The direct effects tend to be pretty obvious, whereas the indirect effects simply get woven into the tapestry of our personalities. These automatic parts of our personalities can be invisible to us, because they are so inherently part of who we are and how we always remember ourselves. This stuff may be more visible to other people and especially to a perceptive therapist. In fact, part of the goal of therapy is to teach clients about themselves so that they have the option to see or do things differently. This is especially true of those with previously undiagnosed ADHD who were not able to do things differently, despite their best efforts.

Untreated ADHD can color every situation someone finds himself in, like doing homework, managing money, and handling interactions with family and friends. Over time, as certain experiences occur much more frequently than other experiences, someone can't help but be affected by the patterns. He may even come to expect certain outcomes—which, of course, makes those outcomes more likely. For example, if he doesn't expect to do well in math, he probably won't study his hardest, which sets him up to not do as well on the next test, but then also not do as well on later material that is built on it. Or, if she expects that her room will always fall quickly to chaos, then she probably won't clean it up all that often. So the past carries forward into the future, sometimes in ways that we're not fully aware of. This can affect how we feel about ourselves, our ability to be successful in various endeavors, and other people. The ripples keep rolling.

Age at Diagnosis

It's worth keeping in mind that someone who is diagnosed with ADHD as an adult probably had a very different life than someone who was diagnosed and treated as a child or teen. Those who were diagnosed later probably had a harder life. Today's kids who are being diagnosed are growing up in a different world. Not only is there greater awareness and acceptance of ADHD, but we have effective treatments and accommodations available at school. The majority of adults out there, however, were born too early and had to find success and happiness the hard way. At least in this regard, your kids and grandkids will have an easier time of it.

Living Without a Diagnosis: Living the Hard Way

Even though ADHD has been around forever, only recently has it been widely recognized (1980s for kids, 1990s for adults). So there were many, many people with ADHD whose obvious symptoms were explained in some other way since ADHD wasn't a possible explanation. There are many reasons why someone's ADHD may be missed, and this was covered in *Missed Diagnoses* on p. 48. But for this article, let's talk about the effect of living without that diagnosis, of having to come up with other explanations for those difficulties.

Our minds automatically seek explanations for things, so when we don't know something for sure, we make assumptions. For someone with ADHD, her symptoms are clear but the explanation isn't, so everyone makes assumptions about why she doesn't do better. Of course, all the old familiar explanations are used—she just needs to try harder, she's irresponsible, she doesn't care enough, she wants to do badly. This very much adds insult to injury. Not only doesn't it help her do better, but it just makes her question herself: "Huh. I thought I tried my best on that, but maybe I didn't." Initially most people tend to fight back against these accusations, but over time the accusations begin to sink in and influence how people see and feel about themselves.

This can then become a self-fulfilling prophecy. Since the ADHD isn't being treated, of course all the same problems keep happening. The person hears these negative comments again and again and eventually starts to believe them. So there goes her motivation to try to do better, since it probably won't work out well anyway. Given her track record, this is a pretty reasonable conclusion. Unfortunately, it also becomes a self-fulfilling prophecy since not trying new strategies, or trying them half-heartedly, tends to bring about those same old failures. So when she is finally diagnosed, she may be guarded in her optimism to try new strategies, even though these have a better chance of being successful.

As time goes on and she doesn't take advantage of opportunities to practice either new or old skills, predictably, she doesn't get better at them. She then starts to fall behind her peers who are using the skills more often. Practice may not make perfect, but it does make better. Seeing this growing gap between what she can do and what she sees others doing only gives her more to feel bad about. Round and round it goes.

Fortunately, this can all change if she is diagnosed and actively seeks treatment. That can open up a whole new life, but it's a tough ride before then. Read sections II, III, and IV for strategies to make your life better.

ADHD at School: Sometimes Intelligence Isn't Enough

When most people think of ADHD, usually the first thing they think about is the effect that it has in school. There's some good reason for this—even if someone is really bright, having ADHD makes it much harder to apply those abilities and be successful academically. This is because success at school requires strengths where many ADHD students are weak—paying attention to sometimes less-than-thrilling lectures, ignoring distractions from classmates, tracking multiple assignments, remembering to bring home all the right books and papers (then bring them all back to school), staying organized, and persisting with repetitive homework assignments.

As a result, the statistics on ADHD students' academic performance are sobering. For example, one large longitudinal study found that one-third of the hyperactive students failed to graduate from high school, compared to none in the control group. In addition, only one-fifth of the hyperactive group had ever enrolled in college, compared to four-fifths of the control group (Barkley, 2006c).

In general, ADHD can affect a person's ability to apply her intelligence effectively in the world and adapt to challenges. These students lose efficiency (some tasks take longer) and also lose effectiveness (they get less done or at a lower quality than they ideally could). Students with high intelligence may be somewhat protected since they have more mental horsepower to spare, so they may not suffer as much from the lost effectiveness. They may be better able to fill in the blanks when they miss parts of the lesson, based on what they did catch. At home, they may also be able to produce strong papers or crank through homework more quickly and easily when they do kick themselves into gear. Even so, intelligence doesn't really offer much protection in the areas of self-control, organization, time management, or exercise of good judgment, so there will still be a price paid for those with hyperactive and impulsive symptoms.

Probably the area of school that is most affected by ADHD is homework. By the time a student reaches middle school, more and more homework is assigned each year. This can feel like rubbing salt in the wound—*I just spent all day at school and now I have to do more work!?* Of course, most daily assignments are not especially hard and are mostly a matter of putting the time in. The biggest challenge is just sitting through them, and this is where ADHD students have trouble. For high schoolers, homework can be the bane of their existence, the thing that they hate more than anything else. Unfortunately, even brilliant students who ace the tests can still wind up with a C, D, or even F if they don't hand in most of the assignments, since homework is often weighted so heavily in the overall grading. Even those students who are motivated to do their best may still miss too many assignments, do the wrong assignments, or turn them in incomplete or late. I call this wide split between tests and homework the unofficial grade profile of the bright ADHD student.

Beyond the daily assignments, the papers and projects become more complex and span larger stretches of time in high school. High school is often a real challenge for ADHD students, since it demands the ability to manage these kinds of longer assignments. This is a completely different set of skills. For example, the student may know the nuts and bolts of how to research and write a paper but have trouble planning his time while taking other demands into account so that it all gets done before the due date. The hard part is the planning and time management, not the writing. Whereas bright students can kind of get by with some minimal effort in earlier grades, this is a lot harder to pull off in high school as the assignments become more involved and can't be done by flipping through the book and scribbling something out on the bus. So being a good student requires lots of skills beyond academic abilities.

Self-Esteem and Motivation Suffer

Unfortunately, for almost all ADHD students, the difficulties they have in performing up to their potential are well known to themselves and others, resulting in frequent comments from parents, teachers, and classmates about those difficulties. It makes most parents and teachers crazy to see how much potential these students have, if only they would "try harder." This then leads to attempts to clamp down on the student to ensure that he does what he needs to. This desire to rescue the student from a bad situation is understandable (at least to me) but often isn't appreciated by the student. Most teenagers want more freedom, not less, so they resist the intrusion and fight like hell to keep their parents out of it, even resorting to lying and hiding work. When the parents discover this, they then clamp down even harder, and the cycle goes around again. Tempers flare, threats and accusations fly, promises are made and then broken, and then it all starts again. It becomes an awful experience for all involved. Getting good grades is a worthy goal, even if the parents' and student's methods don't work that well.

Predictably, these negative experiences often lead to negative feelings toward school and even oneself—the students, parents, *and* teachers can all feel like failures, alternating between blaming themselves and blaming others. Some students protect themselves from these painful feelings by checking out. They stop trying, since they don't have to feel as bad about doing something poorly if they didn't try. It makes sense in a way because it does get rid of the suffering in the moment, except that it is a setup for later troubles. A colleague and friend of mine, Russ Ramsay, Ph.D., got the following responses from an ADHD high school student on a questionnaire the student filled out:

Feelings about middle school: "sucked"

Feelings about high school: "sucks"

Feelings about college: "is going to suck"

Yikes! This kid has had such a hard road that he's given up hope of the future being any better.

Although this disengagement can be protective in the short term, it obviously compounds the problem over time, in that school is a progression that builds on earlier lessons. So whether a student inadvertently missed something because she was lost in thought or intentionally tuned out when the teacher explained it, the student may find future lessons much more difficult without this foundational knowledge. I call this "Swiss cheese knowledge," wherein the student has a general sense of the subject but is lacking bits and pieces. She may know that she doesn't know something or may not even realize that she missed something important. This can create problems later when that missing information is needed. This may be especially noticeable and problematic in math and science classes. So even if someone has the basic abilities to be successful in a class, he may still struggle because he can't make himself practice in subjects requiring repetitive and sustained effort for mastery, such as math and foreign languages.

College Can Be Even Harder

The characteristics of high school that are most troublesome for ADHD students only get worse in college. The parents and teachers who would provide direction and keep the student on track through high school are no longer available in college. Professors don't take that same hands-on approach, figuring that these young adults should be able to manage their own work. For most students, this is probably true, but not for all—as many ADHD college students learn the hard way.

If extra help is needed, it takes much more initiative on the student's part to seek it out. By the time a professor realizes that a student is in trouble, it's often too late to do much about it. So the student has to realize that she is struggling or falling behind, accept the need for help, and then get herself going on seeking that help out. This could be talking to the professor or an advisor or meeting with a tutor. Although some colleges provide excellent support services, generally speaking it is less than what is available in most high schools. Too often a student waits until the final weeks of the semester before getting help, at which point it may be impossible to rescue the semester.

Because college students don't have anyone looking over their shoulders to make sure they are waking up on time, getting to class, and doing their reading, it's up to them to be diligent. Unfortunately, college also provides virtually limitless temptations and distractions, all of which are more interesting than schoolwork. So the students who have trouble resisting distractions will too often be pulled off track, despite their good intentions—like my client who would impulsively jump into an informal Frisbee game on his way to the library. Meanwhile, they're expected to perform at an even higher level. To make matters worse, many of these ADHD students go off the medications that helped them perform well and get into college in the first place. Ironically, they remove something helpful right when things get hardest.

Put it all together and it's not surprising that an unfortunate number do not graduate the first time through. I've seen lots of these folks who fail out and have to move back home, something that neither the student nor the parents are happy about. The student would obviously rather be back at school with friends than living at home but may secretly doubt his ability to be successful there. Mom and Dad are understandably hesitant to send their child back when they have little reason to expect things to be different the second time around. Meanwhile, the student is limited in the jobs that he can get without a college degree. This then puts him in a double bind—suffer with these unsatisfying jobs or risk further failure and frustration by returning to school to get the degree that would give him access to jobs that he's better suited for.

The hard reality is that many jobs and careers are limited to people with certain grades, test scores, or degrees. So those who have the ability but not the credentials, for whatever reasons, may never be given a chance to prove themselves. So trouble in school in one's teens and twenties can carry forward into later life. This is certainly not meant to imply that everyone should go to college or work a white-collar job. Rather, it's that all people should have the opportunity to pursue the paths that would be the best fit for their interests and overall abilities. Those with poor academic records close off some of those options prematurely and have fewer opportunities later in life, perhaps forcing them to settle for careers that are less rewarding, both financially and psychologically.

See chapter 16, *College and Beyond: Teach an Old Dog New Tricks* for information on how to make college a success.

ADHD at Work: More Options Than in School

Most ADHD students feel a great sense of relief when they graduate. After all those years of struggle and strife, they can move on to bigger and better things and hopefully find a job where they can more easily work to their potential. After all those years of being told that they should do better, maybe now they finally can.

Success at work requires some very different skills than success at school. This is both bad news and good news if you have ADHD.

I'll start with the negatives, then give you some cause for optimism. The statistics aren't pretty. ADHD adults are two-thirds more likely to have been fired; three times more likely to have quit impulsively; one-third more likely to report chronic employment difficulties; and 50 percent more likely to have changed jobs in any given time period. Employers rate ADHD employees in more negative terms on measures of meeting job expectations, getting along with supervisors, working independently, and completing work assignments. ADHD employees often get into trouble by not understanding their supervisors' or coworkers' expectations, by choosing an inappropriate career, or by not having the self-confidence to deal with these sorts of dilemmas (Crawford and Crawford, 2002).

ADHD behavior can be difficult for coworkers to tolerate, especially when it affects them, as in a group project or where their work is dependent on someone else's. I have many, many examples from my practice, but one particular client comes to mind. He tended to procrastinate and often missed deadlines. Although he was somewhat bothered by this, his coworkers were far more disturbed by it. He was eventually fired (again) because he was affecting the work of colleagues who depended on his reports to do their jobs.

On the plus side, compared to school, it can be easier for an adult with ADHD to be effective at work. This is mostly because adults have far more options with jobs than students do, so they can find one that is a better fit, whereas most schools are pretty much the same. In addition, work performance may be measured in ways they can better meet, tasks may be more interesting or meaningful, or the job itself may provide more structure. This all makes their ADHD less noticeable.

Some may be lucky enough to have an assistant manage the boring and annoying details so they can focus on better things. This brings to mind an extremely hyperactive client who worked as a day trader to meet his need for constant stimulation and who had enough self-knowledge to hire an assistant to handle the paperwork so that the trades actually went through. Same for the mortgage broker who happily paid an assistant quite well to handle the countless forms required for each loan. On the flip side, employees who were successful when they had administrative support may really suffer if those positions are cut and they need to do that work themselves.

Some ADHD adults may succeed in their first jobs, when the demands placed on them are generally lower or when there is more oversight to keep them on track. However, they may begin to struggle after a promotion to a position that requires them to do the planning and oversight. This new position requires too many skills that they aren't good at and didn't need in their previous position, so the strong performer doesn't live up to expectations after the promotion. Alternatively, even if the person's job doesn't change, she may have a harder time keeping up with it as demands at home increase, like after the birth of a child, since she can no longer make up for inefficiencies at work by staying late.

Adults with ADHD are more likely than non-ADHD folks to use certain bad habits at work. Check out *Unhelpful Coping Strategies* on p. 91 for more information, particularly the parts on pseudoproductivity and abandoning ship. On the flip side, check out chapter 17, *Work: Hopefully More Than Just a Paycheck*, for strategies for finding the right job and making the most of it.

Daily Life Functioning: Doing Everyday Stuff Every Day

It takes a lot of work to keep our lives running smoothly, from paying bills to buying groceries to doing laundry. All of this stuff needs to be completed by at least one person in a family or couple. Few of these necessary activities are exciting or satisfying, and most need to be done again on a pretty regular basis. These are the sorts of tasks where there is no reward for doing them, but there are significant problems or penalties for not doing them or doing them late. It's just expected that adults take care of this stuff without too much struggle or complaint. Most people see them as a necessary evil but not as inherently difficult. Boring and annoying, maybe, but not hard.

Perhaps more so than most people, those with ADHD too often live their lives in crisis mode. With too many of these everyday kinds of chores, they do what they need to, probably at the last minute, just to avoid or stop a painful situation. For example, someone with ADHD will finally get around to cleaning up the living room only to stop his romantic partner from griping. Or he scrambles to get the credit card bill in the mail only to avoid a late fee. Although this may spur the person into action, avoiding pain is not as inspiring as being drawn toward rewards.

Although ADHD can lead to dramatic disasters, like when a blink in attention causes a car accident, most of the time it's the smaller and more frequent problems that cause the most damage to the person's and family's peace of mind and quality of life. It's the constant wear and tear of daily stress that ultimately has the biggest effect. After a lifetime of running from the avalanche, many with ADHD assume that they are forever destined to suffer with this kind of chaos. This actually makes sense since past attempts to get on top of it all tended to fade away to nothing. Over time, they may stop trying to make it better and just roll with it, much to the frustration of others in their lives.

Ground Down by the Daily Grind

What separates ADHD folks from others is their difficulty with handling the daily requirements of life that are not necessarily difficult in isolation but can become overwhelming in total. The analogy is that of snowflakes—pretty one by one, but scary in an avalanche. For too many ADHD adults, much of life feels as though they are running half a step ahead of that avalanche. Just as the snow on a mountain top builds slowly, so do the various tasks and objects in an ADHD household. Then suddenly the ADHD adult is forced into action and scrambles to get it all under control, only to let it all build back up again afterward. These dramatic and sometimes impressive bursts of activity are exhausting and tend to make the person not want to deal with any of it again for a long time.

Unfortunately, keeping an adult life running smoothly requires an ability to keep lots of balls in the air at the same time. It takes a consistent input of energy to fight back the disorder and chaos that are naturally created by living. There are several reasons why adults with ADHD may struggle more than most with these constant demands:

- *Slippery time management.* As our lives get busier and more complicated, there is less wiggle room to take up the slack for those who have trouble creating and sticking with a strong plan. As a result, some important activities simply aren't done because the entire day has passed.
- *Distractibility undermines the best-laid plans.* Even with the best of intentions, the ADHD adult may unintentionally find her attention pulled astray. As one of my clients described to her husband, it isn't that she decided to skip wiping up the spilled syrup; it's merely that she was constantly being pulled to another task, like making the kids' lunches, getting dressed, and feeding the dog. So the syrup spill simply disappeared from her radar screen, even though she knew it would take only a moment to wipe it up, and her husband would be upset to find it on the floor that night. This type of problem repeats constantly in her life, in a million variations.
- *Underdeveloped skills.* Over the course of a lifetime of untreated ADHD, some adults aren't as strong as they could be in certain areas, such as in using a to-do list most effectively. This is usually a small part of the problem, but it can contribute to some situations.
- *Boredom with the current moment.* Some adults with ADHD feel driven to move on to something new before they've finished what they started. This can be a real problem for tasks that take time and are repetitive, which describes many adult demands. So, many tasks are started, but most of them aren't ever finished. For example, the half-folded laundry is still scattered across the couch days later.

When you put it all together, adults with ADHD tend to lead more stressful lives. One consequence of this is that it becomes much more difficult to lead a balanced lifestyle that involves good habits in the areas of diet, exercise, sleep, and relaxation time. This has predictable effects on overall health and well being and efficiency, so tomorrow is worse than today. Check out chapter 14, *Household Management: Stay on Top of the Boring Stuff at Home*, for strategies to make tomorrow a better day.

Money Management: Where Does All My Money Go?

Many ADHD adults struggle with staying on top of their finances. It could be little things, like burning through whatever is in their wallet, or big things, like racking up significant credit card debt or killing their credit with missed payments. Some people lack certain basic skills, like balancing a checkbook or creating a budget, but it usually isn't that simple. As with everything else in life, they usually know what to do but have trouble doing it consistently—not once, not occasionally, but most of the time.

There are many reasons why adults with ADHD run into money trouble. Let's run through them.

- *Impulsive spending.* There are lots of shiny things out there to catch the eye. Those with ADHD are more likely to fall prey to these temptations, whether it's something small or something as large as a car. I had a client who would never leave a store without buying something. Of course, acting in the moment without taking into account the bigger picture tends to lead to unnecessary purchases and later regrets. If credit cards are used, this is especially hard to notice at the time, since you don't see that all your cash is gone (it's really easy to notice, though, when the bill shows up). This is the sort of thing where the person starts out with a full wallet and then somehow the money's all gone but it's hard to say exactly where it all went.
- *Slippery memory.* Even when an adult with ADHD stops to think about a potential purchase, he may still make an unwise choice. Good choices are based on consideration of how individual purchases fit into the whole financial picture. This requires the ability to remember and mentally calculate how much money is coming in and how much is going out. So, for example, if he forgets that he has his car insurance payment coming up, he may incorrectly assume that he has plenty of money to spare for a new (super-cool) TV. This moment of forgetfulness obviously sets up a horrible moment of realization later.

- *Disorganization.* There is often a price paid for not having a balanced checkbook, workable budget, and system for keeping the necessary records for taxes. This stuff is boring but important.
- *Plugging the gaps.* In addition to the big, dramatic purchases, people with ADHD tend to dribble away money in lots of small ways that can really add up, like buying lunch because they didn't have time to make it or buying a duplicate of something they already own but can't find. They use money to compensate for or undo the fallout of their ADHD.
- *Late fees and poor credit.* Writing checks and licking envelopes aren't hard, but remembering to do it is. Even when they have plenty of money, people with ADHD have difficulty getting those bills out on time. I've even had clients drive around for a week with stamped envelopes sitting on the passenger seat before making it that final step into the mailbox. Even though an individual late fee may be no big deal, over time this can drastically affect credit scores, leading to much higher interest rates or rejected loan applications. This is very much a big deal.

Studies have documented that adults with ADHD have pervasive difficulties with most aspects of money management. This can have major consequences not only in terms of financial measures, but just as importantly in the areas of self-esteem, relationship dynamics, life satisfaction, stress, and mood. Money is a common cause of arguments in most couples, but in couples where one person has ADHD, it can really add fuel to the fire. It's too easy for the non-ADHD partner to point to the ADHD partner's financial misdeeds as "proof" of her moral inferiority, requiring the non-ADHD partner to resentfully become the guardian and savior of the family's finances. This lockdown is rarely appreciated.

I had a client who was so overwhelmed by tracking her finances that she simply didn't bother. She just gave up. If she wanted something, she bought it. She knew this was a bad idea when she was doing it, but since she had never been able to manage her finances effectively, she didn't even try. This turning a blind eye to the consequences was partly based in the neurology of her ADHD and partly in her psychological avoidance of dealing with this painful subject. Of course, she later felt guilty and ashamed about spending the money. So, as often happens with ADHD, what starts as a neurological deficit winds up as a complex layer of psychological dynamics.

You can find strategies for managing your money better in *Stay in the Budget* on p. 305.

Social Skills and Friendships

ADHD can have a significant effect on social functioning in both obvious and subtle ways. Social interactions are actually pretty complex, with a subtle and constantly changing interplay between two or more people. A lot goes on moment to moment. To be successful, each person needs to continually monitor where the other person is going in the conversation and adjust accordingly. ADHD symptoms can interfere with this process in several ways:

- *Hyperactivity* can be tiring for others who find the constant activity and need for stimulation hard to keep up with.
- *Impulsive actions and comments* can be off-putting or jarring if they're too unexpected.
- *Distractibility and forgetfulness* can cause the ADHD person to miss or forget important things that the other person said, causing the other person to feel that she isn't being listened to or valued.

Although we all have the occasional social blunder, most people are pretty forgiving if it doesn't happen too often. However, those with ADHD tend to use up their free passes too quickly, causing others to make deeper assumptions about their character. As a result, ADHD people are often seen as irresponsible, self-centered, or rude, even though they're really not. I met a woman at a conference who described how she can come across as brash, but she's really quite caring if someone can see beyond her initial demeanor. Unfortunately, as this woman knows, the other person is left to make assumptions based on what he sees, even if he misinterprets the reasons for that behavior. We're all guilty of this to some extent. We all tend to assign our own motives to others' behavior as a way to understand why they do what they do. For example, if someone without ADHD doesn't pay attention to something, it's usually because he views it as unimportant. Therefore, when the ADHD person seems to not be attending, he assumes that the conversation or his opinions generally aren't important to her. This makes sense in a way and is usually accurate, even though it turns out to be wrong in this case.

Studies have found that ADHD children are not chosen as frequently to be best friends or partners in activities as other children are. Unfortunately, ADHD children tend to be aware of these difficulties and, predictably, generally feel bad about it. They know the phone doesn't ring as much as it could—and that their calls don't get answered as often. Unlike the really oppositional kids who create big, dramatic crises, ADHD kids' social missteps are usually small but frequent. Any one incident is easy to ignore, but in total, other kids choose not to deal with it and to distance themselves. Even if the child is aware of what he is doing that isn't going over well, he still may not be able to reliably behave differently. For example, I met with a fifth-grader and his mother because he was alienating his friends with impulsive actions that too often crossed the line. He went back on his medication and we talked about tricky situations that could come up and how he could better respond to them. Treatment helped him, but this story would have a very different ending without it.

ADHD adults can have many of the same difficulties. As in childhood, they know what they should and shouldn't do but have trouble sticking with that plan. They have trouble with engaging others in conversation and in managing how they present themselves, including tactfulness and adjusting their behavior to be appropriate to the situation, moderating expressions of strong emotions, and controlling nonverbal displays. They too frequently put their foot in their mouth, either saying the wrong thing or having it come out wrong. A fellow presenter on a panel told of literally having to bite her lip to stop herself from blurting out.

ADHD adults also have a tendency to miss the nonverbal cues that are so important in social interactions. They may miss subtle signs about the other person's mood or how that mood changes through the discussion. Or they may not realize that the other person is trying to change the topic or end the conversation. They know how to read social cues, but they don't do so well if they get distracted or caught up in what they are thinking or saying. They may get so absorbed in their next comment that they can barely hold it in until the other person finally stops talking. If they do blurt it out, they may be seen as self-centered or controlling because they don't give the other person an equal chance to talk. Alternatively, they may completely miss what the other person is saying but not even realize it. This may come out only later when it becomes obvious that the two people remember the discussion differently. *(The neighbors are coming over for dinner!?)*

A member of the adult ADHD support group I ran described a job interview where halfway through he wondered to himself, "Have I sounded like an asshole yet?" Everyone laughed knowingly. There are actually two things that are striking about his comment. The first is his pessimism about being able to pull off an interview smoothly. The other is that he knows that he could easily have said something wrong and not even realized it at the time—so even if he walks out feeling good, he might still have blown it.

It should not be surprising that ADHD adults tend to have significantly fewer social acquaintances and close friends than those without ADHD. This isn't necessarily by choice, since they often would like more friends but have trouble keeping them. Sometimes they know why those friendships end; sometimes they don't. This lack of connection is a cause for concern since close, supportive relationships are good not only for our mental health but also for our physical health. See chapter 15, *Relationships and Friendships: Strive for Balance*, for ways to have more satisfying friendships.

Romantic Relationships: Where's Cupid Now?

I get quite a few calls from the romantic partners of ADHD adults to schedule an initial appointment for one or both of them. I think this reveals two important aspects of relationships where one person has ADHD:

- *The partner is also affected by the ADHD.* She therefore has an interest in treatment to improve things (perhaps not fully realizing that she has her own share of the work to do).
- *The non-ADHD partner may not have a lot of faith in the other's ability to follow through with making the call himself.* I had a guy call me twice and leave the wrong number for his new cell phone both times. Fortunately his wife called a few days later (although I don't know if she didn't believe him or was annoyed that I wasn't calling back).

We may also be able to point out a third aspect of these relationships, which is that many ADHD partners are less likely to actually attend that first session if they feel like they are being forced to or are "the problem" in the relationship.

In some ways, ADHD relationships face the same struggles as every other relationship, just more so. It's about balance and fairness and making sure that both partners get their needs met. Unfortunately, despite the best of intentions from both partners, things get off track and neither is able to get them back on. They both get more frustrated and try harder. Some things get better, but other things get worse. When you put it all together, ADHD adults are twice as likely as those without ADHD to separate or divorce and report less marital satisfaction (Barkley and Gordon, 2002).

Although every relationship is unique in its own way, relationships where one person has ADHD tend to fall into a certain pattern, especially before a diagnosis is made and treatment begun. This may be less obvious when the couple is initially dating, although there may be signs that become apparent in retrospect. For every relationship, things are much less complicated before the couple lives together. They don't need to coordinate shopping, laundry, cleaning, and finances, so different styles and preferences are less problematic. In addition, because it's easier to put our best foot forward when dating and harder to hide things when living together, the couple may be surprised by what they learn about each other when they move in. People with ADHD may be especially prone to problems when the thrill of the relationship is gone and consistency is required to maintain the mundane.

Once the couple lives together, it's too easy to fall into a pattern where the non-ADHD partner feels compelled to take on more and more responsibilities to ensure that they are done completely and on time. This is a gradual progression, as the non-ADHD partner slowly adds more tasks to her workload, often after the ADHD partner drops the ball on them for the final time. Initially, this is a good balance, in that she enjoys being needed and doing things her way, and the ADHD partner is more than happy to hand over some of his responsibilities—and not be yelled at for doing them wrong, at least as his partner defines wrong.

Over time, though, the non-ADHD partner begins to realize the full extent of her partner's difficulties and that she will need to carry this extra burden for the duration of the relationship. At this point, she may become increasingly resentful, angry, and demanding, as she tries to whip her partner into shape and lighten her load. Meanwhile, the ADHD partner is once again on the receiving end of that all-too-familiar criticism of not doing things right, of not doing what he's supposed to, and of just generally not living up to expectations.

And so the chase begins. The non-ADHD partner does everything she can to balance the scales and feel less overwhelmed. She will start out by begging for more help and make reasonable requests, like shifting responsibility for paying the bills to her partner. Then when that doesn't work, she will get angry and blame her partner and make unreasonable demands, like pushing him get a second job because "all" of their financial troubles are completely his fault. Initially the ADHD partner will really push himself to rise to the occasion and do what his partner asks, but as you well know, this doesn't last for long, because other demands of daily life begin to intrude. As his partner becomes increasingly angry, he tries to avoid the confrontation, making promises he can't keep and lying about what he's taken care of, all the while resenting being bossed around.

This tug of war continues, as each partner tries to improve the situation. This involves two separate but related areas of the relationship:

- *Emotional.* Love, romance, and caring are crucial to every relationship. It burns brightest in the beginning, then becomes deeper and more subdued over time. This also involves the feeling that your partner is looking out for you and that your happiness is important to him or her.

- *Practical.* Every relationship needs to get some things done. In the beginning, it's relatively easy stuff like meeting at the restaurant at pretty much the same time. When the couple lives together, they also need to pay bills and buy groceries. If they have kids, they have a million more tasks to take care of.

People with ADHD mostly have trouble with the practical aspects of relationships, so their partners often take on more of that burden. However, people with ADHD may also have trouble with showing the emotional aspects. This can be big things, like throwing together a disappointing birthday celebration because they didn't plan ahead. It can also be small things, like giving the impression that they aren't paying attention when their partner is talking.

As much as we all strive for balance and fairness, few relationships are truly fair. Each partner has different abilities, energy levels, and motivations, and these can change over time and circumstances. However, as long as the couple is doing well in the emotional area, they can tolerate some difference in the practical area. Most of us are willing to do some extra work if we feel that our partner is at least trying. Trouble starts in the practical area when one partner feels that the other isn't trying hard enough or if the imbalance is just too big to tolerate. In the emotional area, trouble starts when at least one of the partners feels that the other isn't looking out for him, either by not doing enough or by being too critical.

This is when the couple starts trying both emotional and practical solutions, like more quiet time together or rebalancing the workload. Some of these solutions work quite well, but some of them don't, especially if they don't have ADHD on their radar screen. Eventually, if these strategies don't help enough, they may seek out professional help, hopefully with someone who really understands ADHD. For some couples, there is too much damage done by this time and the relationship ends anyway, but hopefully in a more amicable way. Other couples really work hard both by changing what they do and by changing their expectations for each other.

Given that ADHD affects every other aspect of relationship functioning, of course it also affects sexual functioning. Commonly cited are issues related to the timing and frequency of sex, amount of foreplay, and balancing both partners' sexual needs from moment to moment. More basically, a satisfying sex life requires a certain amount of time and energy. ADHD-based time-management difficulties and lost efficiencies can squeeze out the time for sex. In addition, a romantic partner who is resentful about carrying an unfair share of the household burdens may also be less interested.

Perhaps not surprisingly, an effective medication regimen can improve things in the bedroom, too, by helping the ADHD partner to maintain attention, be more aware of the other's needs, and display an improved capacity to delay gratification. Of course, because the most commonly used medication class, the stimulants, will have mostly worn off by the end of the day, it may be helpful to have sex earlier in the day or evening to take advantage of this improvement.

See chapter 15, *Relationships and Friendships: Strive for Balance*, for strategies to improve all aspects of your romantic relationships.

Parenting: Hard Enough Under the Best of Circumstances

Most parenting books recommend consistency and predictability, neither of which is an ADHD strength. Adults with ADHD have difficulty staying on top of life's demands before having children, and things often get worse as the family grows. Children add a great deal of complication to what can feel like an already hectic life. Compared to work and school, parenting can be quite unstructured. The parent needs to be the one to provide the structure of what happens, when, and how.

As many couples discover, differences between the romantic partners that are easy to ignore before children arrive may become a bigger deal when a child's welfare is involved. So a tendency toward disorganization may be annoying but tolerable until the couple has a toddler getting into everything. In addition, any imbalances in the workload may only become more pronounced as the workload increases. This may push the non-ADHD parent past the breaking point when she just can't do any more and is desperate for assistance.

When it comes to discipline, parents with ADHD may have difficulty setting limits consistently and effectively. This may be partly because they have difficulty being consistent themselves and forget the consequences they are supposed to enforce. In addition, after a lifetime of being punished for their misdeeds, they may hate doing that to their kids. Predictably, the price paid for not setting consistent limits is that the children are more likely to act out, thus making the ADHD parent more prone to emotional outbursts. Contributing to this short fuse, the parent may feel overwhelmed trying to manage children's complicated schedules of after-school activities and ensuring that everyone gets everywhere on time and with all the necessary belongings, a task that sometimes requires the skills of a professional events planner. So the parents race through their days, trying to hold it all together.

Less tangibly, distractibility and forgetfulness may be interpreted by children as a lack of interest in them. Alternatively, parents may miss the subtle and fleeting opportunities to really connect with their children. Hyperactive parents may have greater difficulty enjoying the quiet times that children need or the repetitive play that young children engage in. I had a client with four children who described the agony of playing simple little games with her youngest because she felt she had done it a million times already. Another client spoke of the guilt she felt when she repeatedly brought her son to school late, since he was paying the price for her time-management difficulties. More traumatic are the late pick-ups after school or the times when the parent completely forgets to pick up the child. Finally, growing up in a messy, disorganized household doesn't provide any of the children with a good role model or teach any organizational skills, even if the children themselves don't have ADHD.

The effect of ADHD on a family depends on who in the family has it, how many people have it, how severely they have it, and whether the non-ADHD members have other difficulties. It also depends on what other stressors the family is facing and what strengths and supports the family members can use.

Parents with ADHD are sometimes told to take parenting classes or read books on how to be better parents. Of course, the implications of these suggestions are usually pretty clear. Unfortunately, these parenting resources usually don't help, since the ADHD parents already know what they're supposed to do but can't maintain the consistency to keep the good habits going, as with so many other demands.

Given the continued struggles of the ADHD parent, it isn't surprising that the non-ADHD parent often becomes the overfunctioner. Attempts to shift some of the load to others can result in unsatisfactory performances, or it takes more time to teach and monitor than to do it oneself, so the pattern continues. This dynamic will persist until the non-ADHD parent becomes overloaded, burned out, and resentful.

Parenting a Child Who Also Has ADHD

As with everything else, there are both advantages and disadvantages to ADHD kids having a parent with ADHD. On the positive side, an ADHD parent can relate to the struggles that his child is going through and can offer examples from his own life. He can also serve as a role model for dealing with adversity gracefully and persisting in the face of setbacks. This requires that the parent mostly has his act together. Ironically, some parents who suffered through their own ADHD may be even less tolerant of it in their children, because it brings up too many of their own painful memories. In addition, ADHD children are better at pushing their parents to their limits, so there may be more conflict if the parents are less able to disengage.

Parenting After Divorce

Parents will always be parents together, even if they're no longer married. If the noncustodial parent has ADHD, he is likely to be labeled as the bad guy, irresponsible, and unreliable. This is especially likely if untreated ADHD contributed to the marital troubles that led to the divorce. He may compensate by playing the role of the fun parent who doesn't enforce limits in the same way the custodial parent does. This probably further aggravates the custodial parent, who bears most of the parenting burden when it comes to setting limits and keeping the children on track, leaving her feeling undermined and powerless. As a result, the parents may become even less able to communicate in a civilized manner.

I had a client who complained bitterly about his ADHD ex-wife's unwillingness or inability to ensure that their son completed his homework when he stayed with her. So it fell to him to get the son to make up the missed work the next night, all the while cursing the mother under his breath. She would admit that she needs to do better with the homework, but she also believed that a few missed homework assignments aren't the end of the world, an understandable position given her own academic history. So the battle continued...

See *Parenting* on p. 87 for tips on keeping everybody in the family happy and healthy.

Self-Image and Sense of Effectiveness: A Little Bit Dented

ADHD makes your life harder, especially if you spent most of your life struggling and not knowing why. Over time, this can affect how you feel about yourself and what kind of a person you see yourself as. We like to think well of ourselves, but our experience has to support that positive feeling. If you've had too many experiences of falling short, of not doing what you promised you would, this can also affect your sense of effectiveness in the world. This is the part that adds insult to injury—because you did something badly in the past, you may not try your hardest to do well the next time.

Even when adults with ADHD do achieve some success, many feel like imposters and wait nervously for everything to fall apart. Or if they're successful in one part of their lives, they may work really hard to hide their poor performance in other parts—for example, never having anyone over because the house is such a mess. It may feel like all their energy gets taken up with just keeping that one part of their lives going well, so nothing is left for the other parts. This then undermines their ability to feel good about the places where they are doing well, because they can always pull out the other parts as exhibit A in their case against themselves.

We See Ourselves in Others' Reactions

Especially as kids, but even as adults, we base our feelings about ourselves on the reactions that we get from other people. These reactions tell us a lot—which of our qualities others value (and not), what we are good at (and not), what kind of an effect we have on others. Some people, like parents, close friends, and romantic partners, have a greater effect on us. Granted, different people have different reactions, but over time we see the trends. Mostly this works pretty well, even though it's certainly not perfect.

Because others have this kind of an influence, it's important to understand how people tend to react to ADHD behavior. In general, most people tend to assume that others mean to do what they do, unless there are clearly unusual circumstances. For example, if someone with ADHD forgets to meet her friend for coffee, the friend will assume that the other (ADHD) person didn't really care about the date and blew it off. This is where people with ADHD run into trouble—others make assumptions about their intentions and then reflect those intentions back to the person with ADHD. This is where all that "bad attitude" and "needs to try harder" stuff comes from. After hearing this often enough, it becomes easy to believe it, at least a little.

Even though science has clearly proven that ADHD is a brain-based disorder, it is still invisible, in the sense that ADHD can't be seen directly. Whereas there's no doubt when someone is missing a leg, for example, when someone has ADHD, others assume that the person just isn't trying hard enough and that he can decide to change that. In other words, he has only himself to blame for his troubles. (Would you like some salt with that wound?)

Unhelpful Coping Strategies: Common Habits and Defense Mechanisms

We all experience painful or uncomfortable feelings and use various habits to cope with them. For example, some people find it most helpful to talk a problem out with someone, whereas others prefer to spend some time alone as they think it through. Generally people are aware of these tendencies within themselves.

When these habits are mostly unconscious, we call them *defense mechanisms*, which are mental tricks that we play on ourselves to deal with uncomfortable feelings. Defense mechanisms help us make it through daily struggles, setbacks, and frustrations without getting overwhelmed in the moment. In the right doses and at the right times, this can allow us to continue moving forward. When used too often or at the wrong times, defense mechanisms can bring more trouble later, even if they help us feel better in the moment. These mental maneuvers are usually unconscious, although sometimes we catch ourselves using one of them. A good therapist may help you see which habits or defense mechanisms you tend to use and help you replace less-productive ones with better ones.

At the risk of overgeneralizing, we can say that adults with ADHD tend to have certain unproductive habits. You may realize that you have some of these habits. If so, remember that you're in good company and that everybody has habits like these to greater and lesser degrees. Also remember that with knowledge comes power and that by becoming aware of which habits you tend to use, you're in a better position to replace them with habits that work better for you.

Most of these habits are a combination of both neurology and psychology. ADHD brain wiring tends to set up certain situations that make particular responses more likely. This then means that the most effective way to change these habits is to address both contributors. This may involve keeping an eye out for what you have identified as your most commonly used habits, then consciously working to behave differently when you catch yourself using one.

Let's run through these habits here. There's definitely some overlap between them and in many cases someone will use more than one, so they can also interact. I've tried to put them in a loose order where later habits build on earlier ones.

As a heads-up, I run through these same unhelpful strategies in *Overcome Unhelpful Coping Strategies, Bad Habits, and Defense Mechanisms* on p. 209, so this sets the stage for that.

Rationalization

We all do things that are hard to justify. Sometimes we do knuckleheaded things; sometimes we do things that are self-destructive or vindictive. Hopefully we are able to own up to these less-than-stellar moments. When we can't, we may try to justify our failings and misdeeds so that we don't look or feel so bad. This *rationalizing* makes us feel better in the moment, since we cover our discomfort up with semi-reasonable explanations.

We may use rationalization in the moment when we're doing something that we know we shouldn't, like giving in to an impulse buy, or when we're not doing something we know we should, like starting another load of laundry. We use rationalization to soothe a guilty conscience, even though we know we're setting ourselves up for trouble. We can also use rationalization after the fact to explain away something that has already happened or not happened. For example, someone who showed up late for a job interview may rationalize it by telling herself that it isn't a big deal or that she didn't really want that job anyway rather than admitting that she planned poorly and should have made more time to get there. As a result, she hasn't really learned anything and isn't any less likely to show up late for the next one.

Because people with ADHD tend to make too many of these kinds of mistakes, despite their best intentions, it can feel as though they need to explain themselves too often. This gets old, so it's tempting to explain away some of those troubles without always feeling like the bad guy. (Can't someone else take the blame sometimes?)

People with ADHD are more likely to miss important details or forget them, which often puts them in a position of having to defend themselves (e.g., "You never told me that!"). This is different than rationalizing, since there was no information there to be consciously decided on. An example of rationalization is when the person chose not to do something and then justified it by saying that the task wasn't that important anyway. Or the person may rationalize not writing a reminder note simply because he doesn't feel like tracking down a pen, even though he should know better than to rely on his memory. So it starts with rationalizing and then becomes true forgetting.

Other people may see these rationalizations as excuse making or even copouts, especially if it affects something that is important to the other person. More so than what is actually done or not done, this feeds the idea that the ADHD person is irresponsible—not only did he blow it, but now he won't even own up to it. So it goes from bad to worse.

Rationalization underlies many of the other bad habits that are covered in the rest of this article. This makes sense, since we're usually smart enough to know when we could probably do better.

Externalizing

When things don't work out well, it can be tempting to blame someone else or the circumstances for it—for example, getting to the restaurant late because there was traffic. Obviously, we don't have complete control over our lives, and sometimes external forces or other people do prevent us from doing what we had planned to. However, there are times when we should have known better and planned accordingly. So, if it's really important to get to dinner on time, we can leave early in case something unexpected comes up. This also means that we take partial responsibility for running late if we didn't build in some time.

By contrast, *externalizing* involves blaming other people or the situation for when we drop the ball. *(How should I have known that there was going to be traffic at rush hour!?)* Because people with ADHD can feel as if they too often need to explain themselves, they may try to dodge the bullet in some of those situations. This is especially true for those who are still undiagnosed and untreated. I can understand not wanting to feel like the bad guy all the time; I'm sure that can really wear someone down. Unfortunately, there are two problems with overusing externalization. The first is that it disempowers the person. If he had no responsibility for what happened this time, then that implies that he has no ability to prevent similar problems next time. After all, if he is merely the passive victim of circumstances, then there's little reason for optimism. By contrast, owning up to his part of what happened is actually rather empowering. If he can admit that he didn't expect there to be so much traffic and that he should have left earlier, then the next time he needs to be somewhere on time he might leave earlier.

The second problem with overusing externalization is that it tends to alienate people. Many people will initially give someone the benefit of the doubt, but over time they will likely cease to be so forgiving if there are just too many excuses. It then becomes a boy-who-cried-wolf scenario in which even legitimate explanations aren't believed. They may then distance themselves from the ADHD person because it just feels like too much work to be constantly bailing her out of bad situations. So ADHD adults may cut themselves off from potential resources and allies without fully realizing why people get angry with them or avoid them. Over time, they may quite reasonably begin to assume that everyone will eventually get frustrated with them or single them out negatively, and preemptively keep their distance or assume the worst. This then becomes a self-fulfilling prophecy. Taking ownership for dropping the ball and then offering to address problems go a long way toward keeping people on your side.

It should be noted that externalizing requires that the person has some awareness of the part that he played in creating the situation, but he tries to deny it. As explained in the section on rationalization, this is different from those situations where the person truly wasn't aware of something or forgot it. So, showing up late because he remembered the dinner *only* when he got a call asking where he was is not an example of externalizing. Of course, other people may not believe this if there are too many claims of innocent forgetting—it's that boy-who-cried-wolf thing again. We get only a certain number of free passes before people get skeptical.

Avoiding or Quitting

For all of us, it takes more effort to get going on tasks that are difficult, boring, confusing, frustrating, painful, or otherwise distasteful. However, studies have found that people with ADHD need even more force of will to get going on these difficult tasks (Brown, 1995). Part of this avoidance is neurological because their brains don't fire up as easily for tasks that aren't inherently interesting or rewarding. Part of this is also psychological, if they don't expect something to work out well anyway. (This is covered under *Learned Helplessness*, p. 98.)

If the person does get going on one of these tasks, she may bail out on it before it's done because it has become too uncomfortable. This can also be a combination of neurology and psychology.

We all have to do things that we don't enjoy, both at home and at work. Many of these obligations don't offer much of a reward for doing them, but they certainly offer a punishment for not doing them. For example, the IRS doesn't honor you for getting your tax return in on time, but they sure do penalize you if you don't.

Others in the ADHD person's life may be dumbfounded by the important tasks that he avoids or doesn't finish. They may get anxious about it *(You haven't done your taxes yet?!)* and even get judgmental *(What's wrong with you?!)*. So there can be social fallout from this behavior, in addition to any of the direct consequences. I talk about ways to get going on avoided tasks in *Do It Anyway* on p. 207.

Drinking, drugs, and other addictive behaviors can also serve as a form of avoidance if someone uses them to escape or reduce certain feelings. Adults with ADHD are more likely than those without ADHD to have more trouble with these kinds of behaviors (Barkley, Murphy, and Fischer, 2007), perhaps because a more difficult life may give them more of these kinds of feelings. For more information, see *Substance Use and Addiction* on p. 101.

Procrastination

Procrastination is basically temporary avoidance, but the person does actually get around to doing the task. This is partly based in neurology, in that people with ADHD have a harder time getting fired up for tasks that have a far-off deadline than for tasks with more immediate deadlines. So the report for work that is due in a week doesn't do much to get them going. They may tinker with it a little bit, but most of the real work gets done the last day. This is partly because that last-minute pressure helps them focus in, so they feel that they do their best work right before the deadline. This is one of those habits that works great—except when it doesn't. Doing things at the last minute leaves someone vulnerable to unexpected problems (like empty printer cartridges) or tasks taking longer than projected.

Doing things at the last minute also tends to make other people nervous. I can't even count how many clients have complained about the angst they feel when an ADHD family member waits until the last minute. Although that ADHD person may not be particularly bothered by the stress of waiting for the last minute, it is safe to say that she probably doesn't enjoy the "encouragement" and "helpful suggestions" she receives from those who perceive themselves as being threatened in some way by her procrastination.

Check out *Get Going* on p. 256 for strategies for overcoming procrastination.

Pseudoproductivity

Busy is not necessarily the same as productive. We all have lots of little demands on our time, plus some bigger and more important obligations. Doing the important stuff requires some concentrated effort and persistence, whereas most of the little things are easier to knock out. So it can be tempting to do the little things first (you know, just to clear your desk) but then never get to the bigger things. However, because the person is busily working away, she feels productive, while time ticks down on the items that she should really be working on. Because she isn't indisputably wasting time, like by watching TV, these less-important tasks serve as a great decoy.

I had a client who was in software sales, a business where he had to do lots of research on a potential client and make many contacts before he could make a sale. It took plenty of cold-calling to even get a chance to meet with a potential client. When he was working from home, he was supposed to make fifteen calls a day, in addition to various other activities. Instead he would spend time going through his pile of personal mail, clicking through emails, straightening out that issue with the bank, and so on. These were all important tasks, but not more important than making those calls. He would rationalize it by telling himself that clearing up these other commitments would make it easier to focus on the calls. There's some truth to this, so it makes it easier to justify, but it doesn't change the fact that most of the day would disappear and he still hadn't made his calls. Of course, everyone does at least some of this, but ADHD folks tend to do it more often. (If you want to be amazed by how much of this you can do, try staying on task while writing a book!)

I offer potential solutions to this in *How to Be Productive, Not Just Busy* on p. 251.

Abandoning Ship

Abandoning ship involves jumping to new (i.e., more exciting) projects before finishing the ones that are partially completed and no longer interesting. So the unfinished projects pile up, much to the annoyance of family members and coworkers. (This makes the obsessive-compulsive ones absolutely crazy.) Unfortunately, most projects don't give partial credit—it's either done or it isn't. A room is either completely painted or it isn't. A report is either finished or it isn't. Ultimately, many of these projects are abandoned, never to be completed. If a project is finished, it's often at the eleventh hour when some external pressure forces the issue. For example, the dining room is finally cleared out right before family shows up for Thanksgiving dinner. As with pseudoproductivity, the person gives the appearance of being busy because he's working away on various things, but he isn't necessarily completing tasks or addressing the top priorities (at least as far as some others may be concerned).

More broadly, people with ADHD may become very excited by some new hobby, job, living situation, friend, boyfriend or girlfriend, or other pursuit, getting fairly well absorbed in it. *(Now this is something I can stick with!)* This enthusiasm eventually fades and they move on to something else. This is no big deal for things like hobbies, where the goal is to enjoy oneself in the moment, but it can be problematic in other areas where persistence is rewarded. For example, someone who changes jobs or careers too frequently never earns any seniority and the perks that come with it, including promotions, recognition, and pay raises. Alternatively, someone who gets bored in relationships as soon as the honeymoon glow fades won't build something more meaningful. Predictably, constantly chasing the next big thing leads to upheaval and lost momentum each time they start over.

In some cases, this abandoning ship is based in simple distractibility and forgetfulness—the person doesn't intend to bail on the first project; she just got sidetracked. At other times, though, it's a more conscious or semiconscious decision to seek something more interesting as she gets bored with what she's working on. Tying up loose ends doesn't give people with ADHD the same satisfaction as the thrill of diving into something new, so away they go. They usually have at least some intention of returning to it, even if it never comes to fruition.

This jumping around can become socially expensive if family and friends begin to view the ADHD person as flighty and fickle. Consequently, he may not have a network of longtime friends to provide support during difficult times. Or the friends he does have may not be up for providing support with his struggles because they know he's probably just going to jump to something new, yet again.

Quasi-Obsessive-Compulsive Behavior

People with obsessive-compulsive disorder (OCD) feel anxious and use certain strategies to reduce that anxiety. They may worry that they didn't turn off the stove and feel compelled to go back and check it, even if they just checked it for the fifth time. Or they may perform rituals, like turning the light switch on and off twelve times, for fear that something awful will happen if they don't. They know these fears aren't rational, but can't stop themselves from giving in to them.

People with ADHD may engage in some behaviors that look a little OCD but actually are quite different. For example, people with ADHD may also check the stove, but there is more of a seed of truth to their doubts—there have indeed been times when they left the stove on, so it's good judgment to be sure that it's off this time. For people with ADHD, the checking helps prevent problems because they know that their attention and memory can be blinky. Apart from making a point of trying to be more attentive in the moment (easier said than done), it becomes a balancing act of when it is justified to check and when it isn't.

Some people with OCD engage in hoarding, wherein they keep far too many things, including stuff that has no real use, like used food containers and years' worth of newspapers. They have an unreasonable fear that something awful will happen if they let go of these items.

ADHD folks can also wind up doing some hoarding but for very different reasons:

- *Not taking the time to get rid of things.* They don't have any real desire to keep everything; they just don't want to be bothered with the boring job of weeding out the stuff that they don't need anymore.
- *Not wanting to throw out something they may need later.* This fear may be well justified by prior experiences in which they impulsively or unintentionally got rid of the wrong things. Unlike people with OCD, ADHD people tend to keep things that do have some possibility of being useful later. Unfortunately, because they keep so much, they often can't find what they need when they need it, so all these "just in case" items actually do more harm than good when they interfere with finding more important items.

Controlling or Aggressive Behavior

Some ADHD adults live by the adage that the best defense is a good offense. They work really hard to control the world around them, since they tend to function better under certain circumstances. For example, they need to have the TV off in order to not get distracted during a conversation. This strong need for control makes sense, since if someone has trouble controlling his internal distractibility, it may be easier to control his external distractions. A lot of ADHD interventions involve controlling the person's environment—for example, to reduce distractions or increase the number of reminders.

But exercising control can become too much of a good thing. It's helpful to know what situations you function best in, but it can be problematic if you don't allow others to create the situations that they function best in. Compromise is lost and the relationship suffers. Alternatively, the person may have difficulty adjusting if he can't create the circumstances that he feels most comfortable in. So he doesn't get as much done when the situation is less than perfect. As with many things in life, the difference between good and bad is a matter of degree.

Learned Helplessness

People with undiagnosed and untreated ADHD have more experience with failure than others do. They've had more setbacks and situations where things didn't work out. They've been blamed for their troubles and told that they just need to try harder, even though that doesn't really help much. (If it was really as easy as trying harder, you would just do it, right?) They've been given advice that doesn't work for them but seems to work for other people. It's easy to lower your expectations under these circumstances. Some even give up hope and stop trying.

After a lifetime of struggle, the ADHD adult may become hypersensitive to failure or even the possibility of failure. Rather than seeing a setback as temporary and experience that they can learn from, it may feel like yet another indictment of their bad character. So they don't pick themselves up and keep trying, like others might, since each new failure is so painful. The first signs of trouble may spark such a rush of fear, shame, and embarrassment that they just abandon the project, even if they could have otherwise recovered and made a success of it.

Taking a chance on success requires being able to tolerate failure—if it's too painful, then it just isn't worth the risk. Success is rarely a straight line and usually requires getting back up after getting knocked down. However, it's a lot easier to keep going in the face of adversity if you have some general optimism that it might work out. Based on their track records, many ADHD adults expect trouble, so it doesn't make sense to stick with it.

So when these adults are finally diagnosed and offered the promise of treatment making a difference, they're skeptical. They've been made all sorts of promises before that just didn't pan out—"You just need a different job," "This book will get you on track," "You just need to keep a positive attitude," and so on. If none of those promises helped much, does it make sense to believe this new batch? Even if they're made by some therapist, psychiatrist, coach, or author who seems awfully convinced he's right? Since more of the same tends to lead to more of the same, the trick is for the ADHD adult to determine whether these people really are offering more of the same—or perhaps something different.

I would argue that most of those past promises failed because they didn't take the person's ADHD into account—a crucial missing piece and setup for failure. So it's OK to be skeptical or hesitant. That makes sense. However, maybe with a tiny bit of guarded optimism, give these new ADHD-specific strategies a shot. Not halfheartedly try them, but really try them. I think some of them just might work.

I've seen it go both ways. Some clients take that chance and really make great progress. They stretch themselves and work really hard to stay with the new game plan. Others try initially and then bail out, not ready to take that chance or face the pain and frustration from years past. It's disappointing to see, because I know that they could do better if they really gave it a shot. Of course, then there are all those people who never even call my office in the first place...

For more information on how to change your mindset, see chapter 8, *Self-Esteem and Effectiveness: I Can Do This!*

Impulsively Rushing

There are times when even the biggest avoiders or procrastinators have to bite the bullet and work on something that makes them uncomfortable. After a long stretch of occasional and semiconscious awareness of an impending deadline, they are finally forced into action. So they charge through the difficult or burdensome task with the hope of getting done as quickly as possible to minimize the suffering. The mad dash at the last minute then absorbs their full attention and quiets the chatter of critical inner voices (e.g., it's not going to work out well anyway; you're going to mess this one up as usual). Impulsively rushing can also be an ego-saving technique, if the person rationalizes that it doesn't count as failure if you don't really try or if you whip it out at the last minute. Although this is hardly the ideal solution, those with undiagnosed and untreated ADHD probably have a lower batting average than they would like, so their pessimism is understandable.

I can appreciate the desire to avoid those painful feelings, but when the goal is to get done as quickly as possible, it's hard to produce anything of quality. This then becomes a self-fulfilling prophecy, since it probably works out badly, just as predicted. And so the cycle continues.

Related to this, some adults with ADHD may use *escape into action*, wherein they avoid dealing with difficult emotions or problems by jumping into activity instead. Although the activity may have some benefit for the problem, the real goal is to provide a mental distraction from the uncomfortable feelings. For example, a client told me of her husband impulsively ripping out a bunch of the drywall in the basement after discovering some water damage without considering an overall plan for how to deal with it. Regardless, in the moment, he felt better that he was doing something about it, even though he wound up creating more work for himself later since he removed more than he had to. Those who are impulsive are more likely to leap before looking like this. Although I am all in favor of taking action to correct a problem, there are times when the better (and harder) approach is to stop, hold your reaction in check, and consider the best approach.

Cavalier Lifestyle

Some adults with ADHD live by the slogan "If you can't beat 'em, join 'em." That is, after years of trying unsuccessfully to live a "normal" life like everyone else does, they just embrace the chaos that seems to be their lot in life. They float through life from crisis to crisis, living two steps in front of the avalanche—and sometimes two steps behind it.

They've tried all sorts of strategies that seem to work for others. They've seen therapists and maybe even tried antidepressants to boost their spirits and calm their anxieties. They've read (or at least bought) all sorts of self-help books. They've made more New Year's resolutions than they can count. For all the effort, they don't have enough to show for it. After a while optimism runs thin and they just stop trying, rolling with whatever comes.

As stressful as this can be, it spares them the added sting of feeling like a failure for not living a better life. After all, it doesn't count as failure if you don't try. Of course, defeatism tends to lead to more defeat. They may rationalize it as their not being as stressed out and anal-retentive as everyone else, that they would rather focus on play than on work.

So, despite clear evidence of the cost of these habits, some people may be hesitant to work on changing them, for fear of losing part of who they are, of not being themselves anymore. They may resist getting diagnosed, learning about ADHD, seeing a therapist, or trying medication, so nothing gets any better. Since they have always been this way, they may even have trouble seeing that things could be different.

Some may compensate with *magical thinking*, whereby problems are avoided with the unreasonable belief that everything will somehow work out just fine or that an easy solution will eventually present itself. These rationalizations are reinforced by the relief experienced when they escape the uncomfortable feelings of impending failure, guilt, self-reproach, and negative self-evaluation, even though they haven't actually addressed the problem itself. Meanwhile, time ticks down and things get worse.

This indifference can be mind boggling and anxiety arousing for others, such as parents, romantic partners, friends, bosses, physicians, or therapists, who see the price she pays for this lackadaisical attitude. They may feel compelled to push her to do something to avert the disaster that they see coming. Regardless of whether that disaster actually arrives, these other people feel much more anxious about the situation. This causes a tug of war in the relationship as they try to spur her to action.

For many of these people, the indifference hides a deeper anxiety and fear of failure. They would like to be successful like everyone else, but they don't find themselves able to. So they give up rather than sit with the painful feelings that come from not measuring up. This is fundamentally different than those who make a well-reasoned choice to live a simpler lifestyle and spare themselves the headache of the rat race and keeping up with the Joneses. These people can keep up, but they choose not to. My preference is to help those ADHD folks improve their functioning so they can keep up—and then have the option not to.

Substance Use and Addiction: When the Solution Becomes a Problem

Research clearly shows that those with ADHD are more likely to run into trouble with drinking, drugs, and other addictive behaviors (Barkley, Murphy, and Fischer, 2007). Most of them don't qualify as alcoholics or addicts, but they still engage in these behaviors more than their non-ADHD peers do, and they pay a price for it. Not surprisingly, those with other mental health conditions, such as anxiety, depression, or bipolar disorder, are also at an increased risk for substance use and addictive behaviors. However, those with ADHD are a little bit more likely to run into trouble here. They are more likely to start drinking or doing drugs earlier, to try more drugs, and to drink or do drugs more often.

Perhaps also not surprising is that those who had a history of defiant and law-breaking behavior in childhood and adolescence (technically speaking, those who have oppositional defiant disorder, conduct disorder, or antisocial personality disorder) are at the greatest risk for alcohol and drug abuse. Having the hyperactive/impulsive subtype of ADHD makes someone more likely to qualify for one of these other diagnoses, so ADHD indirectly leads to substance abuse. This speaks to the importance of treating ADHD early so that things don't go from bad to worse.

Research has also found that those who were treated with stimulant medication as children were less likely to get into drinking and drugs as teens and young adults, so there is some protective effect there (Wilens, 2004). Each person is different, but there are several reasons why someone with ADHD may be more likely to drink or use drugs to excess, including the following:

- *Self-medication.* Those with undiagnosed and untreated ADHD have probably had a harder life, so they may have more reason to seek out opportunities to drown those sorrows.

- *Impulsivity.* Some may drink or do drugs without thinking through the potential consequences, either for later that day or over a longer time. Eventually, it can become a habit, and they keep going with it.
- *Thrill seeking and avoiding boredom.* Some may drink or do drugs because they're bored or want to make a good time even better.
- *Peer group.* Many teens with ADHD deal with their difficulties at school by disengaging and finding other kids who aren't into school. This makes them more likely to hang out with kids who are more likely to drink and do drugs.

Although smoking cigarettes is less immediately problematic than drinking and doing drugs, its effects can easily add up over time. Those with ADHD are at a much greater risk of becoming regular smokers, which can produce drastic health and financial detriments over time (Barkley, Murphy, and Fischer, 2007).

Drinking, drugs, smoking, and other addictive behaviors can all have negative effects on various parts of a person's life, including family peace, romantic relationships, friends, school, work, and finances. It's hard to be at your best if you're doing too much of this stuff. It's also hard to get the most from therapy or coaching, which tends to work best with a clear mind. It can also reduce the effectiveness of medication. So, for those who are drinking or doing drugs too much or too often, it is probably worth addressing that directly. Therefore, if this applies to you or someone you care about, you may want to check out *Manage Excessive Substance Use and Other Addictive Behavior* on p. 229.

Driving: No Big Deal, Until It Is

Most adults don't think that much about driving. We just get behind the wheel and go. However, since driving involves lots of attention and split-second decision making, researchers are increasingly looking at the effect that untreated and treated ADHD has on someone's ability to drive safely. Even a momentary attention blink or a single impulsive choice can have profound consequences. As with most other areas of life, people with ADHD know what to do but have trouble being consistent in using those good habits behind the wheel. As a result, research has found that young adults with ADHD are more likely to have greater driving difficulties, including license suspensions and revocations, accidents where the car is totaled, hit-and-run accidents, and accidents where bodily injury is involved (Ellison, 2002).

As much as driving becomes easy and automatic once we get used to it, there is actually a lot going on. Driving requires us to simultaneously attend to what is happening inside and outside the car, predict what other drivers are likely to do and respond accordingly, sustain attention over time when not much happens, and ignore distractions. This doesn't even count all the other stuff we're often doing while driving, like eating, talking on the phone, or changing the music. Because we almost always get to our destination without incident, it's easy to get sloppy and not give driving our full attention. ADHD folks are more prone to this and more likely to wind up in an awful situation.

We also need to consider that driving is affected by other parts of our lives. For example, people who have difficulty managing their time are more likely to speed or drive recklessly when running late. Other people with ADHD purposely drive recklessly due to thrill seeking. I had one client who had racked up twenty-two tickets for moving violations and even wound up spending a few days in jail as a result—and he was only twenty. Even for a sixty-year-old, that would be an impressive collection of driving violations, but it's staggering for someone who'd been driving for only four years.

Crime and Punishment: ADHD and the Legal System

ADHD makes a person more likely to get into trouble. This is more true for those with hyperactive/impulsive symptoms than for those who struggle only with attention. What starts out as kid stuff in elementary school can become much more serious as someone becomes a teen and an adult. The misdeeds get bigger and the punishments more severe.

Research has found that people with ADHD, especially if it's untreated, are more likely to commit crimes and run into legal trouble as a result (Barkley, Murphy, and Fischer, 2007). Having ADHD does not make someone more likely to commit more serious crimes or violent crimes, at least not directly. However, those who have the hyperactive/impulsive symptoms are more likely to develop oppositional defiant disorder or conduct disorder as children or teens and then antisocial personality disorder as adults. People with these conditions are more likely to engage in more serious criminal activity. So indirectly, ADHD does lead to more problematic behaviors.

Although I think it's important to recognize how ADHD can lead to legal problems, we are all still responsible for our actions. ADHD is not an excuse for bad behavior. However, given the potential outcomes of not treating it, it makes it all the more important to address. Given the costs that society pays for these crimes, as well as prosecuting and jailing these offenders, we would be better served to spend more on the early interventions and treatments that we know are effective.

Section II

START WITH EFFECTIVE TREATMENT

Introduction: Integrative Treatment Makes Success More Likely

Section I laid a foundation of knowledge about ADHD. If you read it, you should now understand much better how ADHD affects you and why you do some of the things you do. This brings us to section II, which covers the various treatment options and professionals available to help you get on top of your ADHD. This will help you sort through all those confusing options so that you can make the best decisions for yourself.

As I said before, ADHD does the most damage before it's identified. Once you are diagnosed and begin working on it, it's not nearly as problematic. It's hard to know how much you will benefit from treatment until you try it, but I can safely say that the more effort you put into your treatment, the more you will benefit. This means practicing those new strategies between sessions with your therapist or coach, even when you don't feel like it. If you're trying medication, it means really watching for changes in benefits and side effects as your prescriber adjusts your dosage. Treatment for ADHD isn't like getting a hangnail removed, where you sit there while the podiatrist does all the work.

You may be skeptical about what treatment can really do for you. That's totally understandable. Given the less-than-stellar track record of previous suggestions or even treatments, I can't fault you for having your doubts. So you may need to take it on faith that maybe, just maybe, things might work out better this time—no miracle cures, but some solid and steady progress.

In my first book *(Integrative Treatment for Adult ADHD: A Practical, Easy-to-Use Guide for Clinicians)* I wrote at length about a four-part treatment model for adults with ADHD that includes education, medication, coaching, and therapy. I still firmly believe that the best outcomes are achieved by using all four approaches because each approach benefits the others for a better total outcome. Not every client gets all four, and not every client necessarily needs all four, but I think it's worth considering. So let's run through them briefly.

- *Education.* The more you know about ADHD, the better off you will be—and the more your loved ones know, the better off you all will be. This understanding makes it easier to pick the strategies that will help you be most effective. In addition, it also reduces the unproductive blame and guilt that make you feel bad but don't help you get more done. It can be really liberating to learn that some of your difficulties with attention, memory, and organization are based more in neurology than in your character or bad choices. Reading this book can play a big part in this learning process.

- *Medication.* Although there are no magic potions, generally ADHD medications are safe, have tolerable side effects, and can help you to meet demands more consistently and accurately. They increase focus and concentration, allowing your true abilities to shine through. Adults with ADHD often find that medication provides a sense of clarity, in contrast to a disorganized jumble of thoughts.
- *Coaching.* It's been said that pills don't teach skills, which is where coaching comes in. Coaching can help you to handle daily demands more effectively by finding the strategies that enable you to make use of your strengths, while also taking your ADHD into account. Because your coach or therapist really understands ADHD, she is able to work with you to create strategies that are most likely to be successful.
- *Psychotherapy.* Your therapist's job is to work with you to overcome the effect that a lifetime of ADHD difficulties has had on how you feel about yourself and how you get along with others. He may help you take a more active problem-solving approach and help you reduce avoidance, procrastination, worry, and pessimism.

Getting targeted treatment for your ADHD will enable you to do better in the areas of time management, organization, and remembering. This then sets you up to apply those skills to do better where it really counts—at home, at work, and socially. There are no quick fixes for ADHD. Rather, treatment is an ongoing process that requires a consistent input of energy if gains are to be maintained. This doesn't mean that you need to see your therapist or coach forever, but you probably will need to keep using those strategies and may want to continue taking your medication. Overcoming ADHD is more of a lifestyle than a destination.

You can't leave the past in the past if it's still happening in the present. Fortunately, a good treatment program will enable you to create a future that looks much different from your past.

What This Section Covers

This section contains the following chapters:

5. *Medication: Improve Your Batting Average* (p. 109) Medication is simultaneously the best-known and most-controversial of all the treatment options. We will discuss both the facts and the myths, as well as the relative merits and dosing regimens of the commonly prescribed medications.

6. *Nonmedical Treatment Providers: Pills Don't Teach Skills* (p. 143) Knowledgeable therapists and coaches have a lot to offer an adult with ADHD. They can help you come to peace with the struggles of your past, as well as create a more satisfying future.

7. *Nontraditional Treatments: Miracles or Snake Oil?* (p. 175) Alternative treatments for ADHD abound, but many of them have little or no research showing they're effective. We will review them all so that you can make an informed decision about how to treat your ADHD.

CHAPTER 5

MEDICATION: IMPROVE YOUR BATTING AVERAGE

I'm a psychologist, so I don't write prescriptions. However, it would be impossible to specialize in treating ADHD and not know the medications well. I'm a strong believer in therapy and coaching for adults with ADHD, but the best outcomes are often achieved by using medication along with those strategies. Medication is no silver bullet, and it will probably take some tweaking for you to get just the right regimen, but it can help you build a solid foundation for success. I certainly wouldn't say that you couldn't be happy and successful without medication, but it will be harder and you will probably have more setbacks. Medication makes it more likely that you will be at the top of your game—not just for an afternoon, but day after day.

Whether you're so desperate for something better that you would eat boiled monkey heads if someone said it might help or whether you'd fight to the death before polluting your body with chemically concocted substances, I encourage you to read this chapter to get the facts. If you're already taking medication, this chapter might explain some things that your prescriber didn't have time to cover. The more you know, the better decision you can make for yourself—which may be different from the decision that someone else makes. There are no right or wrong answers about medication, since different people can have different reasons and different responses. It depends on lots of factors, such as what other supports and strengths you have versus how demanding and complex your life is. My hope is that this chapter will help you make the best choice for you.

This chapter contains the following articles:

Make an Informed Choice: The Facts Behind the Medication Controversy (p. 112) There are many myths and half-truths out there about ADHD medications. Whether you choose to try them or choose not to, you owe it to yourself to make a well-informed decision based on the facts.

The Most Popular Stimulant (Coffee, Anyone?) (p. 113) Caffeine is an extremely popular stimulant that doesn't evoke the same kind of comments about morality that the prescribed stimulants do.

To Take Medication or Not to Take Medication: It Depends (p. 113) Some people eagerly choose to take medication, whereas others decide against it. It's a personal decision based on many factors, including how well you can otherwise handle the demands in your life.

Is Taking Medication Like Wimping Out? The Diabetes Analogy (p. 116) Some people see taking ADHD medication as a shortcut, but it's no magic pill. You still have to do the hard work in other ways. Interestingly, people tend to be more accepting of medicating conditions that are seen as more medical, like diabetes.

Potential Medication Benefits: What Does It Do? (p. 117) Adults who take medication for their ADHD tend to find that it enables them to focus on one thing at a time, stick with uninteresting tasks, listen better, and think before acting impulsively.

Realistic Expectations for Medication: Somewhere Between Placebo and Miracle (p. 119) ADHD medications can be quite helpful, but some people are luckier than others when it comes to figuring out dosages and side effects. You won't know until you try them, at which point you can make a fully informed choice for yourself.

Stimulants and Nonstimulants: You Have Two Options (p. 120) The most commonly used medications for ADHD are stimulants, but there are a few other options that aren't stimulants. There are important differences between the two families.

Stimulant Medications: Some of the Basics (p. 120) Stimulants have been around for more than half a century and have lots of good research showing their effectiveness. On the downside, paper prescriptions are required and they can't be called in to the pharmacy.

Commonly Used Stimulants (p. 121) There are essentially two types of stimulants currently on the market—methylphenidate (the Ritalin family) and various forms of amphetamine (the Adderall family). I cover the various brand names that are available, as well as some special considerations regarding some of the specific medications.

How Stimulants Work: Mostly Dopamine, A Little Norepinephrine (p. 124) Stimulants mostly increase the amount of the neurotransmitter dopamine that is available, although they also increase the amount of norepinephrine to a lesser degree.

How Much Should I Take? Finding the Right Dose (p. 124) Your prescriber will probably start you at a low dose and move you up until you find the amount that's best for you. This is a pretty subjective experience that involves balancing desired effects with side effects.

Some People Take More Medication in the Afternoon (p. 126) Although the stimulants generally work quite well, they may not last all day. Some people find it helpful to take a little more in the afternoon to stretch out the benefit into the evening.

Some People Shouldn't Take a Stimulant (p. 127) Although the stimulants are generally safe, some people may have difficulties, including those with bipolar disorder, high blood pressure, cardiac issues, or active substance abuse.

Intentional Abuse of Stimulants: An Unfortunate Reality (p. 129) A small minority of people out there use the stimulants in unintended or illegal ways. I certainly don't condone this behavior, but we shouldn't throw the baby out with the bathwater either.

Medicating Substance Abusers: Balancing the Risks (p. 130) There's an unfortunate irony that adults with untreated ADHD are more likely to abuse substances and that the most-effective medications are potentially abusable. This makes many prescribers nervous, but there are better options.

Managing Stimulant Side Effects: General Principles (p. 131) If your stimulant medication gives you side effects, there are several approaches you can use to reduce them, depending on how and when the side effects occur. Ultimately, you may do better on one of the other stimulants, so it may be worth switching.

Managing Stimulant Side Effects: Specific Side Effects (p. 132) Certain side effects are more likely than others. I offer specific suggestions for addressing each one.

Nonstimulant Medications: Sometimes a Good Choice (p. 136) Although stimulants tend to be the most effective medications for ADHD, some people do better on nonstimulants. I cover those medications here.

Black-Box Warnings: Scary but Rare (p. 138) The Food and Drug Administration sometimes believes that a medication's risks warrant extra attention from consumers, so they place them in a black box. I review them here.

Using More Than One Medication Simultaneously (p. 138) Some people will take more than one medication per day. Sometimes it's just more of the same medication that they take in the morning, whereas sometimes it's a different medication for another condition, such as depression.

Strategies for Remembering to Take Your Medication (p. 139) For forgetful people with ADHD, remembering to take their medication regularly can be a real challenge. I offer some strategies that can help.

Can My Family Doctor Write My Prescriptions? (p. 139) Although psychiatrists hopefully know more about treating ADHD, some people find it easier to get their prescriptions from their family doctors.

Medication Monitoring Form (p. 141) You can use this handy form to keep track of how a new medication or dose is working for you.

Make an Informed Choice: The Facts Behind the Medication Controversy

Even though medication is widely accepted as an effective part of an ADHD treatment program, there is still more controversy than there should be about it. Some of this involves skeptics who don't believe in ADHD at all and just see the medication as part of a larger conspiracy. They may see the medication as an attempt by some people to gain an unfair advantage or to gain access to mood-altering substances. Others believe that ADHD is real but take issue with the medication in particular. They may see the intentional misuse or abuse of stimulants by a small number of people as a reason to deny them to everyone. Rather than get rid of them completely, I suggest that we should try to ensure that the stimulants are appropriately prescribed and taken. As a society, we need to find a balance between denying those who need medication and prescribing it too easily to those who don't really need it.

Let's summarize some of the myths and facts about ADHD medication:

Medication myth	Medication reality
They are addictive.	They are not addictive when appropriately prescribed and taken.
They cause people to abuse more drugs.	They actually can help people with ADHD to abuse drugs less (Wilens, 2004).
They cause heart attacks and sudden death.	After a careful review of the data, the FDA concluded that this isn't true (Connor, 2006).
They are performance enhancers for people who want an edge.	They help those with ADHD to function more like those who don't have it, in the same way that eyeglasses correct poor vision.
They are overprescribed.	Most ADHD adults have never been treated. Medication should be prescribed only to those who have the relevant condition.
Alternative treatments are safer and more effective.	Most alternative treatments have not been proven to be effective for ADHD. (See chapter 7 for more information.)

The decision to take medication is a personal one that is ideally based on accurate information. Medication is neither a silver bullet nor a copout and is only one part of a comprehensive treatment program. Many adults with ADHD find that medication is a valuable contribution that helps them more effectively follow the rest of the program.

I'm a psychologist, so I don't write prescriptions. In general, I tend to prefer other methods of helping my clients. But when it comes to ADHD, I am actually pretty pro-medication. This is based on what the research says regarding effectiveness and safety and also what my clients overwhelmingly tell me—the stuff works. It isn't perfect, but it makes life a lot easier for most people. I usually suggest that clients who are struggling at least try it so they can make a fully informed choice about what medication could do for them. If they then decide that they don't need it, I'm OK with that, because it is a well-informed decision.

The Most Popular Stimulant (Coffee, Anyone?)

For all the controversy surrounding prescription stimulants, most people have no moral issues with caffeine, which is also a stimulant. Caffeine is popular, cheap, and plentiful. The various energy drinks on the market are all loaded with caffeine or compounds very similar to caffeine. Most people in our society use caffeine on a daily basis to feel more alert and to think more clearly. Although some people get huffy about the price of fancy coffees, few become judgmental about caffeine itself. I'm not saying they should, but the casual acceptance of caffeine makes for a puzzling contradiction with the knee-jerk rejection of stimulants for treating ADHD. It's not like we tell caffeine lovers that they should just try to be more awake.

Granted, the prescription stimulants are stronger and have a greater potential for abuse, so they should be taken only by those who have been appropriately diagnosed and received a prescription. So care needs to be taken, but a judgmental attitude is at least a little hypocritical for most people.

To Take Medication or Not to Take Medication: It Depends

There's no objectively correct answer to the question of whether someone with ADHD should take medication, since it depends on each person's circumstances. As a psychologist, I'm interested in the kinds of decisions that people make. This means not only *what* people decide but also *how* they decide. After all, we can sometimes wind up at a good decision with a bad process—like by flipping a coin. The problem is that bad processes are less likely to get you good results. So, my hope is that when it comes to the decision about medication, you use a good process, just as you would for any important decision. This means a well-thought-out process rather than a knee-jerk impulse to never take it or to take it without even knowing the potential side effects.

The majority of my clients with ADHD take medication, at least sometimes. Not all, but most. I very much respect the decision not to take medication—if it's thoroughly considered and informed by facts. For example, I had a client who clearly had ADHD but also had bipolar disorder. This means that she would need to take a mood stabilizer to ensure that she didn't have any more manic episodes. (ADHD medication can set off a manic episode in people who also have bipolar disorder.) Because she had retired from her job and therefore did not need to function at the same high level, she decided that she did not want to take anything for her ADHD. For her, it was the right choice. On the other hand, I have other clients who would practically fight to the death (not really) if you tried to take away their medication because it is so helpful.

In the interest of informing your decision-making process, let's run through the factors that would tend to make someone more or less likely to consider medication. First of all, medication doesn't *make* anyone do anything he doesn't want to do—but it does allow him to more easily, reliably, and accurately do what he wants to do. By way of analogy, wearing glasses doesn't automatically make someone a better student. However, if the student can't see the writing on the blackboard, she doesn't have the option to copy information from it. With glasses, she has the choice to copy the information but may still choose not to. The medicated ADHD adult still has to do the hard work of changing habits, but he has a better shot at being successful. There is a saying of "pills don't teach skills" (which is true) but they *do* make it easier to learn those skills. This is where the strategies from the rest of the book come in. Medications are neither mind control nor a silver bullet, but they do help.

On the other side of the coin, no medication (even aspirin) is perfectly safe, so it's a matter of balancing the potential benefits with the potential risks and side effects—but there are definitely risks and side effects with untreated ADHD, too, as discussed at length in chapter 4. (By the way, if ADHD wasn't significantly and negatively affecting your life, would you be reading this book?) This must also be taken into account to make a fully informed decision. No one would willingly undergo the intense side effects and significant risks of chemotherapy if the risks of untreated cancer weren't so awful. Ultimately, it's a personal decision based on several factors, as the following table shows.

Factors that reduce the need for medication	Factors that increase the need for medication
Strong coping skills and good habits that reduce the fallout of ADHD symptoms	ADHD symptoms that cause significant problems and suffering
Other strengths and abilities, including social skills, that reduce the fallout of ADHD symptoms	Other weaknesses that cause significant problems and suffering
Willingness to work hard to overcome ADHD weaknesses	Desire for more immediate improvement
Supportive social environment	Demands at work or home that exceed abilities
Active engagement in other treatments	Other conditions like anxiety, depression, or substance abuse that reduce happiness and functioning
Willingness to live a smaller and simpler life	High expectations of performance

Keep in mind that different people can have different responses to the same medication—and even to different doses. So someone may have great (or awful) things to say about a particular medication, but that doesn't mean that you will have the same response. The only possible exception is that family members may be somewhat more likely to have similar responses. But generally the only way to know is to try a medication for yourself. You will probably have to try at least a couple of dosages and maybe even try a second medication if the first one doesn't hit the bull's-eye for you. You may get lucky and hit it with the first dosage strength of the first medication, but it will probably take a little bit of tweaking to get it working best.

At the risk of oversimplifying, what it all comes down to is whether the demands on you exceed your abilities to handle them. If so, medication may be helpful. You can also tilt that equation by reducing your demands (like taking a job that is a better fit) or increasing your ability to handle those demands (like using an electronic organizer to remind you of deadlines). There are many ways to change your situation, and medication is only one of them. So it comes down to preferences about what kind of life you want to live and what else you're willing and able to do.

Is Taking Medication Like Wimping Out? The Diabetes Analogy

It's interesting that medicating ADHD brings up such strong opinions, whereas medicating diabetes or other conditions that are seen as more medical doesn't provoke the same debate. Put simply, people are more comfortable medicating physical conditions than mental conditions—even when there is a proven physical basis to these supposedly mental conditions. It essentially comes down to the mistaken idea that we should be able to control how we think and feel, but are given a free pass when any part of the body except for the brain is involved. This seems to be a pretty arbitrary distinction.

When discussing medications with clients, I often use diabetes as an analogy of a condition that can be managed in its milder forms by lifestyle changes, such as diet and exercise. However, these methods aren't enough in more severe cases, so insulin needs to be added to control blood sugar levels. Similarly, medication may be necessary to help manage ADHD symptoms so that the lifestyle changes and other strategies can have their effect. Of course, someone with diabetes who takes insulin can't then eat a bunch of junk and watch TV all day; that person still needs to maintain good habits. Same for ADHD—you can't just take your medication and then do everything else the same.

I also point out that if the client had diabetes, presumably there would be less hesitation, stigma, or feelings of failure associated with taking medication, so perhaps there is no need to feel guilty for taking ADHD medications. After all, it's not like your medication does your laundry for you.

For some people, though, taking medication is seen as an admission of being flawed—it makes ADHD real as a diagnosis for them. Before, they could chalk it all up to just being fun loving or whatever, and now they have to admit that they have a disorder—some weird brain thing that forces them to take medication. I understand that acceptance is a process, sometimes a long process, and that there may be some mourning necessary in order to let go of the dream that it would all just get better by itself. I understand that taking medication can feel awfully official (and maybe even officially awful). But when you get down to it, it's really the daily struggles of untreated ADHD that make the diagnosis real. By the time that medication enters as a possibility, the person has already been suffering for years. The real problem isn't the bandage; it's the cut underneath it.

Others may feel that any successes they do have when taking medication are really because of the medication, not because of their efforts. This robs them of the ability to take credit for anything they do well. If only the medication were such a magic pill! Even if you took a pound of medication, you would still have to make good choices and work hard—it's just that your efforts will be more likely to be successful with the meds than without them. Can I give my glasses all the credit when I don't drive into a tree on the way home?

Potential Medication Benefits: What Does It Do?

As a psychologist, my preferred mode of intervention is talk therapy. However, I've found that for most of my ADHD clients, medication can make such a significant improvement in their lives that I often recommend they at least try them so that they can make a fully informed choice. Medication addresses the core symptoms of ADHD (inattention, hyperactivity, and impulsivity). So, just as these symptoms lead to other problems, which are discussed in other parts of this book, medication can then also lead to improvement in these affected areas. It doesn't make these other problems instantly disappear, but it can make it easier to address them.

Clients have described the benefits of medication in various ways:

- Creates a sense of clarity
- Makes it possible to ignore distractions
- Makes it easier to start and finish uninspiring tasks
- Calms a busy mind
- Brings everything into focus
- Makes it possible to think about only one thing at a time

Medication opens a small space between thought and thought in the case of distractibility, or between thought and action for hyperactivity and impulsivity. This makes it possible to stop and think about the best course of action. With medication, the person with ADHD has the option to make a more conscious choice rather than automatically respond or get pulled by distractions. This doesn't mean that she will necessarily decide to do the "right thing," but now, if she wants to, she can. It may not be perfect, but it's better. So if she is working on a report on the computer and her email alert chimes, she is able to decide to ignore it and keep working on her report rather than get sucked into email. Or if she decides to answer that email, she is better able to remember that she has that report to get back to rather than get lost in her inbox.

Studies with adults have found that stimulants lead to improved attention span and decreased distractibility, restlessness, and impulsivity (Connor, 2006). Stimulants improve vigilance, reaction time, task persistence, work productivity, working memory, handwriting, fine-motor speed, and general coordination. As a result of these improvements, people with ADHD perform better on simple and complex learning tasks. More specifically, medication can lead to improved performance in the following areas:

- Planning
- Organizing
- Prioritizing
- Time management
- Sustained attention
- Attention to detail
- Tolerating repetition and monotony
- Resisting distraction
- Focusing on and retaining reading material

Predictably, this all benefits the person in other areas of life, including how she relates to others. For example, medication improves these areas:

- Frustration tolerance
- Anger management
- Tact
- Patience
- Follow-through
- Listening
- Intimate communication
- Picking up subtle social cues
- Managing restlessness
- Resisting impulses

All of these have significant positive repercussions. For example, it's really interesting that studies have found that ADHD children who are appropriately medicated tend to evoke fewer negative reactions from caregivers and peers (Connor, 2006). In other words, medicating ADHD kids helps their parents do a better job! This presumably leads to bigger gains as time goes on and the relationship improves, and the constant battles are replaced by more harmonious interactions. Although these findings are not as well documented, we can assume that the same can be said for adults and their relationships.

Realistic Expectations for Medication: Somewhere Between Placebo and Miracle

As much as we think that medication just does what it does, there's actually a lot of subjectivity involved when people rate a medication's effectiveness. First of all, it can be affected by physiological differences from day to day, like amount of sleep, diet, exercise, mood, and stress. I actually had a client who kept a notebook when she started medication, and it was interesting to see how these other factors affected how well the medication "performed"—of course, what it showed is that many other factors besides the medication affect attention.

Ratings of a medication's effectiveness can also be influenced by psychological factors, like expectations. Some people unrealistically expect the medication to instantly enable them to do everything they couldn't before. (Go figure: someone with ADHD being impatient.) These people are then disappointed when the miracle doesn't happen, so they rate the medication poorly even when it is, in fact, helping. Medication isn't a silver bullet but rather an aid to help those with ADHD apply their efforts more effectively—but they still have to actually apply their efforts. Some people don't expect instant gratification but still lose patience when it takes some time to find the right dose, so they bail out prematurely or aren't willing to try a second or third medication if the first doesn't hit the bull's-eye.

If someone also has other conditions, such as depression, anxiety, or a learning disability, the ADHD medication may not seem to help as much because these other conditions are also interfering with the person's performance. So some additional treatment may be necessary to unlock her potential.

Whereas most people who try medication are looking for a benefit, some people actually don't want it to help. They may be happy as they are and are just trying medication so that someone else (such as a romantic partner, family member, or boss) will get off their case. Because they aren't looking for benefits, they may not notice them or may even downplay the medication's positive effects. Some of these people may not realize the extent of the effect that ADHD has on their lives, so they don't have much incentive to change it. Others may know it but worry that taking medication is a painful admission that something is wrong with them—so if they don't take medication, then that means that they are normal just like everyone else. I realize that it takes guts to admit shortcomings, but it seems to be better than continuing to suffer from something unnecessarily. In these cases, pride carries a very high price.

Stimulants and Nonstimulants: You Have Two Options

The oldest, best-studied, and most commonly used medications for ADHD are the stimulants, but there are some other options, collectively called the *nonstimulants*. These tend to be less effective, although there are some situations where they can be a good choice. Let's do a brief comparison between the two.

Stimulants	Nonstimulants
Benefit lasts less than 12 hours	Benefit potentially lasts 24 hours
Can be taken as needed	Must be taken daily
Begins to work within an hour	Can take several weeks or more to achieve full effect
Potentially abusable	Not abusable
Generally pretty quick and easy to find the best dose	Slower and more difficult to find the best dose
Must have paper prescription	Prescriptions can be called in to pharmacy

Because the stimulants are much more commonly used, I spend most of this chapter talking about them, followed by some articles on the nonstimulants.

Stimulant Medications: Some of the Basics

Stimulants are the oldest and most commonly used medication for ADHD. They were first used for behavioral problems in children and adolescents in 1937. They are the most thoroughly studied ADHD medications—and also the most thoroughly studied medications in children. The first double-blind, placebo-controlled clinical trials (this is the most rigorous type of research design) were conducted in the 1960s. They studied both dextroamphetamine (the active ingredient in Adderall and Vyvanse) and methylphenidate (the active ingredient in Ritalin, Concerta, and Focalin). Over 200 controlled trials have been completed since then (Connor, 2006), more than fifteen of them in adults (Wilens et al., 2006).

Despite claims that stimulants are overprescribed for children, several professional committees have concluded that there is little evidence of this (Barkley, Fischer, Smallish, and Fletcher, 2003). Although there are certainly some children who were misdiagnosed as having ADHD and thus prescribed a stimulant, there are also many children with ADHD who are not being treated. Although critics focus their attention on the use of stimulants, the real problem is misdiagnosis, in that the person wouldn't be receiving a stimulant if diagnosed properly.

Research has found that more than two-thirds of children and adolescents with ADHD have a good response to taking a stimulant. It may be less in adults (Prince, Wilens, Spencer, and Biederman, 2006). This is probably because adults tend to have other conditions, like anxiety or depression, following a difficult life of untreated ADHD. This complicates the treatment picture.

Paper Prescriptions Are Required

For most medications, physicians can call the pharmacy to place the prescription. This is obviously more convenient and faster than dropping off a paper prescription. Unfortunately, especially for folks with ADHD, who tend to lose things or not notice that they are running low, certain medications are not allowed to be called in. These Schedule II medications, as they're called, have some abuse potential, so the patient has to present a new paper prescription for each month's batch of pills, and the prescribing doctor cannot add refills to the prescription. However, prescribers are now allowed to give patients several one-month prescriptions that are postdated—for example, June 10, July 10, and August 10. Of course, the person then has to be able to find those prescriptions a month later.

Commonly Used Stimulants

There are essentially two types of stimulant currently on the market—methylphenidate (the Ritalin family) and various forms of amphetamine (the Adderall family). All of the brand names within each family have the same or very similar active ingredients, but the ingredients are packaged differently within the pill. The two families are different from each other, but not by much. At the risk of sounding like a product placement, I often use the analogy that one is like Pepsi and the other like Coke—they're mostly the same, but not exactly the same. Also, you can buy each in various sizes of bottles—or buy the pills in various dosage strengths—which last for different amounts of time, but the basic stuff inside is the same regardless of the packaging.

The biggest challenge to overcome since the stimulants were first used in 1937 has been to make them last longer. The older pills last only four to six hours, meaning that someone would need to take them two or three times a day to get a full day's benefit. Not only is this difficult to remember, but it also tended to leave people feeling uneven as the amount of medication in their systems went up and down. So the big advances (mostly) have been to make these short-acting medications last longer by packaging the medication differently within the pills.

I have created the following table to summarize the various medications that are available at the moment. However, the long-acting ones tend to be used most. The short-acting formulations are sometimes used in the afternoon to extend the effect of a long-acting formulation that is taken in the morning. (See *Some People Take More Medication in the Afternoon* on p. 126.)

	Methylphenidate family	Amphetamine family
	Typical adult dose range is 20-80 mg/day*	Typical adult dose range is 10-40 mg/day **
Short-acting formulations (4-6 hours)	Ritalin Methylin Focalin Metadate ER	Adderall
Medium-acting formulations (6-8 hours)	Ritalin LA or SR Metadate CD Methylin ER	
Long-acting formulations (10-12 hours)	Concerta Focalin XR Daytrana	Adderall XR Vyvanse

*Focalin and Focalin XR are prescribed at half the dose of the other methylphenidate products.

** Vyvanse is prescribed at a dose range of 20 to 70 mg/day.

Some Special Considerations

I would like to make a few extra points here about stimulants, since there are some important things to know.

Some Generic Versions Are Available

Most of the short- and medium-acting formulations are available in generic versions, which is helpful for those people who need to pay for their medications out of pocket. Although generics contain exactly the same active ingredients, they may have different inactive ingredients that can cause them to have a slightly different effect. As of this writing, none of the long-acting formulations are available in generic, although Adderall XR is expected to go generic in April of 2009, Daytrana perhaps in 2012, Focalin XR perhaps in 2015, Concerta perhaps in 2018, and Vyvanse perhaps in 2023. (I would be psyched if anyone was reading this in 2023.) The long-acting formulations are generally preferable, but the cost difference may be too much to ignore. Also, it's worth calling different pharmacies for price comparisons, because prices vary at each pharmacy.

Vyvanse

Vyvanse is currently the newest stimulant for ADHD. It is what's called a *pro-drug*, which means that it is actually a precursor that gets converted in the body to the substance that has the effect. Vyvanse is a dextroamphetamine molecule that is attached to a lysine molecule (an amino acid). After you swallow the pill, enzymes in your stomach and blood remove the lysine so the dextroamphetamine molecule can then do its thing. The lysine molecule was added in order to make this medication much less abusable—without it, someone could crush up the pills and then snort or inject the powder in order to get high. (This is one of the reasons that Dexedrine, which is plain old dextroamphetamine, isn't used much anymore.) It turns out that attaching the lysine molecule also makes the dextroamphetamine last longer and gives smoother dosing.

Vyvanse is similar to Adderall and Adderall XR, which contain both amphetamine and dextroamphetamine, sometimes referred to as "mixed salts of amphetamine."

Focalin and Focalin XR

Focalin and the extended-release version Focalin XR are purified versions of methylphenidate. Some molecules exist as two *isomers*, which are mirror images of each other. (Dig back into those dusty memories from chemistry class.) Without getting too complicated, studies have demonstrated that only one of the two isomers of methylphenidate is used by the brain, so the manufacturer removed the other isomer. This is why Focalin and Focalin XR are prescribed at half the dosages of the other methylphenidate products. Nonetheless, this purified form is no better or worse than the regular stuff.

Daytrana Patch

Daytrana is the first skin patch developed for the treatment of ADHD. It contains methylphenidate in a gel suspension that allows the medication to be absorbed through the skin. The patch can be worn for up to nine hours and then provides an additional three hours of coverage once it's removed. This can provide a more predictable off switch, since you can remove it at any point up to nine hours. In addition, Daytrana is also potentially less abusable because the gradual absorption into the bloodstream doesn't produce a rush. One potential downside of the patch is that it can take up to two hours to begin taking effect, meaning that the person goes through half of the morning without coverage, although a low-dose short-acting pill can also be taken as a kick-start.

Food and Stomach Acidity

Adderall XR and Focalin XR use a similar system to make a short-acting medication last longer. (Other extended-release medications use different systems.) Both of them are capsules that contain two kinds of beads. Half of the beads dissolve immediately and give the initial medication benefit. The second half of the beads have a coating that dissolves more slowly, usually about four hours later. This releases more medication as the first beads are wearing off, thereby extending the effect. In other words, one XR capsule essentially provides two short-acting doses without your having to remember to take that second dose.

This outer coating is affected by the acidity of the stomach, in that it dissolves in a less acidic environment. This has two implications. First, drinking acidic juices (like grapefruit) with breakfast can make your stomach more acidic and cause that second dose to release later. This can mean that you get a dip in coverage in the middle of the day and then the medication lasts longer at the end of the day. Second, taking reflux medication that reduces the amount of stomach acid can, in theory, make your stomach less acidic, causing that coating to dissolve more quickly. This can give you too much stimulant in the middle of the day and thereby less at the end of the day. So, you need to be aware of these possibilities, in case it affects how these two medications work for you.

Older Stimulants

Cylert (generic is pemoline) and Dexedrine (generic is dextroamphetamine) are older stimulants that are now rarely used.

How Stimulants Work: Mostly Dopamine, a Little Norepinephrine

Both methylphenidate and amphetamine block dopamine and norepinephrine reuptake in certain parts of the brain. As a result, more of these neurotransmitters are available in the synapse to fire off the next nerve cell, so these areas of the brain become more active. In addition, amphetamine causes the nerve cell to release more neurotransmitter into the synapse.

Because methylphenidate and amphetamine don't work exactly the same way, some people respond differently to the two. To expand the Pepsi and Coke analogy I used in *Commonly Used Stimulants*, some people prefer Pepsi, some prefer Coke, and some like them both. A rough rule with these stimulants is that approximately one-third of people show a preference for one, one-third show a preference for the other, and one-third show an equal response. This preference is based on both how well they work and on the severity of side effects. Since we can't predict someone's response to one based on her response to the other, it's probably worth trying a medication from the other family if you don't get a good enough response from the first medication. I've had plenty of clients who did better on the second medication they tried.

How Much Should I Take? Finding the Right Dose

Most prescribers will start someone on a low dose of stimulant, then move the person up gradually until the right dose is found. You may not feel anything at all at the starter dose, but that doesn't mean that a higher dose wouldn't work. Half an aspirin won't do much for a headache, but two will. So hang in there. You may find that you get some initial benefit that fades over a few days. If you're adjusting well to each new dose, you can go up to the next dose after a few days or week or so.

Some prescribers, especially primary care physicians, tend to be too conservative and will wait a month between dose increases. Unless you're experiencing intolerable side effects that the prescriber hopes will go away, there's no reason to wait this long. Nothing will really change after the first week or two.

You should find that each dose increase works a little better than the one before. You may also find that the side effects increase, although that may fade after a week or so. As long as the side effects are tolerable, wait and see if they go away. If they are more than you want to wait through, you can drop back to the prior dose for another week before stepping up again. Your body may be more adjusted to the medication then. There is a balance to be struck in finding the right dose—higher doses offer greater benefits but also more side effects. You may find that you overshot your ideal dose and then need to drop back to the one that offered the best balance.

Generally speaking, people who are heavier tend to take larger doses than people who weigh less. However, this is a pretty rough rule, so don't make too much of it. There is no blood test to determine what the best dose is for someone. It really comes down to how she rates her experience on each dose. Other people who know her well may also like a vote on that, since they should be able to see some of the effects, too.

Two factors determine the benefits and side effects of a medication:

- *Total daily intake.* The typical adult dosage ranges are based on how much someone takes over the course of a day.
- *Peak blood levels.* Someone may be well within the total daily intake number but experience strong side effects if his peak blood level is too high. For example, someone who takes 30 mg of short-acting Adderall may get intense side effects, but he may do great on 30 mg of extended-release Adderall because it spreads the dose out twice as far, so his peak blood levels will be half as much. (Make sense?) Generally speaking, the total daily dosage of the short-acting formulations should be divided among two or three doses throughout the day.

Although the stimulants don't need to be taken every day to be effective, like some medications do, it's still a good idea to take it every day when you are trying to find the right dose. Once you have that figured out, then you can talk to your prescriber about skipping days where you don't need it.

Do People Develop Tolerance to Stimulants?

Some people worry that they will need to regularly increase their dose to get the same effect, but this has not been found to be the case (Prince, Wilens, Spencer, and Biederman, 2006). The worries are probably based on the tolerance that can develop from intentionally abusing stimulants or illegal drugs. Those who try to get a high take much higher doses, which causes both the high as well as the tolerance. At normal dose levels, this is not a concern.

Some people find that their dose doesn't work as well for them anymore. The most common reason is a significant weight gain, which reduces the dose based on body weight. This is usually more common for kids than adults, since adult weight gains tend to be a smaller proportion of their prior weight.

The other possibility is that the demands on the person have increased, such as after a promotion or birth of a child, and she needs to perform at a higher level. So the dose that seemed to work well before is no longer sufficient to get the job done. Alternatively, stress, sleep deprivation, anxiety, depression, or other lifestyle factors can affect performance, but the person mistakenly assumes it's due to reduced medication effects.

Bring Your Romantic Partner to Medication Appointments

It can be helpful to bring your romantic partner or a family member to your medication appointments. Not that they know more than you do, but they can offer a helpful second opinion on the medication's effects. Sometimes, though, someone else can see us better than we can see ourselves. One guy from the adult ADHD support group I ran said with a smile, "Sometimes my wife asks me if I've taken my meds, and it really bugs me… because she's always right." This got a good laugh.

However, the people you live with may not see the full effects for two reasons. First, if you're taking a stimulant, it may be mostly worn off by the time you get home at night. As a client once told me, quoting his wife, "Your coworkers get medicated Tom, but I don't." So when describing the medication effect, they should perhaps ignore weekdays and instead focus on the weekends when they see you throughout the day. The other possibility is that you may feel more focused, but it may not be completely obvious to someone else. They need to infer the effect based on your behavior, so they may be less aware of your internal experience.

Some People Take More Medication in the Afternoon

One of the biggest problems with stimulants is that they don't last all day, which leaves many people unmedicated for the evening. Even the longest-acting formulations run out after about twelve hours or less.This is especially problematic for adults whose responsibilities don't end at 5:00 or for teens who do homework after sports practice.

If you find that your stimulant wears out too early, this is the general order of how to extend the effect:

1. *Switch to a long-acting medication.* Unless cost is a factor, the long-acting formulations are preferable. This may extend the benefit sufficiently.
2. *Get the morning dose right.* A low dose may wear off earlier. If your medication does what it needs to through the day, it may also last long enough into the evening.
3. *Increase the morning dose.* As long as it is tolerable during the day, this may extend the benefit a little further.
4. *Add in an afternoon dose of short-acting medication.* You can take a small amount of the short-acting version of the medication you take in the morning.

There is always a balance to be struck in having enough medication in your system at night to enable you to do what you need to do, without having so much that it interferes with falling asleep. You may need to work with your prescriber to find the right doses and timing of when you take it, since both affect how much medication is left at bedtime.

Even if you take an afternoon dose, it's still a good idea to try to take care of the tasks that require the most focus or accuracy early in the night while you have more medication in your system. For example, it may be better to pay bills early in the evening and to leave folding laundry for later.

Rebound

Some people experience *rebound*, a crashing feeling or irritability that occurs when their medication starts to wear out. This tends to be less common with the long-acting formulations since the medication leaves their systems more gradually. Rebound can be treated with a small amount of a short-acting formulation to smooth out the sudden drop in blood levels. For more information, see *Managing Stimulant Side Effects* on p. 132.

Some People Shouldn't Take a Stimulant

Although stimulants are generally quite safe and easy to get right, they aren't appropriate for everyone. If you are in generally good health and none of the situations discussed in this article apply to you, then you should consider a trial of stimulants to be an acceptable risk. Granted, there are no guarantees in life, so it comes down to informed decisions. So let's talk about the potentially problematic situations.

Other Mental Health Conditions

Some people are mistakenly diagnosed with ADHD when what they really have is bipolar disorder (which used to be called manic depression). Others have both or have a bipolar tendency that mostly remains hidden but is revealed under certain circumstances, such as when put on a stimulant or antidepressant. It's really important to make sure that someone doesn't have bipolar disorder before prescribing a stimulant, since it can push the person into a manic episode. The person may need much less sleep than usual yet not feel tired, feel intensely irritable or impatient, go on reckless spending sprees, be much more sexually interested and even engage in unsafe sexual activities, or feel excited about a big new project that others see as extremely unrealistic. (If these symptoms occur to a lesser degree, it is called a hypomanic episode.) This obviously makes a real mess of things and highlights the importance of a thorough diagnostic evaluation, because a cursory evaluation can confuse the two conditions. If someone does have both, a stimulant can be safe if the person is first prescribed a mood stabilizer, although many prescribers may still be hesitant, given the risks.

Less problematic is that some people with severe anxiety may feel uncomfortably jittery, revved up, or restless on a stimulant. One solution is to "start low, go slow." In other words, start at a low dose and move the dose up slowly. This will take longer to get to the effective dose, but it will be much more pleasant. Alternatively, one can treat the anxiety first. It can also help to keep in mind that the jittery feeling is simply a safe side effect from the stimulant.

High Blood Pressure

Many primary care physicians are nervous about prescribing stimulants to adults, based on the potential cardiac and blood pressure effects. Although I understand their desire to avoid problems (and, let's be honest, lawsuits), these fears tend to be overblown, especially when you balance the medication risks against the negative effects of untreated ADHD.

As with all stimulants, the stimulants prescribed for ADHD can cause a small increase in blood pressure and heart rate. For healthy adults, this shouldn't be a concern. For those who use medication to normalize their elevated blood pressure, a study found that Adderall XR leads to only minor and insignificant increases. If an elevation does occur, it will often return to baseline within a week, so it should be monitored, but medication should not automatically be withdrawn (Wilens et al., 2006). Although methylphenidate wasn't tested in this study, the results presumably apply equally.

We should also keep in mind that untreated ADHD makes it much harder for someone to create the stability required to exercise regularly, plan healthy meals, resist the temptation of junk food, and manage stress—in other words, all the stuff that contributes to high blood pressure. So ADHD medication may actually help someone to reduce blood pressure naturally.

Severe Cardiac Issues

There have been dire reports in the media about a possible connection between prescription stimulants and sudden cardiac death. This is certainly dramatic enough to warrant additional research. Careful review of the data revealed that in all of the small number of cases, there had been undiagnosed or untreated cardiac issues or other complicating factors, such as heat exhaustion, near drowning, or fatty liver. In addition, the incidence of these unfortunate events among thirty million Adderall prescriptions written between 1999 and 2003 were not significantly greater than they were in the general population not taking Adderall, and therefore were probably not due to the medication (Connor, 2006). So additional caution should be exercised by those who have serious cardiac issues or a family history of them—but these people should seek appropriate evaluation and treatment regardless of whether they take a stimulant.

Substance Abuse or Addiction

Because this is a larger topic, it is covered in *Medicating Substance Abusers* on p. 130.

Intentional Abuse of Stimulants: An Unfortunate Reality

Some people snort, inject, or otherwise take large doses of prescription stimulants to get high. Some of them have legitimate prescriptions, whereas others obtain the pills illegally. I've had at least three clients (that I know of) who intentionally abused their prescribed stimulants. This is clearly a bad idea, for all the obvious reasons: excessive doses pose health risks, medication is quickly used up that could be helpful through the month, abuse destroys the prescriber's trust, and so on. Although I certainly don't want to defend the actions of those who do abuse prescription medications, I also wouldn't throw the baby out with the bathwater by saying that all stimulants should be banned simply because a few people use them inappropriately.

It's possible that most of the abuse of stimulants is used to improve performance or to stay awake rather than to get high (not that this is any better). This is probably especially true on college campuses, where students may be more willing to take something to help them stay up all night (hence the popularity of energy drinks).

The fact that some people will fake the diagnosis solely to gain access to the medications speaks more to the need to do a thorough evaluation than it does to anything inherently problematic with the stimulants. By the same token, the fact that teens will try to get alcohol shouldn't lead us to ban it entirely, so much as it should motivate sellers to be more careful about carding their customers. The same goes for those who divert their medications to others who don't have ADHD—they should first be educated about the dangers of giving away or selling prescription medication, and then they should be punished if they do it anyway. Once again, this is more about individuals' decisions to subvert the prescription process than it is about the medication itself.

Medicating Substance Abusers: Balancing the Risks

Because prescription stimulants can be abused by those who choose to do so, many prescribers are leery of giving them to patients with a history of substance abuse—and especially to those who are currently using. This is sometimes due to a fear of intentional misuse, but prescribing doctors may also be concerned that the stimulant will give the patient a craving for illegal drugs again. The patient may have the same fear, as one of my clients did after several years of being clean. It was a real dilemma for her whether she wanted to try stimulants, even though her ADHD was really making a mess of her life. Although the stimulants are abusable when taken at excessive doses, they will not create a high when taken at the dosage prescribed. Additionally, the longer-acting formulations tend to give a slower onset and therefore very little rush.

Unfortunately, there is a pretty big overlap between ADHD and substance abuse, so there are a lot of people out there who may potentially be denied access to the most effective medication treatment. Some prescribers like to see the patient stay clean for a certain length of time before starting the stimulant. While understandable, the untreated ADHD can undermine that sobriety. Conversely, medicating the ADHD may better enable the person to stay clean. This is a judgment call for both the prescriber and the patient. One option is to have a reliable family member dispense the medication, thus ensuring that it's taken only as prescribed. This family member would then be authorized to communicate with the prescriber. While not ideal, it may be better than nothing. If substance abuse is an issue for you, it may be worth treating it directly, either through a twelve-step group or more formal treatment, in addition to whatever you do for your ADHD.

If you disclose at a twelve-step group that you take medication for your ADHD, you may want to be prepared for someone saying that it is similar to abusing drugs. It actually isn't if you are taking something as prescribed, but you may want to think up a brief canned response to give.

Some Formulations Are Better Options

All stimulants are not created equal. In increasing order, here are the options for those with a history of substance abuse:

- *Long-acting formulations are less abusable than short-acting ones.* All three of my clients who admitted to abusing their prescription stimulants were taking one of the short-acting formulations. However, where there's a will there's a way, so even the long-acting ones may not be totally safe.
- *Daytrana patch.* Because the methylphenidate needs to absorb through the skin, it has a gradual onset, even if someone were to use several, so it gives very little rush.
- *Vyvanse.* Vyvanse needs to be activated by enzymes in the stomach and bloodstream, so it doesn't give a high when snorted or injected because that enzymatic conversion regulates how quickly the active medication is created.
- *Strattera.* Strattera is a nonstimulant ADHD medication and therefore completely nonabusable (i.e., not worth abusing), although it tends to not work as well. But it can be just the right thing for someone who is locked out of taking stimulants.

So there are some options to consider and discuss with your prescriber. It really comes down to being completely honest with yourself about whether you are ready to handle the responsibility of managing a medication like this. If you aren't sure that you are, that's OK. Work on your ADHD in other ways and maybe you'll be more ready later.

Managing Stimulant Side Effects: General Principles

Fortunately, the stimulants' side effects generally are tolerable and often subside within a couple of weeks as you adjust to the medication. Any side effects that linger can usually be managed by adjusting the dose or changing the timing of when you take it. As with most medications, higher doses tend to bring on more side effects.

If you do get side effects, pay attention to when they start and go away. Generally speaking, if they're from the medication, they should occur at around the same time, relative to when you took your medication.

- *First hour or two.* It's likely that the medication is entering your system too quickly, so you may be able to slow that down by taking it with food, preferably a meal with some fat in it.

Alternatively, you can take part of the dose later in the morning, but this is a setup for forgetting.

- *Middle part of the effective period.* It's likely that you have too much medication in your system, so you can either lower the dose or change to another formulation that will spread out the medication further and more smoothly.
- *Last hour or two.* It's likely that the medication is clearing out of your system too quickly, a situation called *rebound.* You can either switch to another formulation that will fade out more slowly or add in a small amount of short-acting medication at this point in the day.

Some people may feel that the medication makes their ADHD worse at the end of the day. Apart from rebound, what's most likely going on here is that the benefits of the medication during the day make the untreated symptoms at night seem worse by comparison. Ironically, the success of the medication during the day is misinterpreted as a failure. This can be fixed by extending the medication's effective period so it covers more of the evening (see *Some People Take More Medication in the Afternoon* on p. 126).

Intolerable Side Effects? Try the Other One

Because the medications in the methylphenidate and amphetamine families are somewhat different, some people respond better to one than to the other. (See *How Stimulants Work* on p. 124.) Therefore, if you are getting intolerable side effects from your current medication, you may have better luck if you try one from the other family. Unless the problem is that your current medication is wearing off too quickly or is too uneven in how it spreads out the dose, it's unlikely that trying another medication in the same family would have a different effect. For example, since both Concerta and Focalin XR are in the same family, they would probably work about the same for you. One possible exception is Adderall XR and Vyvanse, since they are in the same family but are a little different.

Because the medications are mostly worn off by the end of the night, there's very little left in your system by morning. As a result, you can safely try the other medication the very next day. This makes it very easy to make quick adjustments and compare the relative benefits and side effects.

Managing Stimulant Side Effects: Specific Side Effects

Although stimulants are quite safe and generally well tolerated, you may experience some side effects. Some of these may disappear on their own over a few days or a couple weeks as your body adjusts to a new medication or a higher dosage. If the side effect isn't too bad and the medication works well, you may want to hang in there and see if it gets better or goes away over time. Otherwise, most side effects can be reduced by lowering the dose, but then you may not get as much benefit, so a balance needs to be struck.

In addition to this general advice, you can try the following strategies for each specific side effect. If none of these strategies are helpful enough, then you may do better by switching to a stimulant from the other family (see *Managing Stimulant Side Effects: General Principles*, p. 131).

Trouble Falling Asleep

You may have trouble falling asleep if you have too much medication in your system at bedtime—it's like having a big cup of coffee late in the afternoon. However, many people with ADHD will have preexisting sleep difficulties, so if you feel that the medication is making that worse, then make sure that it isn't just more of the same.

- Take your medication earlier.
- If you take a second dose at midday, then reduce that dose or take it earlier.
- Reduce the morning dose.

Appetite Suppression

This is probably more of a concern in children, in whom reduced caloric intake may have some connection with a possible growth suppression effect. Most adults probably wouldn't mind losing a few pounds. Nonetheless, it's important to eat often enough to keep your blood sugar up.

- Take your medication with or after breakfast.
- If a big lunch is too much, then eat several smaller meals throughout the day.
- Make up for lost calories at lunch by eating a larger breakfast and dinner or a healthy snack at night.

Elevated Blood Pressure or Heart Rate

A small increase in blood pressure or heart rate is acceptable in healthy adults.

- Treat preexisting cardiac issues before starting a stimulant, then adjust as necessary.
- Drop down to a lower dose and increase it slowly.
- Monitor to see whether side effects subside over time.
- Stop medication and consult physician if excessive.

Stomachache and Headache

These side effects can occur if the medication is taken on an empty stomach or absorbs into your system too quickly.

- Take medication with food. Foods with fat may cause the medication to absorb more slowly.

Rebound

This occurs when the medication wears off too quickly and can make some people irritable or emotional for about an hour. It is more common with the shorter-acting formulations.

- Switch from a short-acting formulation to a long-acting formulation.
- Add in a small amount of a short-acting formulation one hour before rebound tends to begin.

Nervousness

People who are prone to anxiety are more likely to feel anxious, amped up, or jittery when starting a stimulant. Others actually feel less anxious when the stimulant helps them focus better, causing them to feel more on top of their demands.

- Start on a low dose and increase it slowly (start low, go slow).
- Keep in mind that these feelings are probably just a safe and temporary adjustment to the medication. Don't get anxious about feeling anxious.
- Reduce caffeine intake since that can make this worse.

Spaced Out

Too much medication can make some people feel like a zombie, spaced out, or emotionally flat. They don't feel like themselves anymore, and others may notice that they seem withdrawn.

- Lower the dose.
- Change the timing or type of formulation you are taking in order to reduce the peak blood levels of medication.

Edginess, Agitation, or Irritability

Some people feel edgy when the medication is wearing off, which is called rebound, as explained previously. However, the edginess can also occur when the medication is at its peak. Sometimes the person just needs to get used to a new dose. Other times, the dose needs to be reduced.

- Reduce the dose and then perhaps increase it again more slowly.
- Seek evaluation for bipolar disorder if it is extreme.

Hypomania or Mania

Some people are diagnosed with ADHD when they are actually bipolar. Others have both ADHD and bipolar disorder. If someone with a bipolar tendency is put on a stimulant, he can go into a hypomanic or manic episode. He may have much less need for sleep, have lots of energy, spend money recklessly, engage in dangerous activities, feel very irritable or impatient, and have a strongly elevated sex drive. This behavior is notably different from his usual self, although at the time other people may see it as more problematic than he does.

- Immediately stop taking the stimulant and contact your prescriber.
- A mood stabilizer may be necessary to control these symptoms. Once your mood is stabilized, it is possible to start the stimulant again.
- Reevaluate whether ADHD is the appropriate diagnosis.

Tics

Stimulants tend to make tic disorders worse. Some people have a tendency toward developing tics but don't really have many tics until they start taking a stimulant. The tics then go away when the stimulant wears off.

- Evaluate the degree to which the stimulant is making your tics worsen.
- Reduce the dose to find a better balance between improving the ADHD and tolerating the tics.
- Treat the tics with another medication. <end BL>

Dizziness

If you feel dizzy when the medication is at its strongest, then either reduce the dose or switch to an extended-release formulation that has a lower peak blood level.

Withdrawal

Withdrawal symptoms are unlikely to occur at normally prescribed dosages, but any symptoms should be temporary as your body readjusts.

Depression

Some people actually feel kind of depressed or overwhelmed when the medication helps them see more clearly how much they need to work on. The improved clarity that comes from the medication is mostly a good thing, but it can be depressing when you fully realize how much fallout a life of untreated ADHD creates. Remember that it took a long time to create your current circumstances, so it will take you some time to clean it all up. Focus on one thing at a time so you can see that you are indeed making progress.

Psychosis

This is a very rare side effect at normally prescribed dosages, but it is serious when it does occur. It usually reflects a tendency toward more severe mental health conditions. However, others may become temporarily psychotic if they abuse the medication by taking much more than the prescribed amount.

- Immediately stop taking the stimulant and contact your prescriber.
- Another medication may be necessary in order to control these symptoms.
- Reevaluate whether ADHD is the appropriate diagnosis.

Nonstimulant Medications: Sometimes a Good Choice

Although the stimulants are the best-known and most-prescribed medications for ADHD, there are a few options that are not stimulants. The good news about the nonstimulants is that they are often seen as less controversial and less problematic than the stimulants because they are completely nonabusable. This makes nonstimulants potentially a good choice for patients with a strong history of substance abuse. Unfortunately, they are less effective for most people. They can be great for some, but overall you're more likely to get a good benefit from a stimulant, so these should be considered a second choice behind the stimulants.

Unlike the stimulants, which begin working within an hour and then fade away over the course of the day, the nonstimulants need to be taken every day for four to eight weeks to achieve full effect. The downside of this is that you need to wait for the nonstimulants to start working. This delayed response also makes it harder to notice improvements that take place slowly, making it more difficult to get the dose just right. It also means that these medications can't be taken on an as-needed basis, and you must be consistent about remembering to take it every day. On the plus side, the nonstimulants provide twenty-four-hour coverage once their effect kicks in, which is a distinct advantage over the stimulants.

Strattera

Strattera (atomoxetine) was the first nonstimulant to be approved by the FDA for ADHD and the first medication of any class to be approved for adults with ADHD. (To give some sense of how recently ADHD was recognized in adults, this was only in 2002.)

Strattera works a little differently than the stimulants. It mostly affects norepinephrine, whereas the stimulants mostly affect dopamine. This is why some people have a different response to one than the other. It may be a good choice for people with ADHD who are also very anxious and therefore may feel more revved up from a stimulant.

Common side effects are dry mouth, insomnia, decreased appetite, constipation, decreased libido, dizziness, and sweating. Males may also experience difficulty attaining or maintaining an erection. As with the stimulants, it can be problematic for those with a bipolar tendency.

The bottom line on Strattera is that it just doesn't seem to be as effective as the stimulants. For some people it works very well, but not with the same frequency that the stimulants do. An informal survey of therapists and psychiatrists whom I know matches my experience and also what the research shows—it is just not as likely to be of significant benefit. Therefore, in my opinion, it should be prescribed only for people who don't do well on stimulants or who have specific reasons why they shouldn't try a stimulant. If your physician wants to try Strattera first, you may want to ask what her rationale is.

Antidepressants

Strattera is a second-line medication for ADHD, and antidepressants are a third-line choice; but they do seem to have some benefit for some clients. They can be helpful for someone with mild ADHD and also depression or anxiety, with the hope of killing two birds with one stone. They can also be considered for people with cardiac abnormalities that rule out the use of stimulants.

Wellbutrin, Wellbutrin-XL, or Wellbutrin-SR (bupropion) inhibit the reuptake of both dopamine and norepinephrine. The typical adult dose range is 150 to 450 mg/day. Its side effects include excitement, agitation, increased motor activity, insomnia, tremor, tics, and a potential for increased seizures in those with that tendency.

Effexor (venlafaxine) inhibits the uptake of both serotonin and norepinephrine. More research is needed to determine whether there is an actual benefit for ADHD, but it is sometimes mentioned as a possibility. Therefore, it should probably be considered a last resort for ADHD at this time.

Some of the old antidepressants seem to have some benefit but are rarely used because they are generally not as effective.

Some adults with depression or anxiety and undiagnosed ADHD are given one of the newer antidepressants that affect mostly serotonin (called the SSRIs). These work well for depression and anxiety but do nothing at all for ADHD. However, since depression and anxiety can also affect attention, it can seem like it is helping the ADHD, but it actually isn't. Unfortunately, this partial treatment response can give the impression that the medication is kind of working, so the prescriber doesn't look any further.

Black-Box Warnings: Scary but Rare

When you fill a prescription, the pharmacist gives you a sheet of information about the medication, including the side effects and potential risks. Some medications have risks that are deemed by the Food and Drug Administration to be especially serious and deserve extra attention. These are highlighted on the sheet and called black-box warnings. The risk is not considered likely enough for the FDA to pull the medication off the shelves, but it is still important to be aware of.

Stimulants

Stimulants have a warning about cardiac issues, particularly for people with structural abnormalities and high blood pressure. In addition, the methylphenidate products are cited as being problematic for those with other mental health conditions, such as bipolar disorder. The amphetamine products have a potential for dependence if misused.

Strattera

Strattera's warning concerns reports of potential liver toxicity, so you should contact your prescriber immediately if you develop jaundice (yellowish tint to skin or eyes), excessive itching, dark urine, right-upper-quadrant tenderness, and/or unexplained flulike symptoms. Most likely your prescriber will take you off the medication. Despite this rare possibility, routine liver functioning tests aren't necessary.

Using More Than One Medication Simultaneously

People with ADHD often find themselves on more than one medication. This may be as simple as taking an extended-release stimulant in the morning and then taking the same stimulant in a short-acting form in the afternoon to extend the effect. However, some take medication to treat other conditions, like depression or anxiety. Fortunately, the ADHD medications do not tend to have problematic interactions with other medications. The one exception is the old antidepressants known as MAOIs, which are now rarely used because they have dangerous interactions with too many things.

Most of the antidepressants used today are in the class called SSRIs, and they primarily increase serotonin levels. ADHD medications have no effect on serotonin, so there is no interaction (this, indirectly, is also why the SSRIs do nothing for ADHD). However, there may be some small interaction effect between the stimulants, Strattera, Wellbutrin, Cymbalta, or Effexor, since they all increase norepinephrine levels to varying degrees. So if you are already taking one, you may need to adjust the dose if you start another.

Some people may take a mood stabilizer to treat bipolar disorder or strong emotional reactions. This, too, is a safe combination. Usually the mood stabilizer is prescribed first.

If you have any concerns about possible drug interactions, ask your pharmacist.

Strategies for Remembering to Take Your Medication

"I need a pill to help me remember to take my pill!" This was said by a client who was having difficulty taking her medication consistently. Although washing down a little pill isn't that hard, remembering to do it can be, especially when it's a new habit. Of course, we could almost say that anyone who has no trouble remembering to take an ADHD medication probably doesn't need to take it!

That's obviously an overstatement, but there are some strategies to make it much easier. The problem is that taking a pill, especially when done every day, becomes a completely unmemorable event, making it too easy to remember yesterday's pill as today's (so you don't take a pill today) or forgetting that you already took today's pill (so you take another). A missed dose and a double dose are both problematic. To solve both possibilities, I strongly encourage clients to buy one of those inexpensive plastic weekly pill cases, so they can look to see if they did indeed take their pill today.

I also encourage my clients to place the pill case somewhere that they can't miss seeing it. Putting it in a drawer dramatically decreases the odds of remembering. The converse of "out of sight, out of mind" is "in sight, in mind," so leave the pill case next to your toothbrush, on the kitchen counter, or somewhere else that you will see it without having to remember to go looking for it. As a woman from my adult ADHD group joked, "The biggest problem with the meds is that they don't work if you don't take them."

As a failsafe, I also recommend that clients keep a few extra pills at work, in the car, or on a key chain so the day isn't an uphill climb if they realize after leaving the house that they forgot to take one at home.

If your prescriber has you taking a short-acting medication in the morning and then again in the afternoon, it may be simpler to take a long-acting medication so that you don't need to take that second dose later in the day (unless you are taking the short-acting medication because of cost considerations). That was one of the problems with the old, short-acting medications—it was really hard (and disruptive) to have to remember to take those later doses. Mornings, before your day has taken off, are often easier. I recently saw a client who had been put on three doses a day of a short-acting medication, which he was supposed to increase in strength through a complicated progression. The whole thing made me wonder how much the prescriber really knew about ADHD.

Can My Family Doctor Write My Prescriptions?

Most parts of the country have a shortage of psychiatrists to prescribe medication for ADHD and other mental health conditions. Many neurologists also prescribe for ADHD, but there aren't a lot of them, either. As a result, much of this prescribing is done by primary care physicians (PCPs, such as internists, family physicians, OB/gyns, and pediatricians). When my wife and I went out to dinner with another couple, my wife asked the woman, who is an internist, what kind of work she tends to do. Her husband joked, "Mostly psychiatry!"

My preference is usually that a psychiatrist write the initial prescriptions, since they can take more time and hopefully have more expertise in this area, so they're more likely to get it right. However, if a therapist has done a thorough evaluation and is confident that the person has ADHD and not some other condition (like bipolar disorder), then a PCP who is familiar with treating ADHD can do a good job, too. A number of local PCPs send me patients to evaluate and will then prescribe if necessary. They feel comfortable prescribing but not diagnosing. This is really my preference, too, since most PCPs just don't have the time to do a thorough evaluation, even if they have the knowledge. Other PCPs will write prescriptions, but only after the patient has already been prescribed by a psychiatrist or someone else, so they will maintain prescriptions but not start them. This is usually easier, especially if not much has changed in the patient's life.

There's no black-and-white answer about whether it's better to see a psychiatrist or a PCP. It really depends on your preferences and what services are available in your area. This table can help you compare the two, even if exceptions do exist:

	Psychiatrist	**PCP**
Appointment length	Longer	Shorter
Expertise	More	Less
Cost	More	Less
Ease of appointment scheduling	Less	More

Generally speaking, it's worth the extra cost and wait for a psychiatrist if the following are true:

- You really want to be sure that you get the right medication and optimal dosing.
- Your situation is more complicated, such as you have (or suspect you have) more than just ADHD.
- You have tried several medications for ADHD but feel that you're still not getting enough benefit or are getting too many side effects.

It's been my experience that PCPs are much more likely to prescribe doses that are too low than too high. This is probably based either on overcautiousness or on using childhood dosage ranges for adults who weigh significantly more. As a result, the adult may get some benefit so the PCP doesn't increase the dose, even though the patient might do even better. So if you feel that you're doing a little better and the side effects are tolerable, it may be worth asking your physician to try a higher dose.

The other tendency I've noticed is that many PCPs seem to prefer the nonstimulants for adults, often based on concerns about cardiac effects of the stimulants for their adult patients. Unfortunately, their concerns tend to be overblown for patients who are generally in good health, especially when we consider the clear risks associated with ADHD that is only partially treated by a medication that isn't doing a great job. They may also be more likely to prescribe the short-acting medications rather than the preferable long-acting versions.

Medication Monitoring Form

You can use this sheet, one per day, to record how a new medication or dosage is working. This can help you and your prescribing doctor find the right medication regimen. This monitoring sheet is short enough so you can fill it in quickly, but it still covers enough important areas to help you judge the benefits that you are receiving from the medication. (See Medication Monitoring Form on page 142.)

Medication Monitoring Form

Name:________________________________Day: ______________Date: __________

Was this a typical day in terms of the demands placed on you? If not, then how was it different?

Inattention Symptoms	Improvement (0 = none, 4 = significant)				
Distractible	0	1	2	3	4
Disorganized	0	1	2	3	4
Poor time management	0	1	2	3	4
Forgetful	0	1	2	3	4
Careless mistakes	0	1	2	3	4

Hyperactive/Impulsive Symptoms	Improvement (0 = none, 4 = significant)				
Feel restless	0	1	2	3	4
Tendency to blurt things out	0	1	2	3	4

Are you experiencing any side effects? If so, write down those effects to keep as a record for your prescriber.

CHAPTER 6

NONMEDICAL TREATMENT PROVIDERS: PILLS DON'T TEACH SKILLS

More of the same tends to lead to more of the same. In this chapter, we talk about the various professionals who can help you change what you do and hopefully thereby change how things work out for you. Regardless of whether you take no medication or a pound of it, you will probably benefit from meeting with a therapist, coach, professional organizer, career counselor, or support group. Whereas medication tightens up how your brain works, these other interventions help you clean up the fallout of a lifetime of untreated ADHD and teach you new skills to make a better future.

Let's use the analogy of the student who can't see the blackboard and falls behind in class. Once he is finally given glasses (i.e., prescribed medication), he may still be skeptical about his ability to be a successful student and not apply himself fully, even if he can now see perfectly. He may also need someone to go back and fill in the blanks of what he didn't learn the first time around.

A clinician who really understands ADHD can offer you strategies that are much more likely to work for you, because she understands how your ADHD affects your performance. This is fundamentally different from the million and one bits of advice that you've gotten over the years. The problem with uninformed advice is that it can often feel like there is an unspoken "you dummy" at the end of it—"you should get a schedule book to help remember things (you dummy)." An informed clinician will not only give you better strategies but will also explain them in a way that you don't have to feel bad about. This makes you much more likely to keep coming back, even after you've addressed the easy stuff and now need to trudge uphill on the harder stuff. It also makes it much more likely that you'll actually give the proposed strategies your best shot.

As a quick side note, I decided to put information about career counselors in chapter 17, *Work: Hopefully More than Just a Paycheck*, because it seemed to fit better there.

This chapter contains the following articles:

You Need an Expert: A Little Knowledge Isn't Enough (p. 145) Adults with ADHD need therapists, coaches, and other professionals who really understand the complexities of the condition. Here are some Websites where you can find someone local.

Talk It Out: Therapy Can Offer Clarity and Peace (p. 146) Therapy can be especially helpful for adults with ADHD who spent most of their lives undiagnosed. It can be helpful to understand yourself in a more accurate and less pejorative way.

Why Was Past Therapy Not Helpful Enough? (And Why You Can Expect Better This Time) (p. 148) Many adults have seen a therapist who missed their ADHD and instead tried to work on other things like relationship issues, anxiety, or depression. This therapy was probably not as helpful as it could have been, whereas therapy that is informed by your ADHD should work out much better.

Get the Most Out of Therapy (p. 150) Unmedicated ADHD can affect many parts of your life, including getting treatment for it. I cover a number of the ways that this can happen as well as what you can do to minimize these effects.

Goal Setting in Therapy (p. 154) Therapy is often more helpful if you have some specific things to work on. I talk about how to set these goals and adjust when necessary.

ADHD Coaching: More Than Obvious Advice (p. 155) Coaching can be quite helpful for adults with ADHD, as long as the coach is well informed. The trick is coming up with solutions that really work, not just once, but consistently.

What's the Difference Between Coaching and Therapy? (p. 157) It can be hard to know where the line is that separates coaching and therapy. There's definitely some overlap between them, but there are also some important differences.

Coach and Therapist: One Person or Two? (p. 160) Some people see both a coach and a therapist, whereas some just see a therapist who also does the coaching. Both can work, depending on your circumstances.

Coaching Certification: Is This Coach Any Good? (p. 162) Although there is currently no licensing requirement for coaches, there are various coaching certifications available. However, some of these certifications are more meaningful than others, so it's important to know what you're getting with a potential coach.

Changes on the Outside Create Changes on the Inside (p. 165) Helping an adult with ADHD be more successful and consistent in her daily demands can have a powerful effect on how she sees herself. This is important stuff.

How Coaching Helps: A General Coaching Theory (p. 166) Coaching helps mostly by preventing problems from developing but also by helping clients to clean up problems after they occur.

Goal Setting in Coaching (p. 167) Initially coaches tend to help clients come up with better solutions to their current difficulties, but the process should move toward teaching clients how to solve future problems themselves.

Create Structure and Schedules: More Guideline Than Jail (p. 170) A good coach will help you come up with the routines, plans, time commitments, and reminders that will most effectively keep you on track (and that you hopefully won't hate too much).

Professional Organizers: Move That Mountain (p. 170) A professional organizer can help you not only tackle your current mountain of stuff but also create better organizational systems so that you don't wind up with another mountain later.

Don't Underestimate the Power of a Support Group (p. 172) Support groups can offer ideas and reduce the feeling of being alone. This can be especially important right after you've been diagnosed and have lots of questions, but it is good for old-timers too.

Group Therapy: Learn With and From Others (p. 173) Therapy groups can be a great opportunity to learn about how you relate to other people and to work on your relationships. Some groups are specific to ADHD, whereas most have a variety of participants, each working on different issues.

You Need an Expert: A Little Knowledge Isn't Enough

If you are an adult with ADHD, you need treatment providers who really understand ADHD in adults. Whether it's a therapist, coach, prescriber, organizer, or career counselor, you need someone who understands ADHD beyond the basics—and beyond the classroom. It's not that someone without that background can't be helpful at all to you; it's just that they won't be as helpful as you would want them to be. For example, you just won't get enough benefit from a therapist who specializes in depression but doesn't take into account the untreated ADHD that is giving you good reason to be depressed. If I get a call from someone who needs experience in an area that I just don't know that well, I always refer that person to someone who can do a better job. No one can be an expert in everything, so I don't even pretend to be. Besides, I'd be quickly found out to be winging it, anyway.

It takes work to find treatment providers who have the necessary level of expertise, but it is well worth it. Otherwise you may feel like you're spinning your wheels with someone who just doesn't get it. There are many ways to find that right person. Often the best is a personal recommendation, but even then it's still a matter of finding the right chemistry. Try asking friends and other professionals you know, such as therapists, physicians, coaches, or tutors, to see whom they recommend.

Many websites include listings of professionals. However, you should keep in mind that these professional directories carry no guarantee of the person's abilities.

They are merely offered as a service to collect this information in one place. The professionals pay a fee to be included in that list; it's your job to feel them out and make sure that they offer what you need. The good news, though, is that they at least have an interest in ADHD in adults, so that weeds out those who have no interest or training. Here are the sites that I tend to recommend when someone outside my local area is looking for a referral:

- www.add.org
- www.chadd.org
- www.addresources.org
- www.addconsults.com
- www.psychologytoday.com

It's perfectly acceptable to interview several candidates before deciding on one. I strongly feel that if someone takes more than a day or maybe two to return your calls or isn't able or willing to spend ten minutes on the phone to tell you about his practice, then that's probably a bad sign. Here are some questions you may want to ask each candidate:

- How long have you been practicing?
- What kind of general training do you have?
- What kind of training do you have in ADHD specifically?
- What percentage of your practice involves adults with ADHD?
- Do you ever write or present on ADHD in adults? If so, are those resources available?

You also want to find out about logistical matters like fees, potential insurance reimbursement, scheduling, and communication between appointments. After that, it's all about chemistry, that feeling that you click with this person and that she can be helpful to you.

Talk It Out: Therapy Can Offer Clarity and Peace

Therapy doesn't help your ADHD directly so much as it helps you clean up some of the fallout from your ADHD. It also helps with lots of stuff not directly connected to your ADHD—the kind of stuff that everyone wrestles with, to some degree. As someone who does therapy all day and has spent a fair amount of time in the other chair, too, I'm a big fan of it. However, I can say definitively that the harder you work at it, the more you will get from it. Related to this, I can also say that clients who go to therapy mostly to appease someone else tend to not get very much from it—unless they decide that they want to. I'm not saying that you have to know exactly what you want to work on; I'm saying that it really helps if you are open to the process and willing to see what develops. I myself have benefited in ways that I didn't predict or didn't initially intend to work on. This is especially true if you find a therapist who is good at what he does, clicks well with you, and has the knowledge base that you need him to have.

Generally speaking, if you are an adult with ADHD, a therapist can help you in the following ways:

- *Understand how living with undiagnosed ADHD affected who you became and how you approach situations.* You don't need to delve into dirty secrets, but living with ADHD definitely affected the path that your life took. It can be helpful to understand that and perhaps replace some of the other explanations you are using (mostly negative ones, like not being smart enough).
- *Separate what is you and what is your ADHD.* Many people find this to be an important question (and so do their romantic partners!). This can sometimes be a blurry line, but it's important, especially right after someone is diagnosed. ADHD is a part of who you are, but not all of who you are.
- *Understand how ADHD currently affects your life.* If you can identify how ADHD is affecting your life, you are in a better position to make desired changes. It may also help you beat yourself up less.
- *Work on other conditions that currently affect your life.* If you are an adult who was diagnosed not too long ago, there's a good chance that you also have at least some anxiety or depression. Not only does this make life less fun, but it also reduces your ability and willingness to try new strategies that can make your life better.
- *Understand how you think, why you tend to feel certain ways, how you approach challenges, and how you relate to others.* For all of us, the better we know ourselves, the more likely we are to feel fulfilled, successfully pursue our goals, and have more satisfying relationships.

Being diagnosed with ADHD, especially as an adult, can be a life-changing event (see *The Four Stages of Adjustment to a New Diagnosis* on p. 195). It explains a lot, which is a relief, but it also forces you to rethink a lot of things about yourself and your life up to this point. Things you thought you knew maybe now you're not sure of. It can be a big help to have a therapist you see regularly, even for just a few sessions, who can help you make sense of and integrate all this new information.

A knowledgeable therapist will be able to disentangle and explain what is neurological ADHD stuff, personality preference, and general life circumstances so that you gain a more sophisticated understanding of it all.

A potential side benefit of this is that they can send you back to your prescriber to tweak your medication regimen (if you're taking any) when your struggles seem more neurological than psychological. Even though therapists don't prescribe medication, they should still know about the commonly used medications, side effects, and dosage ranges. Since clients often see a therapist more frequently than they do their prescriber, therapists are often in a position to answer general questions and recommend a call to the prescriber if necessary.

Why Was Past Therapy Not Helpful Enough? (And Why You Can Expect Better This Time)

Many adults have seen therapists before being diagnosed with ADHD. They probably went for the usual reasons that most people go—stress, unhappiness, relationship issues, maybe drinking a little too much. If you've seen a therapist before, perhaps it was helpful, even if it didn't completely address why you were having the troubles that you were. It can feel as if there is a missing piece that isn't being identified or addressed. It's not that what the therapist was saying is wrong; it's just that it isn't right *enough*. This can actually have a subtle but powerful effect on how you feel about yourself—*Here is yet another person who doesn't quite get me, and it's his job to understand people! I must be really different from everyone else if even a professional therapist can't explain why I do some of the things I do!*

The feeling of being truly understood is crucial for newly diagnosed adults with ADHD after their lifetime of inexplicable difficulties and standard solutions that didn't really work. This crucial experience may not happen even with a great therapist if she doesn't understand and address the ADHD piece of the puzzle. The moment of receiving the diagnosis often involves a sense of relief, of finally being understood and understanding oneself. It's as if all the random pieces suddenly fit together. Now you have an explanation for why you've always felt different. In my diagnostic evaluations, I make a point of leaving time to educate clients about ADHD in general and to tie together the events in their lives with the diagnosis—for example, "No wonder you did so badly and got depressed when you were promoted up to team leader. There were way too many details for you to manage effectively because of your ADHD."

It's really important that a therapist acknowledge clients' deep feelings of distress caused by the undiagnosed ADHD and to frame those feelings as a normal response to a lifetime of unexplained struggle. This allows clients to let themselves off the hook of guilt, shame, and self-blame. Without this, it's hard to feel good about yourself if you're still making all the same mistakes that made you feel bad about yourself in the first place.

It's not that people with ADHD don't want to do better or be "more like everyone else," they just can't figure out how. They're not being self-defeating, defensive, or oppositional when they get stuck, any more than someone with bad eyes is choosing to not see things more clearly. Interpreting neurologically driven symptoms as being primarily psychological implies that the person could change it, if only he addressed those psychological issues. This can feel like adding salt to a lifelong wound, even if it's said in a well-intentioned and friendly way.

Treating only anxiety and depression while ignoring the underlying ADHD is like painting over the water stains on the ceiling without fixing the leaks in the roof—a short-term solution at best. By contrast, identifying the real source of the difficulties allows the therapist and client to more effectively address the problems.

Part of this involves identifying and celebrating your successes in life despite having undiagnosed ADHD. This contributes to a sense of competence and hope that you can be successful when you apply yourself in better-informed ways. I once had a client who never finished college, despite several attempts, but managed to run a successful lawn service business that was a pretty good situation for him in many ways. He still felt bad about not yet having a college degree, but I pointed out to him that, given his undiagnosed and untreated ADHD, it was hardly surprising. I also stressed, however, that he should give himself credit for being smart enough to create a work situation that was a good fit for him and enabled him to be successful without a degree. Celebrating successes may also involve smaller achievements, like forming the habit of always putting your keys and wallet in the same place at home, or other good strategies that you have already come up with on your own.

These achievements may seem too trivial if the ADHD is left out of the equation and can feel like pandering (e.g., "What a big boy you are, remembering to put your keys in the same place!"). I get really turned off by those overly simplistic "Everyone is special" kind of affirmations. Of course I want everyone to feel good about themselves, but I prefer that they have reasons with more substance. Partly this is because it's too easy for less-generous people to take away the fluffy feel-good statements—and let's face it: everyone has heard plenty of those kinds of comments, too. By contrast, no one can take away the reasons that are based on legitimate successes. So, for someone with ADHD who tends to have certain weaknesses, finding strategies to work around them is something to feel good about. It shows self-knowledge and a commitment to improving his life. A therapist who doesn't fully appreciate ADHD will probably miss these opportunities to help his ADHD clients recognize those strengths.

Get the Most Out of Therapy

We are who we are, wherever we are. As a result, you bring your ADHD and other issues with you wherever you go. This includes a therapist's office. This can actually be a good thing, since it allows you to work on some of these matters in the moment rather than merely discuss things that happened over the course of the week. So it's important to be yourself in therapy—the goal is for the therapist to really get to know you. Not just the polite you that knows all the social rules, but also the private you that you try to not show too often.

In the interest of getting the most out of therapy, let's run through some suggestions that would tend to apply to people with ADHD. (Other people get other suggestions.) Some of these are symptoms of ADHD, whereas others are outgrowths of living with ADHD. In either case, by keeping these potential snags and their solutions in mind, you're more likely to get the most bang for your buck.

Dig in and do the hard work.

Going to therapy isn't like getting a hangnail removed, where you show the doctor where it hurts and she does all the work. You need to be actively involved in the process, both in session and in between. The harder you work at it, the more you will get from it. It won't always be easy, but it will be good for you.

Get to appointments on time.

Most therapists make a point of starting and ending their sessions on time, to prevent their schedules from snowballing over the course of the day. So, showing up late will cut into your available time. However, it is also an opportunity to explore in detail where your time management got off track. This may shed some light on what happens in other parts of your life and offers strategies that can be applied elsewhere too. It also provides an opportunity to work on not beating yourself up so much, if you tend to do that, and instead see it as a learning opportunity.

Remember that you have an appointment.

It's hard to get much from therapy if you don't show up. Missed appointments offer an opportunity to figure out what happened that can benefit you in other parts of your life. If possible, many therapists will try to reschedule a missed appointment for later in the week. However, if it has been a consistent pattern or if they're not able to find a replacement time, then many will charge for missed appointments. They do this for two reasons. First, the rest of the world expects adults to be reliable, so why should the therapist be any different? Ultimately, that wouldn't be a favor. Second, to highlight that what they are doing in therapy is important, the appointment times should be respected.

Remember that change takes time (and is sometimes boring).

It's easy to get excited about something new *(This therapy stuff is awesome!)* and just as easy to grow bored with it later *(We just talk about the same stuff every session).* Unfortunately, change takes time and even a little patience. Try to keep this in mind when you're looking for that quick answer. You've already answered all the easy questions in your life, so now you're left with the ones that will take time. Patience, Grasshopper, patience.

Sometimes you need to talk before doing anything.

Some ADHD people would rather do things than talk about it, yet therapy is mostly talking. They may want the therapist to just tell them what to do, as if it was a football huddle—*Feel better about yourself and listen to your wife more. Break!* It comes down to that old adage of giving a man a fish and you feed him for a day; teach a man to fish and you feed him for life. Most therapists prefer to help you figure out *how* to figure things out, so that you're prepared for whatever life brings next. You may want to ask your therapist for specific things to practice between sessions to reinforce what you're talking about in session.

Focus on what you can do to improve your situation.

Some people see therapy as an opportunity to complain and blame everyone else in their lives. As fun as this can be, it really isn't productive. Even if you do have really difficult people in your life, there are always some things that you can do differently to make the situation at least a little better. You may not see how you are contributing to your situation, but a good therapist can help you see it more fully, which clarifies your options for changing it.

Think your decisions through.

Life presents many interesting opportunities, most of which we shouldn't pursue—for example, the cool new gadget that's on sale in an eye-catching display. As fun as it can be in the moment to run with our impulses, they have an unfortunate tendency of getting us into trouble. Your therapist may work with you on resisting those impulses or even avoiding those too-tempting situations in the first place. Therapy involves learning why you do what you do—and then perhaps pushing yourself to apply that knowledge to do things differently. Granted, it's harder and less fun than giving in to temptation, but if it were easy, you wouldn't have to work on it! It's a lot easier to leap without looking if you don't have a plan for where you are going, which is covered next.

Create some plans.

Planning can be complicated and boring, so many people with ADHD tend to avoid it. Instead, they kind of meander through life, reacting to whatever comes up next, taking whatever options are available to them in the moment. This can lead them into some strange places, like a job that is a really bad fit for them. Your therapist may push you to think about these things and then even (gasp!) follow that plan. You may still not like doing it, but hopefully you will see the value in it.

Remember that your therapist is there to help.

After receiving more than your fair share of criticism and nagging, it's easy to assume that people are doing that to you, even when sometimes they aren't. You may have gotten good at ignoring nagging, which, of course, makes the person nag you more. Or maybe you've become extra sensitive to hearing anger or disappointment in someone's tone. If you feel that your therapist is being critical or nagging, ask about it, because that perception can really undermine your relationship. It may be that you are being overly sensitive or have a guilty conscience about something, but are putting that onto your therapist as making you feel that way. (This is called *projection*.) It can be really interesting and informative to explore those feelings. Of course, it could be that your therapist is in fact expressing those feelings more than she should and can hopefully admit to it (we're all human, after all).

The key to being an effective therapist is to care about your clients without caring too much—that is, I want my clients to do well, but I can't care more than they do about it, since that puts me in a position of pushing them more than they want to be pushed. Of course, I may point out some things that I see that perhaps they don't, but when it comes to actually doing things, I need to let them make their own choices. I may tell them that I disagree and why, but it isn't my job to tell them what to do. This means holding back my anxiety if the client wants to do something that I feel will lead to trouble. That's how I keep my own sanity after a long day, which is a good lesson for all of us in all of our relationships.

Try to remember your main points.

It's easy for ADHD adults to tell long, rambling stories that quickly move away from the main point. This can definitely be entertaining, but it tends to use up a lot of session time on less productive matters. You can minimize some of this by bringing in some brief notes about what you want to talk about and maybe even share that with your therapist at the start of the session so he can redirect you, if necessary. When we're hanging out with friends, it's OK to let the conversation take us where it may, but in therapy the clock is ticking down, so you want to be sure to get in the intended topics.

Try to remember what happened between sessions.

Good therapy tends to rely on details—what happened, how you felt, what you did next. If you have a hard time recalling enough of this, you may want to write some notes after something happens, then be sure to bring those notes to session with you. Rather than being a sign of a bad memory, most therapists will see it as a sign of your commitment.

Work on things between sessions.

Just as with school homework, ADHD adults will often forget to do therapy homework assignments, do them halfway or at the last minute, or forget to bring things back to the next session. Sometimes the problem is that the client didn't really understand what the assignment was but felt awkward asking—it's always better to ask! If you're worried that you might forget what you're supposed to do, then be sure to write it down on paper or in your PDA.

Focus more on building skills than on getting help.

Perhaps after a lifetime of not being trusted to do things because they may not do it right, some people with ADHD may get used to others doing things for them. Or maybe they've gotten into the habit of others being responsible for the reminders and the pushing to finish projects. As a result, they may now be good at getting others to do things for them, either by charming them into it or by playing the incompetent who needs to be rescued. As tempting as this is, it really limits your options in life, since not everyone will be so accommodating. If your therapist is really doing you a favor, she will call you on this and encourage you to do these things yourself rather than be dependent on her or others to do them for you. This can be a hard lesson to learn, but it is important and a big favor.

Conclusion

My hope is that you find a therapist who challenges you but who is also comfortable being challenged. I want you to be able to work together and to push each other to make the therapy as effective as possible. A good relationship of any kind can tolerate and grow stronger from respectful honesty. Don't assume that your therapist is psychic and knows exactly what you need. Tell him when you feel that you're not focusing on the areas that you want to focus on or if it's not as helpful as you want. As a therapist myself, I would much rather hear that from a client and have an opportunity to fix it rather than have her bail out without my knowing why. If I don't know about something, I can't do anything about it. Besides, if I'm asking my clients to be open and direct and willing to take constructive advice, I need to be, too!

Goal Setting in Therapy

Some clients and therapists find it helpful to structure the sessions by creating specific goals to work on and using a specific process. This isn't for everyone, and some people find it too constrictive, so find the amount that works for you. Then either find a therapist who offers that amount of structure or ask your current therapist if he can adapt his style. Some therapists run their sessions very tightly, whereas others are wide open. Generally speaking, therapists with a psychodynamic tilt tend to be more open, whereas those with a cognitive-behavioral tilt tend to be more structured, but ask to be sure.

Goal setting can be helpful to reduce the amount of session time spent wandering or dealing exclusively with the day's crises or entertaining events. These can pull you away from more important but less dramatic topics that require ongoing effort. You may want to create both short-term and long-term goals; ideally the short-term goals will lead into or support the long-term goals. Many ADHD folks have difficulty or feel overwhelmed breaking long-term projects into the necessary parts, so this can be a good skill to work on with your therapist.

Create and pursue your goals in this order:

1. **Select a few goals to work on first.** Start with a manageable number of goals. It can be tempting to work on everything at once, but that just becomes confusing and leads to too much jumping around. You may want to start with a few things that you can make some quick progress on, even if they aren't the most important projects in your life. This quick success will hopefully give you some momentum and keep you motivated to work on harder items.

2. **Develop workable plans to reach those goals.** Thinking up your goals can be more fun than figuring out how to pursue them. This is where you get into the details that make or break these plans. If your therapist is doing his job, he will present you with situations that could derail your plan so that you can create solutions ahead of time. We tend to come up with better solutions when not in the heat of the moment.

3. **Decide how to measure success or failure**. It's helpful to know whether a plan is working well so that you can decide whether to keep using it or come up with something different. Some goals have concrete measures, such as the frequency of working out, whereas others are more ephemeral, such as "a better relationship with my girlfriend."

4. **Create a plan B.** Even the best-laid plans encounter unexpected obstacles. Sometimes it just takes some tweaking to make the old plan work. Sometimes you need to scrap it completely and start over. That's OK—sometimes we need to learn by doing. So if your

plan bombs, take it as a learning opportunity to figure out why it bombed and what you can do differently. I've had very few successes in life that didn't involve some sort of initial failure on which those later successes were built.

5. **Change the goals when necessary.** Some goals seem reasonable but turn out to be too ambitious, overlook obstacles, or don't take into account new developments. Actively choosing to drop a goal is a sign of strength and wisdom, fundamentally different from flaking out or wimping out because it got too hard. As the saying goes, sometimes wisdom is the greater part of valor; so it's wiser to drop a project than to pursue it past the point of good judgment. Stubbornly holding onto an unworkable goal is just as problematic as abandoning it prematurely or failing at it due to insufficient planning. After all, it wasn't his bravery that made Colonel Custer famous; it was his stubbornness. By contrast, flexibility is a sign of healthy problem solving.

6. **As goals are reached, add new ones.** As successes begin to fall into place, you will find that your new habits take less conscious effort, freeing up some mental energy to pursue a new goal. Just don't let the thrill of novelty lead you to take on more than you can handle.

ADHD Coaching: More Than Obvious Advice

At the risk of oversimplifying, I would define ADHD coaching as helping clients with ADHD to make their intentions happen. Or maybe closing the gap between intention and action. This is easier said than done. If you're an adult with ADHD, you've gotten tons of generic advice, like "Buy a schedule book to remember appointments." As if it were really that easy. Of course, none of these advice givers also say, "Then buy another one when you lose it a week later" or "Handcuff it to your wrist so it's always there with you." That would actually take the ADHD into account. The first part of the advice, to buy an appointment book, is easy. The hard part is figuring out a way to be consistent about using it. That's where coaching comes in—offering strategies that go beyond the obvious and unhelpful.

To be truly helpful, the coach has to know ADHD inside and out. Not just the obvious symptoms, but also the more subtle information-processing tendencies that people with ADHD employ, as well as some of the personality traits that often grow out of a lifetime of untreated ADHD. This is one of those situations where more is better—the more a coach really understands ADHD, the better she will do with creating strategies that will really work for the client, not just in the short term, but also after the shine has worn off. A fact of human nature is that we are all much more likely to stick with habits that are easy or a good fit, so strategies that don't really work for us are quickly lost.

The coach also needs to learn about the client's situation—strengths, weaknesses, preferences, demands at work, and people in the client's life. There are no one-size-fits-all strategies. Success requires customization.

Success also requires collaboration. You need to work with your coach to create strategies and to really give those strategies a fair test. Even the most brilliant strategy will take some effort on your part to stick with it. The difference is that, unlike the strategies that don't take your ADHD into account, it shouldn't be a Herculean effort to stick with them. After you try the strategies, then you need to report back with the results of what worked, how well, and perhaps why something did or didn't work. The more details you provide, the more your coach has to work with to help you fine-tune it all.

In addition to this collaborative brainstorming process, a coach may also teach clients specific skills, like how to use a schedule book most effectively or better ways to do filing. Perhaps because their untreated ADHD got in the way, many clients will never have really learned some of these skills or need a refresher to solidify their knowledge.

Let me give an example of how a coach might work with a client. Notice the level of detail that the coach gets into and how much it is tailored to how the ADHD brain processes information.

Client: I keep losing my keys. I was late to work today because it took me twenty minutes to find them.

Coach: Where were they?

Client: I don't know if I should laugh or cry about this, but they were in the fridge! I stopped at the grocery store on the way home last night. So I went straight to the fridge to put things away and must have laid my keys down on the shelf. It makes sense now, but I was pretty frantic this morning.

Coach: Do you have a designated place for your keys?

Client: Sort of. Well, a few places. But my keys are usually somewhere else entirely.

Coach: It may be better to have one specific place. What would be a good place for them?

Client: Maybe the kitchen counter, in a basket.

Coach: Do you mostly come in the same door?

Client: Pretty much.

Coach: Is that near the kitchen?

Client: Not really. It's at the other end of the house.

Coach: Hmm, that sounds like a setup for trouble—too many places to get distracted before you make it to the kitchen. The closer the designated place is to the door, the less you need to think about it and the more likely the keys will wind up where they should.

Client: Good point. I know I'll have trouble remembering sometimes when there's too much going on.

Coach: Let's find a place that is as close to that door as possible, in as noticeable a place as possible, so you don't need to think too hard about it. The more automatic it is, the better.

A coach who doesn't fully appreciate the difficulty that someone with ADHD will have with resisting distractions between the front door and the kitchen may have been satisfied with putting the keys on the counter. Unfortunately, it wouldn't have worked as well as finding something closer. This is what separates the great coaches from those who merely mean well.

Coaching is much more than just giving clients obvious advice like "Get to appointments on time," and "Don't forget to mail in your mortgage payment." ADHD folks already know this stuff, but they have trouble carrying them out consistently. Coaching can improve their odds of success.

What's the Difference Between Coaching and Therapy?

To be completely honest, it can be hard to tell the difference sometimes between coaching and therapy. I've seen various descriptions that are supposed to distinguish them, but I still notice a lot of overlap between the two. This is partly because both coaching and therapy are very broad fields, so that makes it easy for them to overlap in the middle. It's easy to point at the coaches who are at one extreme and the therapists who are at the other extreme and describe how they are different from each other, but it's those people in the middle who use a lot of the same techniques that are harder to differentiate. This may be especially true for therapists who are well versed in working with ADHD adults, since they probably incorporate more coaching techniques than your average therapist.

Let's talk first about the similarities between coaching and therapy (just to muddy the waters further). Both ADHD coaching and therapy:

- Require a strong understanding of ADHD
- Require a good working relationship based on trust and openness
- Assist the client to find greater success and happiness

I've listed here some differences that are often cited, even if I feel that there are often exceptions to these loose rules. So they aren't written in stone but may help you get a clearer sense of the differences.

Therapy	**Coaching**
Treats diagnosable disorders	Is strength based rather than pathology based; although clients should not have other mental health conditions, they do have ADHD
Often considers how the past affects the present	Stays focused on the present and the future
Generally does not get into practical problem solving	Focuses on how the client's ADHD affects his ability to get things done and how to overcome those challenges
Seeks understanding (why someone has certain feelings or does certain things)	Seeks tangible accomplishments (how to achieve them)
Explores complex emotional and relationship experiences	Focuses on pragmatic strategies and necessary steps to meet goals; may create customized systems to help the client function better

There are many therapists who would mostly fit the bill for coaching described in the table, at least with some clients. And there are also coaches who slip into therapy territory, either intentionally or unintentionally (see *Coach and Therapist* on p. 160). So these descriptions of what each profession does in theory tend to blur together in reality. I suppose at its simplest we could say that coaches do coaching and therapists do therapy, but that feels like copping out.

Perhaps we could say that coaches help clients to clarify and pursue their goals, with an emphasis on moving forward. They don't get too much into why a client's belief systems about issues have held him back, which may be more of a matter for therapy if a client isn't able to overcome those obstacles with coaching. A coach will focus on what needs to be done and how the client can do that. This may involve creating some systems that take the client's ADHD more into account or exploring some of the beliefs that the person has about himself, to the extent that it affects the pursuit of these goals. A good coach, though, won't delve too deeply into the client's beliefs for fear of drifting into therapy territory. A good coach will identify the unique ways her client processes and learns in specific situations, to help him pursue goals more effectively. She may also explore exactly what is happening in the situations where the client is successful, so he can repeat and generalize from those successes. In this way, ADHD coaching focuses more on clients' strengths than their weaknesses.

One big difference, perhaps, is in how the logistics of sessions are handled. Most therapists see clients in person for 50 minutes every week or two. Coaches tend to meet by phone and may do some email check-ins between calls. Some coaches will also do brief check-ins by phone. As a result, a therapist will be local, whereas a coach doesn't have to be. Coaching sessions may also be more structured in how the time is used, although some therapists are also very structured.

Because coaching in general is pretty new (about twenty-five years old) and ADHD coaching in particular is even newer (about fifteen years old), coaches are still defining what they do and how they do it. Even therapy, which has been around for a century, is continuing to evolve. As a result, members of both fields borrow techniques from the other (if it works, why not?), so some convergence can take place. The various coach training programs are working to create more consistency within the field, so we should see more clarity develop over time.

The Boundaries Are Different

There is one distinct difference between therapy and coaching, and that is how the boundaries are handled. Licensed therapists have very strict limitations on how they can interact with clients, whereas coaches have no such legally enforceable restrictions. For example, I am not allowed to go out to lunch with current or former clients or engage in business dealings beyond our therapy relationship. The licensing boards worry that these extracurricular activities could lead a therapist to intentionally or unintentionally take advantage of a client. For example, a client may worry that if he didn't pick up the tab for dinner, his therapist would be angry with him and feel compelled to make the offer. This then is a setup for bad blood. By contrast, coaches have no such restrictions and may have contact with clients outside of the coaching sessions. They have their own good judgment to rely on, as well as ethical standards put out by professional organizations, but neither is legally enforceable.

You can make arguments both ways about which is better. The restrictions on therapists can feel unnecessarily rigid at times, but it does offer some real clarity about the nature of the relationship, so there is no confusion on anyone's part. Because coaches have more freedom on these matters, they can take advantage of mutually beneficial opportunities. This carries a risk, but it also offers rewards.

If you are considering expanding your relationship with your coach to beyond the predefined limits, or if your coach suggests it, you need to think seriously about it beforehand. Probably the most crucial factor that determines whether this is a good or bad experience is how strong each person's boundaries are. That is, can you each see the situation clearly, come to mutually agreed-upon expectations, and resolve differences of opinion peacefully? Most important, can each person walk away from the interaction without bad feelings? If you can truly answer yes to these questions, then it may be worth discussing possibilities with your coach. As when friends start dating, the danger is that your initial relationship may be lost or damaged by these additional activities.

Coach and Therapist: One Person or Two?

Do you need a coach *and* a therapist, or can one person do both jobs? It depends. Or maybe you don't need therapy at all and just need a coach. Some therapists are happy to work on practical problem solving and strategies, whereas others prefer to focus on more traditional therapy matters. A therapist may say that he employs a more action-oriented style but not call it coaching, even if that is what he is kind of doing. So don't get too hung up on the labels (speaking of labels, these therapists may tend to practice *cognitive-behavioral therapy* or CBT).

We can't say across the board that it's better to have one person or two. It all depends on your circumstances. So let's talk about the relative merits of each.

Here are some reasons why it can be better to have your therapist also do the coaching:

- There's something to be said for the efficiency of one-stop shopping. It's one fewer professional to schedule and pay.
- A therapist can help you look more deeply into why certain strategies aren't working as expected, which can make the coaching more effective. For some people, there are complex psychological reasons beyond their ADHD that prevent them from moving forward or breaking old patterns.
- It can be hard enough to find one professional who really understands ADHD and who you feel comfortable with, let alone two.
- There is less risk of repetition or of hearing contradictory advice. There is also then no need for coordination between therapist and coach.
- Because therapists are licensed healthcare professionals, their services are potentially reimbursable by insurance, whereas coaching is not. This may influence the ultimate cost of the services.

This of course all assumes that your therapist feels comfortable dealing with practical matters and is knowledgeable about how your ADHD affects your effectiveness. Some will be quite competent, whereas others won't be but think they are, so you need to use your own judgment. For this reason, as well as the following, it may be better to have a coach who isn't your therapist:

- Some people need both therapy and coaching. It can be more effective and less confusing to separate them rather than mix them together.

- Since most coaches interact with clients by phone and email, they don't need to be local. This gives you a much bigger pool of knowledgeable professionals to choose from, especially if you live in more rural areas. By contrast, many therapists are leery of doing phone sessions. This is even more so with clients from other states, because of concerns about being charged with practicing in a state where they aren't licensed.
- Coaches tend to have more flexibility in how they work with clients—such as types of contact and frequency of communication. Most therapists do 50-minute sessions, which can impose limits on how they can schedule. Because of these logistical matters, a coach may better fit your needs.

Maybe You Just Need a Coach

Whereas some adults with ADHD would benefit from both therapy and coaching, some primarily need coaching. If you're thinking about this, you need to be honest with yourself about your situation. A good candidate for ADHD coaching would find the following to be true:

- Generally is doing well in life (except for the ADHD-related struggles), but would like to do better. He may or may not know what is getting in his way.
- Generally knows himself well but wants to better understand how his ADHD affects his functioning.
- Can be honest about himself. Takes constructive feedback well, doesn't get defensive, and can apply it effectively.
- Has a pretty good sense of what he wants to work on and what his goals are, but he can't figure out how to make the desired progress.
- Has manageable anxiety, depression, and substance use and is free of other mental health conditions that could interfere with progress.
- Has stable relationships.

If all of these criteria don't apply to you, then you will probably find that the coaching is not as effective as it could be until you have done some good therapy. It also potentially puts the coach in a situation of practicing beyond her areas of training and competence. Although professionals have a responsibility to refer clients who they can't work with effectively, consumers also have a responsibility to seek the right professional.

Coaching Certification: Is This Coach Any Good?

ADHD coaching is still a new field, but it's growing up quickly. As with any new field, lots of people have jumped in, printed up business cards, and called themselves coaches. While this is good news, in the sense that it makes it easier to find a coach if you want one, it has also been bad news because standards about who can call themselves an ADHD coach have not been established. This leads to concerns about quality control, where a would-be coach may have more enthusiasm than training.

Fortunately, the tide is turning. There are more and more training programs offering comprehensive education on coaching generally and also ADHD coaching in particular. The programs vary greatly in how rigorous their requirements are, though, and there is not yet an accepted standard they all must meet. It should also be noted that someone who is well trained as a life coach may not be all that effective working with an ADHD client, just as an underinformed therapist or psychiatrist wouldn't be.

The Institute for the Advancement of AD/HD Coaching (IAAC) was started in 2005 with the goal of creating a set standard for the certification of ADHD coaches. They created two levels of certification, the main difference being amount of experience required. The Certified AD/HD Coach (CAC) must have two years of ADHD coaching experience, as well as other educational requirements. The Senior Certified AD/HD Coach (SCAC) must have five years. (More information can be found at www.adhdcoachinstitute.org.) This is a real step forward for the field because it creates a uniform standard.

However, although the credentials CAC and SCAC are legally protected and can be used only by coaches who have been approved to use them, the term *ADHD coach* can still be used by anyone. This is different from titles that are legally protected, like *psychologist* or *certified public accountant*, which can be used only by professionals who have met certain criteria and been approved to use them by the state they are licensed in.

Just to keep it interesting, a second group has formed to create requirements for ADHD coach certification—the Professional Association of ADHD Coaches (www.paaccoaches.org). They will perhaps release their standards at the end of 2009. They felt that ADHD coaching had not been sufficiently distinguished from general coaching. In addition, PAAC intends to develop a rigorous assessment process that will clearly ascertain an ADHD coach's competence before she can be certified.

Also, there is now a nonprofit association that represents ADHD coaches and seeks to advance the profession, the ADHD Coaches Organization. Its goals are to establish professional and ethical standards, promote awareness of ADHD coaching, provide resources to its members, and serve as an informational link to the general public and other professionals working with people affected by ADHD. You can find more information at www.adhdcoaches.org. Their website also includes a searchable database of member coaches.

There are other private accreditation organizations, but not all of them are worth much—as in every field, some of these vanity credentials seem to have as a primary qualification the ability to make the payment correctly. So you may want to find out what is required to earn some of those letters after someone's name.

If you are thinking about getting a coach, ask some of these questions:

- What manner of coach training have you had? Did you complete a training program? If so, what was the curriculum? Did it include supervision of your coaching work? Did you need to pass a test to graduate?
- What manner of training about ADHD and ADHD coaching specifically have you had?
- What did you do before coaching, to the extent that it informs your coaching work?
- How many ADHD clients have you coached? How many years have you been coaching?
- What professional organizations do you belong to?
- What other professional activities, mentoring, or peer supervision groups are you involved with?
- What sorts of continuing education activities do you engage in?
- How do you tend to work with ADHD clients? What is your philosophy of coaching individuals with ADHD?
- What do you do in the event that more serious psychological issues come up?
- What is your opinion about medications?
- Have you ever been coached yourself?

There are no right or wrong answers. It comes down to your level of confidence that this potential coach has the skills and knowledge to help you accomplish your goals and to make it worth the investment of time and money. Many coaches offer a free initial session to give prospective clients a test drive. This gives you an opportunity to present the coach with a problem area that you would like to work on and ask him how he would handle it. Obviously, his answer will have to be general since he doesn't know you that well yet, but you should be able to get a feel for how he works with clients. You should also get a feel during this initial conversation about the chemistry between the two of you. Since every coach has his own style, it's often a good idea to interview a few before committing to one. This small investment of time will be well worth it.

Coaching Is Serious Business

I'm now going to get on my soap box: I take my work very seriously. People come to me in distress, looking to make their lives better. That carries a tremendous responsibility, so I've worked hard in school and since then to be as prepared as possible. By the same token, coaching shouldn't be a hobby. Given the current lack of licensure requirements, it's really easy to become a coach—maybe too easy. I don't doubt that all these new coaches mean well, but good intentions are not a substitute for thorough training and solid skills.

If you're looking for a coach, you deserve one who knows what he's doing. If you are a coach, your clients deserve your best—even if that means more training. With insufficient training, a coach puts his clients at risk if they both get in over their heads—for example, with a client who has a history of abuse, bipolar disorder, a personality disorder, substance abuse, or other mental health conditions. He may take on more than he can handle and encourage his client to do things that aren't in her best interests or are downright dangerous. At best, a poorly trained coach wastes the client's time with unhelpful but benign advice—but even this carries a cost, too. It means more time goes by where the client continues to suffer before hopefully seeking a more effective professional. Some of these clients may wait a long time before trying again, if ever. This means months or years of additional and unnecessary suffering. It can also validate the client's deep-seated feelings of being defective and incurable.

So, to all the would-be coaches out there—go for it, but get your training first. It's not just that you owe it to your clients to ensure their safety and give them their money's worth. You also owe it to yourself. Coaching, like most professions, is much more satisfying when you really know what you're doing. Perhaps the greatest danger of insufficient training is that you may not even know what you don't know. So be honest with yourself about the extent of your training. To be blunt about it, does anybody else think you're qualified? That is, did you have to pass any exams to earn your coaching credential? If so, did the exam set the bar high enough that you would feel comfortable being coached by someone who passed it? I spent five years, full time, in graduate school to get my degree, was supervised for another year, and had to pass a lengthy exam in order to call myself a psychologist, so I'm not holding others to a higher standard than I hold myself.

Changes on the Outside Create Changes on the Inside

I have a saying: You can't leave the past in the past if it's still happening in the present. This is where coaching comes in—it helps adults with ADHD to make the present look better than the past. Success in the present can go a long way toward undoing much of the damage to their self-esteem because it helps them feel more effective in their lives. One vindication for past failures is to learn to overcome them in the present. You may not be able to change your past, but perhaps you can create a better future.

Ultimately, this sense of effectiveness is more beneficial than simply lowering expectations for adults with ADHD, because that can feel like it confirms that they are damaged and shouldn't be held to the same standards of personal responsibility as other adults. In contrast, coaching provides tangible successes and improvements, so they have some legitimate reasons to feel good about themselves. Granted, they may have to climb uphill to learn these habits that don't come naturally, but they can still improve if they work at it. I sometimes tell clients exactly that. I say, "This is stuff that won't come as easily for you as it does for some other people, but that doesn't mean that you can't do at least somewhat better."

Of course, this entire process is easier if you have the right medication. Not everyone needs medication, certainly, but for those who do, it can be quite helpful. Pills don't teach skills, but skills do come easier with the right pills.

Beyond the effect that it has on the rest of their lives, typical ADHD difficulties such as disorganization, chronic lateness, and forgetting important events can also interfere with ADHD adults' ability to get the most from therapy if they miss appointments or show up late. The irony is that the very symptoms that they are looking for help with are also the symptoms that will interfere with their getting the help they want. For that reason, a therapist who is well informed about ADHD will do at least enough coaching to get clients into his office for the full session. Otherwise, missed therapy appointments can feel like yet another failure experience and spark a lifetime of old shame, causing clients to drop out early.

Most ADHD adults have the most trouble on the sorts of maintenance activities that offer no reward for doing them, but there is a punishment for not doing them or for doing them late, like laundry, grocery shopping, paying taxes, or showing up on time. Friends don't give out plaques for showing up on time, but they do get angry if someone frequently runs late. Therefore, many ADHD adults need to find rewards elsewhere to keep them motivated to stay on top of these important but sometimes uninspiring tasks. A coach can provide that enthusiasm and motivate the client to keep pursuing these goals. Eventually, these successes begin to replace the all-too-frequent failures of the past, perhaps changing the way an adult with ADHD sees herself.

It's interesting that most of my clients with ADHD seek my services not to *feel* better, but to *do* better. They want both, but they're smart enough to know that they won't feel better unless they actually start doing better. This is fundamentally different from the anxious or depressed people who call me—for them, it's more about feeling than doing. So a therapist who focuses too much on the feeling and not enough on the doing may do a good job for the anxious and depressed clients, but will be missing the boat for the clients with ADHD. This is where the coaching part comes in—helping clients do better so that they can legitimately feel better.

How Coaching Helps: A General Coaching Theory

At its simplest, folks with ADHD run into problems when they don't do the right thing at the right time. This can happen because they do the right thing at the wrong time, don't do the right thing at all, or do the wrong thing. Coaching aims to help in two ways:

- *Prevent problems.* Help clients do the right things more often at more right times, as well as do fewer wrong things. A coach who really understands ADHD will know how to craft strategies that improve clients' batting averages. There are no guarantees in life, but a good coach will help clients to improve their probabilities.
- *Clean up problems after they occur.* Situations can either go from bad to worse or bad to better, depending on what the person does next. For example, after realizing that he forgot about a project at work, how does he reprioritize his time? Salvaging situations is an important skill for everyone to learn, but especially for those who are more likely to make mistakes in the first place. This may also become something to work on in therapy as issues of self-esteem and self-image get triggered by these situations.

Preventing problems usually entails helping the client set himself up for success beforehand because he can't reliably trust himself to do the right thing in the moment. I had a client who was a college student and decided that he would leave his laptop in his room when he went to the library to study, because it was just too tempting to start messing around online. A more generic example I often use with clients is that you shouldn't bring home a box of doughnuts if you don't want to be tempted to eat them—the more powerful choice point occurs when you're standing in the supermarket aisle contemplating their purchase, not when you're standing in the kitchen. For my client, the more powerful choice point was when he was standing in his room, not when he was sitting in the library staring at his computer bag.

The theory is for the ADHD adult to act at the moment when the goal is on her mind rather than wait for later when the goal is more likely to have been squeezed out by more recent events or ideas. To succeed, the client may need to learn new skills or habits and consciously push herself to use them, like my client did. Some of this may also involve changing things at home or work, such as getting rid of clutter so that important items are less likely to get lost or putting up a whiteboard to write reminders when the thought comes.

You May Involve Others in the Process

Some of these strategies involve changing how the adult with ADHD interacts with other people, in that it can be helpful or necessary to get significant others or coworkers on board with the changes. This can take two forms:

- *Direct assistance.* You may ask others to take on certain tasks that you are just not good at, such as having your romantic partner do the bills. Alternatively, you may ask people to give you reminders or other assistance so you can do it yourself. Balance still needs to be maintained in the relationship, but things work out better for everyone when the other person provides some help.
- *Expectation management.* Since most adults don't have ADHD, most people assume that others will be reliable and consistent in their performance. Related to this, they tend to make assumptions about someone's intentions and character if she falls short. Therefore, she can save herself and others a lot of trouble from the get-go by being up front with them about what they should and should not expect from her. Creating this kind of clarity is an important skill for everyone, especially for people with ADHD or other limitations that may not be immediately obvious. (For more information, see chapter 15, *Relationships and Friendships: Strive for Balance*.)

Goal Setting in Coaching

The first step in coaching, as in most treatments, is to identify the problems to work on. Sometimes, though, a client's stated goals are actually other people's goals. For example, it may be more important to other people in her life that she get more organized or run on time better. In these cases, it may be more accurate to say that her goal is to have less strife with this other person, but she doesn't see any other way to do it. The problem is that it's not as motivating to work on someone else's goal as it is to work on our own. So if you find yourself in this position, be honest with yourself and your coach about whose goal it is. Together, you may be able to find a goal that you can get into more. You may also want to check out chapter 15, *Relationships and Friendships: Strive for Balance*, since there may be some benefit to trying some noncoaching strategies, too.

Once the client's true goals are identified, the client and coach work together to brainstorm possible strategies and how best to implement them. This will depend on what is causing the problem in the first place. There are two reasons why someone with ADHD might have trouble with particular situations or habits. It's important to figure out which one (or probably both) is contributing to the particular difficulty. If someone is weak in a particular area, it could be due to neurological dysfunction or skills deficits.

- *Neurological dysfunction.* Someone may have trouble because his brain doesn't reliably or accurately process certain kinds of information—for example, the ability to remember to do something later that day. If this is the case, the coach and client need to find workarounds to enable the client to get the job done in other ways. In this example, getting into the habit of setting alarms might work better than relying on memory.
- *Skills deficits.* Someone may also have trouble because she never learned necessary skills, such as the ability to create and maintain an effective organizational system. In this case, the coach may teach the client how to do this, keeping in mind that some approaches tend to work better for people with ADHD.

In some cases, it will be obvious which one of these is causing your difficulty—remembering to remember is more of a brain-based ability than a skill that can be taught, whereas knowing how to organize requires both a brain-based ability to remember what goes where, plus the knowledge of what makes for an effective organizational system. Because both of these causes can play a part in your difficulties, you may need to work with your coach to figure out how much each contributes. At the risk of oversimplifying, we might say that whatever weaknesses are improved by medication are probably neurologically based. Of course, it's possible that the medication has less than a total benefit, so some neurological dysfunction may remain even with a generally effective medication regimen. So, if you take medication, once you and your prescriber feel like you've optimized the benefit, you're left with a smaller pool of difficulties to deal with and try to explain.

Fortunately, medication will probably also make it easier to learn those weak or missing skills in a way that wasn't possible without the medication, just as wearing glasses will enable a student to get more out of what's written on the blackboard. So, in our previous example, medication may not give you the knowledge of creating an organizational system, but it should help you use that system more reliably and effectively.

Coaching's Short-Term Goal: Give a Man a Fish...

As the saying goes, "Give a man a fish, feed him for a day. Teach a man to fish, feed him for a lifetime." Although the longer-term goal of coaching is the latter, the client needs to get beyond the current situation for that to matter. Most people tend to seek out a coach when things are not going well for them. This could be a crisis, such as an impending job loss or divorce, or it could just be that they have finally had enough of being worn down. A coach can kick-start the turnaround in a way that would be much harder or slower for the client by herself. By offering more effective strategies, the coach helps the client make the desired changes. The coach can also help to maintain a sense of optimism that this time can be different than the times in the past when things didn't work out well. To help make this success more likely, the coach may help the client to stay focused on the agreed-upon goals rather than impulsively jump to something else before finishing the first.

Even if the client has big things to work on, it may be best to start with some smaller problems that have more immediate benefit. For example, a client may need to exercise more and improve his diet because of coronary risks associated with his unhealthy lifestyle. This is a worthy goal but also a somewhat lofty one, so a better goal to start with may just be to create a shopping list of healthier foods to buy, then to leave copies of that list in the car so they are always on hand at the supermarket. If he can get some momentum going on that, he may be more inclined to work on the bigger and harder changes.

Coaching's Long-Term Goal: Teach a Man to Fish...

Once the client is in a more stable situation, the coach should work on handing over the reins to the client. The longer-term goal of coaching is to teach the client a process of creative problem solving that can be used to deal with future difficulties. Essentially, this is an adaptation of the experimental method that we all learned in science class—identify the problem, brainstorm possibilities, try some strategies, evaluate the results, make small or large corrections as necessary, stay focused on the goal over time, and then use the strategy until it needs to be changed. Over time, the client should know himself and his home and work situations well enough that he can begin to do his own coaching. It may still be helpful to have occasional check-ins with the coach, but he should be able to handle most things himself, at least until significant changes occur in his life (such as promotion to a more demanding job or the birth of a child).

Create Structure and Schedules: More Guideline Than Jail

A coach often helps clients to create the structure necessary for them pursue their goals more consistently and become sidetracked less often. Most ADHD folks have a love/hate relationship with structure and schedules—they know they need them, but they still hate being constrained by routines, plans, time commitments, and reminders. Therefore, a coach may work initially with a client to see that the benefits will outweigh the costs, including the emotional costs of feeling closed in and claustrophobic. Over time, as the client begins to rack up some successes, she may see the benefits more clearly without the coach's encouragement and buy into it all more fully.

Unfortunately, for most people with ADHD, structure has tended to be something that was imposed by others and usually in a way that didn't feel like a good fit, so they have learned to hate it. What's worse, there was probably often a righteous tone to it, that the person with ADHD should automatically know about creating structure and should want it. This then makes many people with ADHD want to avoid structure all the more, even beyond the fact that their brains don't easily take on these habits. If this is you, try to remember that it may be a good idea to increase the structure in your life, even if some people in your life have done a crummy job of explaining why. Don't let their bad delivery and maybe your own stubbornness prevent you from using some tactics that could prove helpful to you.

As with any other strategy, the best kind of structure for you will be the kind that takes into account your general preferences, life situation, strengths, weaknesses, and information-processing style. Blindly adopting someone else's strategies may not do much to improve your situation if it isn't a good fit. We're looking for strategies you can maintain over the long haul, which tend to be strategies that work well for you and how you tend to process information. A good coach will work with you to find the kinds of structure that will work best for you.

Professional Organizers: Move That Mountain

It's probably safe to say that most Americans have too much stuff. We live in a time of plenty where it's easy to acquire things and hard to keep some things away, like junk mail. Everyone needs to expend more energy dealing with all this stuff. However, those who are weak at organizing and getting rid of the overflow will spend a lot of time drowning in their belongings. The field of professional organizing has sprung from this growing societal trend, promising to impose order on the chaos and rescue us from all of our stuff.

Beyond the struggles that everyone faces, many ADHD adults are disorganized not just because they hate organizing and don't spend enough time doing it, but also because they're not good at creating an effective and workable organizational system. As a result, they wind up moving stuff around and put some things away, but overall the space may still not be organized well. Because every item doesn't have a designated place, things tend to get stuffed away somewhere, but not necessarily in a place that makes it easy to find. As a result, lots of extra time is spent later trying to find those items, some of which are never found when they're needed.

An organizer can help in two ways:

- *Help clients dig out from under the accumulated chaos.* Once the disorganization gets bad enough, it's easy to feel overwhelmed and hopeless about ever turning the tide. It can be a real morale boost to work with an organizer who has probably seen worse and is able to offer encouragement. Plus, just having someone work next to you can push you to stick with it longer than you otherwise might have.
- *Create a more effective organizational system.* Many adults with ADHD are disorganized because they don't have a good system for what goes where. An organizer who knows ADHD will be able to work with you on creating a system that makes it easier to find what you need and also to put things back again afterwards. Organizing may never be fun for you, but it can be less awful. This is important, because it's really about creating a system that is maintainable.

One common problem among disorganized people is that they hang on to too many things, which makes everything worse. The extra clutter makes it harder to find the important items and adds to the feeling of chaos. An organizer can help clients go through everything and make the hard choices about what to keep and what to toss, often freeing up a surprising amount of space. The remaining items may then be easier to organize.

Hiring an organizer periodically may be money well spent. If you have the money to do it, then it becomes a personal choice of whether it brings enough happiness or peace of mind to justify the expense. Even if they can afford it, though, some adults with ADHD feel guilty about bringing in an organizer to do something that everyone else seems to do so easily, so they continue to suffer with their secret shame. My response to this is that I could change the oil in my car myself if I had to, but the hassle isn't worth saving twenty bucks, so I have the people at the garage do it for me. In other words, the choice to bring in an organizer comes down to a decision about the relative merits of spending the money rather than to self-esteem issues. It may also save you a lot of family strife if the disorganization is a frequent cause of arguments.

The National Association of Professional Organizers (www.napo.net) is the national nonprofit organization that represents organizers. They provide a searchable directory as well as classes for organizers. Ideally, an organizer should be a member. I would also want to know that the organizer has some knowledge of ADHD so that she doesn't create a system that you just can't maintain.

If you don't need a complete reorganization, there's something to be said for a plain old cleaning service. It's not that you aren't capable of cleaning, but it may just be that it is more likely to be done reliably if someone else does it. If you have more peace of mind when the house is clean, then it may be worth the expense. However, as with any financial matter, it gets more complicated when you are part of a couple. A member of the audience at one of my seminars on adult ADHD told a story of a client with severe ADHD whose husband refused to allow her to hire a cleaning service. His opinion was that she should be able to do it herself, despite the fact that she had never managed to keep the house clean and orderly over all the years of their lengthy marriage. Obviously, the dynamics in this relationship created a situation where a simple solution wasn't so simple. Hopefully your situation isn't quite so contentious.

Don't Underestimate the Power of a Support Group

Many adults with ADHD feel alone in their struggles, like they're the only one who has these problems. Of course, we know that's not true, but it can certainly feel that way when you don't really hear anyone else talking about it. (By the way, lots of other people have ADHD too; they're just not talking about it.) This is where a support group can prove invaluable.

I ran a free monthly adult ADHD support group through Northern Virginia CHADD for five years and found the attendees' appreciation really gratifying. Many of them came up to me afterward to tell me that it was such a relief to finally feel understood and to be surrounded by others who have similar struggles.

A support group can be something formal and structured, such as those offered by one of the many local chapters of CHADD (Children and Adults with AD/HD, one of the national ADHD advocacy organizations), or maybe a stand-alone group offered through a local hospital or university. Or it could be an online forum or just a few people who meet regularly to talk. The group may have a designated leader who takes care of sending out meeting announcements, reserving the space, and running the meeting, including offering information about local resources. Some support groups have speakers present on various topics or have a designated topic to discuss at each meeting, whereas others are purely discussion groups with no set topics. Some groups allow or encourage family members to attend as well, whereas others are closed. None of these formats are inherently better or worse than any others, so it depends on what you are looking for and what is available.

In addition to the usual asking around and Web searching, you can find listings of support groups on CHADD's website (www.chadd.org) as well as the Attention Deficit Disorder Association's site (ADDA; www.add.org). If you are thinking about starting your own support group, you can find a manual on ADDA's website.

Group Therapy: Learn with and from Others

Therapy groups involve one or two therapists and then two to ten clients. Loosely speaking, there are two kinds of therapy groups. Standard therapy groups, also sometimes called *process groups,* use the interactions between the group members to reveal more facets of members' personalities than would happen if it was just one client and a therapist in the room. This can make for some interesting and useful situations that offer opportunities for participants to learn about themselves that can be hard to come by in other settings. For adults with ADHD, it may be one of the first times that they get totally honest yet constructive feedback on how they come across to others—for example, how their tendency to interrupt makes some people feel like withdrawing. Members also get to learn vicariously from the other group members. Process groups may have a diverse membership in terms of diagnoses or issues, age, and sex or may be centered on a particular diagnosis or situation, such as ADHD, postpartum depression, or retirees.

There are also psychoeducational groups, which tend to focus less on the interactions between the group members and instead have a structured program of topics to be covered in each meeting, such as time management, organization, or social skills. As a result, group members tend to all have the same diagnosis or situation.

Both kinds of groups can be helpful, depending on what you're looking for. If you're looking to learn more about yourself or to deal with relationship issues, then a process group may be a better fit. However, most process groups probably won't deal directly with your ADHD. On the other hand, if you want to focus primarily on learning about your ADHD and building skills, then a psychoeducational group may be a better choice. In either case, talk to the therapist beforehand to find out how the group works and to describe what you are looking for.

CHAPTER 7

NONTRADITIONAL TREATMENTS: MIRACLES OR SNAKE OIL?

There has been growing interest in nontraditional, complementary, alternative, holistic, or natural treatments across all of the medical and mental health disciplines. Given all the controversy and hype that have surrounded stimulant medications, perhaps it isn't surprising that ADHD seems to have more than its fair share of these treatments on the market, including many that claim to cure the disorder. Although numerous nontraditional treatments are available and touted as effective, there is still much research to be done to determine whether any of these treatments live up to their promised benefits. The fact that people spend as much as they do on these untested treatments speaks to their suffering and clear desire for relief. It unfortunately also speaks to the success of those who are waging a campaign of misinformation about the diagnosis and its treatments.

When it comes to nontraditional treatments, I'm willing to listen but skeptical. I don't want to miss out on potentially effective treatments, but I also don't want to blindly recommend every new flash in the pan. I want to see some real data from real studies before I will recommend anything. I take my role as a psychologist, author, and presenter very seriously—my advice can have profound effects on people's lives, and not always for the positive. It's my job to use my knowledge and intellect to evaluate these new treatments so I can share those informed opinions with others. I don't claim to always be right, but you can be damn sure that I will be honest, including when I don't know something. It's not my job to protect others' feelings or incomes if they are providing a product or service that isn't helpful—because that doesn't protect the people who are wasting their time, money, and hopes. I assume that most of the people touting these nontraditional treatments mean well, but good intentions don't remove the burden of proof or the need to show effectiveness.

So let's review the proposed treatments that are most available or known. There are far too many lesser-known proposed treatments to cover them all, but we'll hit the biggies.

This chapter contains the following articles:

Nontraditional Treatments: Separate the Wheat from the Chaff

Despite the grand claims made by the people who sell nontraditional treatments, there is absolutely no cure for ADHD. As with diabetes, treatment means lifelong management. Most people see at least some improvement in symptoms with age, but getting older isn't really a treatment.

As for the various nontraditional treatments, I've seen little evidence to give me much faith in their effectiveness. The research that does exist for most of these treatments could be called pseudoscience at best or junk science at worst. It's possible that some of these interventions may work for a few people, but that doesn't mean that they will work for other people. And let's face it: most of us don't care if some treatment supposedly helped the people in the study group. We want to know how likely it is to help us. So if a study is poorly designed, they may find that the treatment helped their participants, even though there is a very low probability that the treatment will be effective for anyone else. Alternatively, the proposed treatment had some small benefit but didn't address the ADHD specifically, so much as it affected something else that looks like or exacerbates ADHD. For example, getting a good night's sleep can help everyone be more attentive at work, but I would hardly call that a treatment for ADHD.

A Little Skepticism Is Good for You

We can use the following as red flags to strongly suggest that a proposed treatment may not be everything that it promises to be. If you see any of these, you should start asking questions and really consider the answers that you get. You may also want to do more research before committing to anything.

- *Miracles.* If it sounds too good to be true, it probably is.
- *Cure-alls.* My facetious rule of thumb is that if something treats more than ten unrelated conditions, then it's probably bogus.
- *Testimonials.* Legitimate healthcare professionals don't solicit testimonials or use them as the primary basis to show effectiveness or as the centerpiece of their marketing materials.
- *Conspiracies.* If the manufacturer or service provider makes claims that the treatment is being unfairly attacked or suppressed by the medical establishment, then perhaps there are legitimate reasons why the new treatment is being attacked. Valid treatments tend to be embraced, not scorned.
- *No evidence.* Effective treatments have the results of research studies published in reputable, peer-reviewed journals, not in company-owned publications or sham journals.
- *Money-back guarantees.* Legitimate professionals don't have to rely on this gimmick.
- *No side effects.* Anything that has no side effects will have no main effects. Nothing is so precisely targeted that it will have absolutely no side effects. Anything that is gentle enough to have no side effects will not have sufficient power to treat something as serious as ADHD.

If a proposed treatment has any merit, it should be able to show those results in a double-blind, placebo-controlled study (and preferably in more than one of them, actually). This is the gold standard for proving that a treatment has benefit. These studies aren't easy to pull off, but they produce results that are much more reliable. If proponents of a proposed treatment can't offer at least one of these studies, then we need to remain skeptical or at least defer judgment until they do.

However, we can make informed predictions about which proposed treatments have a better or worse shot of ever being proven effective. To be taken seriously, a proposed treatment needs to be consistent with what we already know about ADHD specifically and neurology in general. For example, some chiropractors say they can treat ADHD by doing spinal manipulations. However, it doesn't make any sense to think that spinal manipulations could change the functioning of specific areas in the brain—and, by the way, also not change the functioning of other parts of the brain if it really was that powerful an intervention. That's not how our brains work. If a proposed treatment is inconsistent with what we know about brain functioning, then that means that we need to change the entire field of neurology in order to believe that this new treatment could work. It seems much more likely that this new treatment is wrong rather than the broader field of neurology. So it isn't a matter of waiting for the studies to be completed, since no study will ever prove some of these theories.

Some of these proponents of new treatments face a fundamental problem of plausibility. Given the billions of dollars of research and thousands of talented and educated people working in this area, is it reasonable to believe that someone outside of or new to the field could suddenly find a cure or treatment that nobody else did? For example, the packaging on one product claims to have been invented by a schoolteacher. Although she may be familiar with the effects of ADHD in the classroom, it's hard to see why this would enable her to create an effective treatment for it. Just because I've been driving for twenty years doesn't make me qualified to invent a revolutionary engine. A little common sense should go a long way in helping you sort out what sounds legit and what sounds questionable.

What's the Harm in Trying Something? Plenty

Some people say there is no harm in trying these nontraditional treatments first, since someone could always try more accepted treatments if they don't work. I would disagree. Trying a treatment with dubious or untested effectiveness has several potential disadvantages:

- *Bets on the long shot.* If we have treatments that are proven to work and proposed treatments that haven't been proven, it seems unreasonable to start with the long shot.

- *Delays better-established treatments.* Even if a nontraditional treatment were completely free and had no side effects, there is still a price paid in terms of additional struggles and suffering that could have been prevented or reduced by employing more-effective treatment during that time. This price needs to be factored into your decision making. Are you willing to tolerate being essentially untreated for this period of time?
- *Wastes money that could be better spent.* Whatever gets spent on less effective treatments isn't available to be spent on more-effective treatments.
- *Creates unfounded pessimism about better-established treatments.* Getting little or no benefit from an untested treatment can be demoralizing to some people, causing them to delay or avoid trying treatments known to be more effective. This can be a real loss.

When you put all of these reasons together, there is indeed harm that can come from untested treatments. I'm not saying that you shouldn't try them, but if you do, you should be clear about the potential costs.

Final Thoughts

My advice to clients is to start with what we know works, then experiment with some of these other interventions if they feel they want to give some alternative options a try. If you do try one of these nontraditional treatments, you should make a point of paying attention to the kinds benefits it's providing, then weigh that against the cost, inconvenience, side effects, and risks. As I've said before, I'm all about making well-informed, thought-out decisions—if you do that, you will be most likely to be successful.

Natural = Safe (Except for Radon, Lead, Arsenic. . .)

I will freely admit that this is a pet peeve of mine, but it makes me crazy when people say that some remedy is safe because it's natural. This makes absolutely no sense, since there are millions of naturally occurring substances that are incredibly dangerous or even lethal. For example, cyanide compounds are produced by certain bacteria, fungi, and algae and even found in trace amounts in apple seeds, mangoes, and almonds, yet I wouldn't recommend eating much of this natural substance.

The implication that these proponents use is that natural substances are somehow superior to those manufactured by humans, but that's clearly not always true. Just to beat a dead horse, if natural substances are so wonderful, then our cities are wasting a lot of time filtering and purifying our drinking water and thereby depriving us of all sorts of interesting natural substances.

Some substances occur in nature that are also manufactured by humans, such as certain vitamins and supplements. Even here, natural sources aren't necessarily better. If the two substances are chemically identical, then there is no difference between the naturally derived one and the one made in a lab. There may be purity differences, though, since both methods of obtaining a substance can leave behind other substances, although I don't think we could say that one is better than the other across the board. That's more of a quality-control issue.

I will certainly not say that I defend every practice of the pharmaceutical or chemical companies (seriously), but I become instantly skeptical when I see something that says that a product is superior because it's natural. It's a naïve logic that makes me wonder about every other claim associated with this product.

As for the various herbal remedies that are available, none have been found to have much of an effect on ADHD. However, they can affect other body processes or how you metabolize other medications or even other herbal supplements, so you should keep your physician up to date on what you're taking.

Diet, Nutrition, and Supplements: Try to Eat Well

There was a lot of press in the 1970s about the effects of food additives on behavior. Thus the Feingold diet was born. The premise is that hyperactive children are sensitive to a variety of food additives, colorings, and artificial products that cause their symptoms. The theory is that removing these problematic additives from the diet will lead to an improvement in symptoms. Unfortunately, scientific studies have disproven any connection between these additives and ADHD symptoms. It may be that some small percentage of kids (more than adults) do have some food sensitivities or difficulties with blood sugar regulation such that they do behave differently after eating certain foods. But then the problem is more about allergies or diabetes than it is about ADHD.

So the bottom line is this: if you notice that you feel or perform worse or better after eating certain foods, then tailor your diet accordingly. Without making yourself completely nuts about it, try to eat a healthy diet, since that helps all people perform at their best.

Vitamins, Minerals, and Supplements

Several nutritional supplements purportedly treat ADHD. Unfortunately, none of them have been proven to have any specific benefit for ADHD. Sure, we all do better with a balanced diet that provides the right amounts of all the necessary nutrients—the key word here is the *right* amounts. As with so many other things, when it comes to nutrients, too much of a good thing is no longer good. Nutrients that are good for us in small doses can be dangerous in higher doses—for example, taking excessive quantities of fat-soluble vitamins can lead to poisoning. More is definitely not always better. Our bodies work really hard to keep a very complex and careful balance among thousands and thousands of compounds, so adding too much of any one thing can throw the whole system out of whack. As a simple analogy, plants need water to live, but you can definitely kill most plants by giving them too much (I've proved this myself).

In a related example, I could spray my garden hose against the window all day, but it won't get any water into the plants in my living room. By the same token, taking neurotransmitter precursors like L-dopa or other amino acids like tyrosine and phenylalanine won't have much of an effect on how much dopamine or norepinephrine is created in the brain. Just because something passes through your stomach doesn't mean it winds up in your brain or corrects a deficiency there. As a result, these supplements haven't shown much lasting benefit.

If there is a single nutritional supplement that may possibly have some benefit for ADHD, it's the essential fatty acids. However, more study is needed to determine effective doses and whether some kinds of fatty acids are more effective than others. Some very expensive versions are available, but it is premature to say that they are inherently superior to the cheap stuff. If nothing else, essential fatty acid supplements are generally cheap, safe, and easy, so there isn't that much harm in taking one.

Given the increased prevalence of processed foods with less nutritional value, my general advice to everyone is to take a good multivitamin and an essential fatty acid supplement. This is especially true for ADHD folks whose poor planning makes them more likely to eat on the run, which means that they eat more junk and less good stuff. It won't cure your ADHD, but it will help you perform at your best in other ways.

Does Neurofeedback Work? Maybe

Audience members at presentations often ask me what I think about neurofeedback, a form of biofeedback where clients are taught to alter their brain waves. People with ADHD are taught to make certain changes that correspond to more focused attention. The idea is that the client should eventually be able to consciously control brain waves when not hooked up to the neurofeedback equipment. As the brain waves change, so too should the symptoms—at least that's the theory.

At this point, I put neurofeedback in the maybe column—it might work, but I want to see some better research proving that it does. Unfortunately, most of the studies on neurofeedback that show its effectiveness have been crummy ones that don't answer the question definitively. There were too many problems with the study's design, size, or data analysis for me to trust the results. Proponents of neurofeedback claim that after treatment, most clients will be able to reduce or go off their medications entirely since they will have trained their brains to function better. Although this would be great, more research is needed to really answer the question of whether there is any benefit from it, how long it lasts, and what kind of booster sessions are needed.

Strange as this sounds, I think that neurofeedback's biggest supporters have also been its biggest problem. Their overly enthusiastic claims of neurofeedback's ability to cure a long list of ailments makes them sound like snake-oil salesmen. A bit of restraint would give them a lot more credibility.

Typically, neurofeedback involves twenty to forty sessions or maybe more, usually two or three times per week, which can be a significant investment of time and logistically difficult for many clients. Fees tend to be similar to those of standard therapy sessions, but because insurance reimbursement for this service is often inconsistent, it can become expensive.

It's relatively inexpensive to set up shop as a neurofeedback practitioner—some systems cost less than $5,000. Training programs also certify, at least by their standards, practitioners in less than five days. This makes me worry about the competence of some of the people out there offering a service that can be potentially dangerous when applied incorrectly or used with the wrong clients. If you're interested in trying neurofeedback, ask a prospective practitioner if she is certified by the Biofeedback Certification Institute of America. To qualify, the applicant must demonstrate certain didactic training and supervised hours and then pass a test. (More information is available at www.bcia.org.)

Even if neurofeedback were to instantly rewire an ADHD person's brain so that it worked just like a non-ADHD brain, the person may still benefit from coaching and therapy. He may still need to learn more effective ways to organize, set priorities, keep a schedule book—in other words, all the life-management skills that he never got along the way. He may also need to work on his self-image after a lifetime of ADHD-based struggles and failures.

Computer-Based Training Programs: Most Won't Upgrade Your Brain

Several computer programs claim to train the brain in a way that is beneficial for ADHD. Despite their grand claims, there is very little reason to think that these programs will have any benefit. Sure, someone with ADHD may perform better on the program after practicing it for a while, but that doesn't mean that he will perform better in his actual life—which is presumably what actually matters. Going to a basketball camp may make someone a better player, but it won't make her *taller*. By the same token, practicing these computer games won't change the brain wiring that is causing her ADHD. If the sellers of these computer programs want legitimacy, let them earn it by publishing studies that show the benefits. Until then, I remain highly skeptical.

As negative as I am about most of the computer programs, there does appear to be one that might actually work. The Cogmed working memory training system seems to improve users' working memories, which leads to reductions in overall ADHD symptoms. It appears that the crucial difference between Cogmed and the other programs is that Cogmed constantly adjusts to the user's performance, so it is neither too easy nor too hard. With practice, this leads to improvements in working memory, not just on the program but also in the person's actual life. This in turn leads to measurable reductions in ADHD symptoms. This improvement in life functioning separates treatments from games.

The Cogmed inventors have tested its performance using reliable methods and published the results in respected journals, so there is reason to be optimistic that they may be on to something here. Other researchers are repeating their studies to make sure they get the same results. This is standard practice in research. Replication is required if we are to have faith in the results. So stay tuned and let's see what happens.

Mindfulness Meditation: We Could All Do with Being Calmer

There has been growing interest in the use of mindfulness meditation to treat a variety of mental conditions, including anxiety, depression, sleep problems, and addictions. Therefore it shouldn't be surprising that it is also being used for ADHD. I know many people with ADHD would rather eat dirt than sit silently and try to not think. Fortunately, it's possible to alter the meditation techniques so that they are shorter or involve walking in order to make them more tolerable for the restless.

Mindfulness involves intentionally focusing on your current experience without analyzing or judging it—just noticing. It tends to involve three basic steps:

- Bringing attention to an attentional anchor, such as breathing or walking
- Noticing when a distraction occurs
- Refocusing back to the attentional anchor

This sequence is repeated many times during the course of each meditation session. As the individual becomes better able to maintain his focus on the attentional anchor, he hopefully also becomes more aware of his attention generally. This of course is the central question: does learning to control your attention better when meditating generalize to when you're not meditating? If so, then we'd really be on to something good. Meditation proponents claim that it can help people with ADHD to regulate their attention better, become more self-aware, feel less overwhelmed, act less impulsively, and have fewer racing thoughts and emotional outbursts.

Brain scans show that meditation affects activity levels in multiple parts of the brain, both during meditation and also (with practice) when not meditating. The question that remains, though, is whether it can change the specific brain areas involved in ADHD and thereby reduce its symptoms. More research is needed, but there appears to be some cause for optimism. Even if meditation has no direct benefit on ADHD symptoms, it can still be generally beneficial in terms of stress, anxiety, and mood. It also has no real side effects, except perhaps boredom, so there is little harm in trying it. Therefore, because it potentially offers at least some sort of benefit, unlike most other nontraditional treatments, my opinion is that it's worth trying if you feel so inclined.

Other Nontraditional Treatments: Don't Hold Out Hope

Lots of other nontraditional treatments are out there. If I didn't mention something specifically in this chapter, you can assume that it has very little chance of being effective for ADHD. However, just for the sake of clarity, I will mention a few more of them here.

The Dore program involves vision, balance, and sensory exercises for cerebellar developmental delay, a generic term that could mean virtually anything but sounds impressive in the company's marketing materials. Despite the website's claims, there are absolutely no data to suggest that these exercises accomplish anything other than enrich the company's owners (Ingersoll, 2006, October).

No benefit of any sort has been found for optometric vision training, applied kinesiology, interactive metronome, auditory training, antimotion sickness medication, or treatment for Candida yeast (Ingersoll, 2006, October). Since none of these fit the current theories of ADHD and brain functioning, it's unlikely that any evidence will ever be found to show any of these as effective treatments.

Section III

BUILD THE NECESSARY SKILLS

Introduction: Address ADHD's Core Deficits—The Means to Better Ends

The chapters in this section offer specific strategies to help you be more effective. These are the building blocks that you will apply in the various parts of your life covered in section IV: household management, relationships, college, and work. This section covers the means you will use to achieve those better ends. For example, time management doesn't really matter by itself—what matters is that you pay a price at work and with friends if you don't manage your time well. So managing your time effectively helps you do better in these other areas.

In these chapters, I list tons of strategies that you can use to overcome whatever ADHD-based challenges you face. Pick and choose among them, starting with the ones that best seem to fit your situation. There's some overlap in the strategies I offer because the problems share common causes, so some of the same strategies will work for multiple problems. Knowing that some readers will read only parts of each chapter, I would rather repeat a few things than have them miss the ideas completely.

By this point in the book, you might have gotten the impression that I like to understand things. I want to know why some things work and others don't. It's not just because it can be interesting. More important, it can be really helpful—with this understanding, you can make adjustments on the fly and adapt smoothly to new situations. It's that old adage, "Give a man to fish, feed him for a day. Teach a man to fish, feed him for a lifetime." I would rather feast forever, and I want you to do the same.

Therefore, I've created a small general theory for how to overcome typical ADHD challenges. This is simplified and won't always work, but it can be helpful most of the time. If you have this in the back of your head, you will be in a better position to create effective ways of dealing with whatever life throws at you.

Three Weaknesses, Many Problems

ADHD has three core deficits: inattention, hyperactivity, and impulsivity. Some people have all three, whereas some people have only the inattentive part. The various symptoms of ADHD cluster under each of these three headings. Each of these core deficits leads to all sorts of difficulties when you try to function in our complex world. For example, being inattentive and distractible can lead to problems with the following:

- Time management and following your stated priorities, if you drift to other tasks

- Memory, if your attention gets pulled away from what you're trying to remember
- Organization, if your attention bounces around between the things you're trying to organize so that you struggle to maintain a consistent system
- Social blunders, if you miss important nonverbal cues

So, from three core deficits come many different kinds of problems. That's the bad news. The good news is that you can use the same basic strategies to overcome these struggles. We can create some general guidelines for how to address each of the core deficits. For the most part, the strategies that are most successful for people with ADHD will be consistent with these guidelines because they take into account the way that people with ADHD typically process information.

You will still need to customize each strategy to your own particular situation, but this general theory provides a good place to start. It can also help you feel less overwhelmed when looking at all the possible strategies, because you will see the common threads that run through them all. You will be able to see that they are all just variations on a theme. In addition, if you keep this general theory in mind, you will be able to create better strategies of your own.

Overcome Inattention

People with ADHD have difficulty keeping their attention on the most relevant part of their environment. They tend to get pulled off by other stimuli that may be flashier but aren't as important. This could be distractions in the world around them or distractions from within their own thoughts. The goal, therefore, is to reduce the odds of getting off track and thereby increase the chances of doing the right things at the right times. We can do this by working it from both sides:

- *Reduce extraneous stimuli.* The fewer distractions that are competing for your attention, the more likely you are to stay focused where you should be. You can assist this process by reducing clutter, noise, visual stimuli, or reminders of tasks you shouldn't be engaging in, such as by turning off your phone or email alert. By eliminating these sticky stimuli, you would have to make a conscious choice to get off track, as opposed to getting drawn off before you even realize it.
- *Amplify relevant stimuli.* The stronger and stickier the desired stimuli are, the more likely you are to notice and stay on them. So setting an alarm when it's time to leave for a meeting makes that moment in time stand out much more than when relying on

yourself to notice the passage of time. Similarly, a big reminder note taped up on the wall is much more noticeable than a note written in a schedule book. The general idea is to prevent the desired stimuli from fading into the background and to instead bring them forward, front and center.

This is why the very first accommodation that is suggested for students with ADHD is to seat them at the front of the class. It reduces the distraction of seeing their classmates and also makes the teacher loom larger in their attention. We can increase the relative intensity of the relevant stimuli by both decreasing the strength of undesirable stimuli as well as by increasing the strength of the desired ones.

Overcome Hyperactivity

Hyperactive kids tend to grow into less obviously active adults. Much of the overt activity will settle down, but it is often replaced with a more internal sense of restlessness—they can make themselves sit still if they have to, but it takes mental effort and they would rather not. The key to dealing with the remaining hyperactivity, if you ever had it, is to do the following:

- *Seek out situations that allow for the safe expression of hyperactivity.* If you have a hard time sitting still, then don't expect yourself to. If you need to move to satisfy that internal restlessness, then look for times and places where you can. Many ADHD adults will wisely select the situations that they put themselves into. For example, they will watch movies at home where they can move around easily rather than feel trapped at the theater. Others may need to counterbalance the mental efforts and demands for restraint at work with more active pursuits at night and on weekends.

- *Minimize or avoid situations that require more restraint than you can muster.* There's little to be gained from putting yourself into a situation that will force you to do something you're bad at. For example, someone who hates sitting still shouldn't take a desk job that doesn't allow frequent breaks. You may find that you have greater tolerance for repetitive or boring activities if you allow yourself some breaks, remind yourself of the benefits of doing the task, or build in a reward. It may still take some real mental effort and you may never be great at it, but it's still worth working on.

Overcome Impulsivity

I tend to define *impulsivity* as actions that precede conscious thought. Or more simplistically, leaping before looking. It's easy to say "Don't act impulsively," but that just doesn't work (as you undoubtedly already know). The problem is that you will have already leapt before realizing that you didn't look. Apart from inventing a time machine, you will do better if you set yourself up for success before you find yourself in certain situations. There's less to think about this way, and less willpower is needed. The key to dealing with impulsivity is to do the following:

- *Create barriers to problematic actions by reducing tempting stimuli.* This is the "lead me not into temptation" approach. For example, if someone knows that she is far too likely to spend too much money in certain stores, she shouldn't even go into those stores in the first place, because any good intentions will be quickly lost. It's much easier to not be tempted if there is no temptation.
- *Set up cushions to reduce the potential damage.* Sometimes you can't remove temptations completely. However, you may still be able to find ways to minimize the potential costs of impulsive acts. For example, if this same woman has to go into one of these risky stores, she could bring a specific amount of cash with her and leave her credit cards at home. This way she can't spend more than planned, even if she gets really excited about something. Although there's some potential benefit from working on self-control and reminding yourself in the moment about the consequences of an impulsive act, you will probably have greater success with setting yourself up correctly beforehand.

What This Section Covers

This section contains the following chapters:

8. *Self-Esteem and Effectiveness: I Can Do This!* (p. 191) It's hard to prevent a lifetime of ADHD from affecting how you feel about yourself and your sense of being able to be effective in the world. Some solid successes in the present can do a lot to vindicate struggles from the past. They also make it easier to not feel so bad about the places where you're still having a hard time.
9. *Memory Management: What Was That Again?* (p. 237) There's a lot to remember in this complicated life. These strategies can enable you to more reliably remember everything from little details to momentous occasions.
10. *Time Management: What Should I Be Doing Now?* (p. 247) If you have a lot to do, then you need to manage your time well to get it all done. These strategies will help you not only get more done, but get more of the right stuff done.

11. *Get Organized, Stay Organized: Wrestle the Avalanche* (p. 263) It's easier to find what you need when you're at least a little bit organized. We will talk about how to whip your stuff into shape so that you can be more effective and less overwhelmed.

12. *Using Tools and Technology to Stay on Top of Your Life: Gizmos* (p. 273) There are lots of great tools out there, from sticky notes to PDAs, that enable us to get more done. The trick is to use the right tool for the job and to use it consistently.

13. *Achieve Your Goals: Take the Long View* (p. 285) Short-term goals lead into long-term goals. These strategies can help you get on top of both of them.

CHAPTER 8

SELF-ESTEEM AND EFFECTIVENESS: I CAN DO THIS!

ADHD is clearly a neurological condition. Over time, though, all sorts of psychological fallout starts showing up. Perhaps most insidious, untreated ADHD starts to affect how someone sees himself and how hard he is willing to work toward goals that he's skeptical of achieving. This then creates a self-fulfilling prophecy that is difficult to escape.

I've seen far too many adults who are battered from a lifetime of struggle and inexplicable failures walk through my door. There's still a part of them that wants something better (otherwise they wouldn't show up), but they're understandably hesitant to get their hopes up again. I give them a lot of credit for being willing to take that chance. And there are plenty of adults who will never show up in someone's office, the ones who've given up hope. They've decided that their fate is sealed and there's no point in fighting it. These are the ones who suffer the worst, especially as the problems begin to pile up—job loss, chaotic relationships, substance abuse, other mental health conditions, and even jail time. Even if you have been fortunate enough to avoid these major pitfalls, you've probably paid a price at school and work and with family and friends.

Medication can change the symptoms of ADHD, and PDAs can compensate for organizational weaknesses, but neither directly changes the psychological fallout. That's where understanding your ADHD and getting some momentum going in your life comes in. Happiness comes from both achieving real successes to feel good about and altering how you feel about the setbacks. We'll talk about both of them in this chapter and a whole lot more.

This chapter contains the following articles:

Fully Accepting the Diagnosis (p. 197) Coming to a full understanding and acceptance of your ADHD isn't easy, but it is empowering.

Personal Responsibility: You Can't Control What You Don't Accept (p. 199) Accepting your ADHD gives you much greater control over what happens in your life. It offers you a short list of strategies that are more likely to be effective for you.

Rewrite History: Understand Your Past (and Yourself) in a Different Way (p. 200) Being diagnosed with ADHD not only enables you to create a better future, it also changes your understanding of your past. It explains all sorts of events in your life in a much less pejorative way.

Is ADHD an Excuse or an Explanation? (p. 201) Using ADHD as an excuse for poor performance is disempowering because it betrays an expectation that the person can't do any better. By contrast, using it as an explanation helps the person understand how and why things go badly and, more important, what she can do differently to increase the odds of success.

ADHD Is Bigger Than Good Intentions (p. 202) People with ADHD usually have good intentions but have trouble reliably turning those desires into action. There are important neurological reasons for this, so it's important to use the right strategies when trying to close the gap.

Calling All Frauds, Fakes, and Actors (p. 204) Many adults with undiagnosed ADHD work really hard to hide the extent of their struggles. They also tend to minimize their good qualities. Success requires honesty, which includes giving yourself credit for your successes.

Is the Problem ADHD or Motivation? (p. 205) Many ADHD struggles can look like problems of motivation. After enough failures, what starts out as purely neurological can quickly become psychological as motivation begins to slide.

Just Do It! (p. 206) Adult life involves lots of mundane activities that aren't especially hard but still need to be done. The trick is getting yourself up and moving on them.

Do It Anyway: Avoid Avoidance (p. 207) It's tempting to avoid dealing with those projects that make us uncomfortable, even though this tends to make things worse. Therefore, it's better to push ourselves to approach those challenges.

Change Your Mindset, Change Your Life (p. 208) Adults with undiagnosed ADHD tend to adopt certain mindsets that limit their ability to be successful. These mindsets are pretty reasonable given the person's history, but they can also be quite limiting. So keep an eye out for when you find yourself thinking in these ways.

Overcome Unhelpful Coping Strategies, Bad Habits, and Defense Mechanisms (p. 209) I cover ways to overcome rationalization, externalizing, avoidance, quitting, procrastination, pseudoproductivity, abandoning ship, quasi-obsessive-compulsive behavior, controlling or aggressive behavior, learned helplessness, impulsively rushing, and cavalier lifestyle.

Failures Lead to Successes (and Better Self-Esteem) (p. 217) Most challenges in life involve some setbacks before success comes. The trick is to get up after getting knocked down.

Can I Trust Myself? (p. 219) People with ADHD learn that they aren't as reliable as they want to be. This makes sense when their ADHD is still untreated, but you can learn to legitimately have more confidence in yourself once you do get on top of your ADHD.

Take Charge of Your Life (p. 220) Many people with untreated ADHD feel as if they don't have enough control over what happens in their lives. It works out best when you shift your mindset to see that you do have control over some things, while accepting that there are other things that you don't have control over.

Is ADHD a Gift? (p. 222) Some people claim that ADHD also has positive qualities. I don't doubt that people with ADHD have all sorts of positive qualities, but I wouldn't say that those strengths come from their ADHD. Fortunately, you don't have to attribute them to your ADHD in order to feel good about yourself.

Build Healthy Self-Esteem (p. 224) Strong self-esteem comes from what we do and what we make of those experiences. Solid self-esteem comes from doing better as well as learning to accept certain weaknesses and setbacks.

Adversity Makes You Stronger (Hopefully) (p. 226) Adversity takes many forms. If ADHD is one of your struggles, then perhaps you can learn some important life lessons from it.

Is Life a Journey or a Destination? (p. 227) People with ADHD are good at enjoying the moment, but not as good at bringing projects to completion. I cover some of the strategies you can use to get more done while still enjoying yourself.

Roll Back Anxiety and Depression (p. 228) Adults with undiagnosed ADHD are more likely to be anxious or depressed. Fortunately, treating your ADHD may also help you feel better in unexpected ways.

Manage Excessive Substance Use and Other Addictive Behavior (p. 229) People with untreated ADHD are more likely to have addictive behaviors, for several reasons. Getting on top of this will benefit you in other ways, too.

Anger Management: Lengthen That Fuse (p. 231) People with untreated ADHD are more prone to angry outbursts. This anger is usually a symptom of other things, so addressing the causes will give you a double benefit when you find it easier to control your temper.

Perfectionism: Almost Always Overrated (p. 238) Some adults with ADHD compensate for their failures by going for perfection. Although this makes sense in a way, it tends to make things worse.

ADHD, Eating Disorders, and Weight Management (p. 234) Some new research is showing that people with ADHD are more likely to develop eating disorders or at least have trouble controlling their weight. Although this may bring some extra challenges, getting on top of your ADHD may also benefit your eating habits.

I'm Only Getting Treatment to Shut You People Up

When one person has ADHD, his whole family kind of has it too. They're the ones who need to tie up the loose ends, give the reminders, and deal with the tasks that aren't done by the person with ADHD—*and* deal with their anxiety and frustration over all these things. As a result of this impact, family members and others are often the ones pushing the person with ADHD to seek treatment. This is most common for young adults who are receiving strong pressure from frustrated parents, but it could also be romantic partners doing the pushing. Even if they don't know that the person has ADHD, they know there's *something* going on that needs to be improved. This is a natural setup for the person with ADHD to, at best, not feel invested in the process or, at worst, be downright resentful about it. He may then give some halfhearted effort, secretly hoping that the treatment doesn't help so he can tell everyone that he tried and now they need to leave him alone. Of course, this lack of effort becomes a self-fulfilling prophecy.

I can understand that hesitation, since nobody likes to be told what to do, especially if it's about a sensitive topic. However, your family might be on to something that's worth checking out. Like I tell my teenage clients who are dragged in by their parents, "Since you have to come here anyway, you may as well get something out of the time, even if it isn't exactly what your parents want." By the same token, although you should take your family's concerns seriously, your treatment is really for you. If you have ADHD, or whatever, it affects you more than it affects anyone else, so you have the most to gain from working on it. Your family also stands to benefit, but that shouldn't be the only reason to seek treatment—let *them* see someone if it is.

You should also know that there's something really interesting that happens when someone begins to get on top of his ADHD: it becomes clear that other people in the family also have their own things to work on. Before that, the chaos of untreated ADHD serves as an excellent smoke screen to hide other people's issues. So, family members may need to work on managing their anxiety when things aren't the way they want, on feeling more comfortable with loose ends, or on taking care of their own needs in the relationship. (See chapter 15, *Relationships and Friendships: Strive for Balance*, for more on all this.) I feel that this is a good thing because the family members can be happier and better off by working on their own issues anyway. So everybody benefits.

It can be a real sign of love and caring to call someone on her issues and blind spots, at least if it's done in a constructive way that isn't too obviously self-serving. It's usually easier to ignore things, so the person is choosing to take the harder path and address the problem. This usually works out best when done in a collaborative manner where each person agrees to work on his own part, since it's almost never the case that only one person has the ability to improve the situation. Even if it is more one person's fault than the other's, still both of them have the ability to contribute to the solution.

The Four Stages of Adjustment to a New Diagnosis

Receiving a diagnosis of ADHD can be a life-changing event. Everyone reacts in his own way, but I've noticed some general trends that people tend to follow. I've broken it into four stages. Don't get too hung up on exactly what stage you're in, so much as use it as a way to understand how this process may unfold for you. Some people feel more comfortable knowing where they've come from and where they're going.

1. Getting Excited

By the time they're finally diagnosed, many people react excitedly with, "This explains everything!" They finally have an explanation that isn't pejorative, that they don't have to see as an indictment of their character. They now have an explanation that ties together all sorts of issues in their life, from getting in trouble on the school bus to feeling bored during long movies. This clarity can be pretty exciting.

Others, however, find that the diagnosis confirms their feelings of being defective. It's just further proof that there's something wrong with them—and now it's official.

Regardless of their initial reaction, some people may also experience intense feelings of anger, sadness, and regret for all the wasted time, lost opportunities, and unnecessary struggle. As one of my clients put it, "I spent most of the weekend crying, pissed about how hard things were and how bad things got sometimes. I was mad at my parents for not realizing, and then mad at myself. Finally, I was able to come to some peace with it." This can be a time of mixed emotions, all of which make sense, even when you feel completely crazy.

This is the time when people gather their treatment team, buy too many books (which they don't finish—I won't take it personally), join support groups, and get involved. They may see everything through the ADHD lens and use ADHD to explain everything that happens in their lives, even when it's a bit of stretch.

2. Getting Down to Business

After the initial rush fades, they get to work. The motto during this stage is, "OK, now I know what I can do to make my life better." The rush of discovery is replaced by a more sober attitude of responsibility. They start trying some of the tips and tricks they've learned, work to get their medications adjusted, and explore the psychological manifestations generated by a life of ADHD. Pieces continue to fall into place. Although this can be a very positive time, it sometimes represents the calm before the storm that occurs once they start hitting some roadblocks and that initial enthusiasm starts to burn off, which brings us to the next stage.

3. Getting Overwhelmed

As with many big habit changes, the real challenge comes after that initial enthusiasm but before consistent effort has yielded some tangible results to maintain motivation. It's this middle time that's the hardest. Adults with ADHD often run into the hard reality that, even with a good medication regimen, it still takes a great deal of hard work to make and maintain the desired changes. The motto here is, "Damn, there sure is a lot to do. Maybe life was better without the diagnosis." They may feel frustrated that everything doesn't magically fall into place. They got their hopes up once again, only to be disappointed. In some ways it's worse now since they know so much better what their problems are, including perhaps some problems that they didn't know they had. At this point, they will have more problems than solutions.

They probably discovered that medication isn't a cure-all or that it has side effects that might have required starting all over with a different medication. The stress and demands of daily life began to interfere with those perfectly crafted plans and strategies, causing some slipping back to old habits (which is what we tend to do in stressful times). In an effort to counteract hopelessness, I often remind clients that they've already solved all the easy problems in their lives so, by default, they're left with the harder problems that take more time and effort. So remind yourself of this when you're tempted to abandon your new good habits and give in to pessimism. Rome wasn't built in a day, and neither will your new, successful life be.

Some people may feel angry about the injustice of the universe that gave them this condition. I understand that anger and the wish for an easier life. Unfortunately, life isn't fair and *everyone* has his own limitations, issues, sacrifices, and annoyances. Awful things sometimes happen to good people. ADHD is one of the crummy cards that you were dealt, but presumably you were dealt many good cards, too. You may need to work on accepting that you need to do things differently than others in terms of the strategies, therapy, and medications that you need to function at your best. With acceptance comes a greater ability to create success.

4. Getting on Top of It

Ideally, over time people will settle into a fuller understanding of their ADHD and how it fits into their life as a whole—it's a part of their life, but not their whole life. The motto for this stage is, "I can do this. It's hard work, but there are real rewards for it." They understand that they will have more work to do in some areas than most people, but they also know that that work will pay off in reasonable ways. They have become automatic with some of the good habits that are especially helpful to them, making those habits less consciously driven (and requiring less effort). They recognize their imperfections and know that sometimes they will fall short. They can accept that it's difficult to live in an information age when one has information-processing deficits. They may not be happy about this, but they can accept it.

Some people have an easier time of this than others. This is more an ideal to strive for than a mark to fall short of. True success is usually a combination of doing better and accepting it when you blow it occasionally. You'll still mess things up sometimes, probably more than you would wish, but you can see it in perspective and maybe even laugh at it. That's what real success looks like.

Fully Accepting the Diagnosis

Coming to a full acceptance of your ADHD is neither quick nor easy. It involves really understanding the effect that your ADHD has on your life and then integrating it into how you see yourself. This is that happy middle ground between denying your struggles and feeling overwhelmed by them, between feeling that nothing is wrong and everything is wrong.

Part of fully accepting a diagnosis of ADHD, or any other condition, involves mourning the lost potential for the future and letting go of the hope that one day these troubles will go away. It also involves accepting past losses and failures without crumbling into despair or self-hatred. This process goes far beyond clichés about never giving up or whatever. It may involve accepting the need to change your environment or strategies in order to be more successful, even if other people don't need to go to these lengths. It may also involve changing your goals to minimize avoidable struggles—if at first (and second, and third...) you don't succeed, then maybe you need different goals. Persistence is admirable, but only before it reaches the point of stubbornness.

Someone who fully accepts his ADHD can advocate assertively, but appropriately, for himself. He can sort out what is his responsibility and what is others' and negotiate a mutually agreeable compromise. When he runs into resistance from people who are unwilling to be understanding, he doesn't have to take it personally because his self-esteem isn't overly dependent on others' opinions or validation. He knows that you can't please all the people all the time, so he does his best but doesn't make his happiness overly dependent on others' opinions.

This is an important realization, because there are some people who just can't be won over. He recognizes which battles are worth fighting and which are best abandoned. For example, he may be able to pull off keeping the lawn immaculately trimmed in order to please the critical neighbors, but at what price to his peace of mind? And what else won't be completed while he's mowing the lawn? Is a perfect lawn worth less time with his kids? Is it worth it within the context of his whole life? If he is secure within himself, he will be able to answer these questions with much greater clarity and less regret and self-recrimination.

Some people try to shortcut this difficult acceptance process by touting ADHD's positive qualities. This is a well-meaning attempt to rescue ADHD folks' self-esteem from becoming swamped by the painful feelings stemming from their ADHD deficits. The supposed positive qualities are the sugar that makes the bitter pill go down easier—"Sure, I'm forgetful and disorganized, but I'm also creative." This may make it easier for some people to accept their ADHD, but it also gives the ADHD credit that it doesn't deserve. I'm not denying that this person is creative, but I would disagree that it comes from his ADHD. I just don't think that we need to sweeten the deal in order for people to come to a full acceptance of their ADHD. I talk about this in detail in *Is ADHD a Gift?* on p. 222. Finally, touting ADHD's positive qualities also subtly undermines the need for treatment, because why should we treat something that also has all these good qualities? Wouldn't the treatment be likely to take away these good qualities, too?

Whether one touts the positive qualities or not, it's important that he keeps his ADHD in its rightful place, without making it too big a part of his self-definition. It's the difference between "being ADHD" versus "having ADHD." Or, in other words, it's the difference between seeing ADHD as a *part* of who he is and as *all* of who he is.

This full acceptance allows the person with ADHD to experience feelings of shame, embarrassment, defectiveness, anger, resentment, guilt, and fear at appropriate times without becoming flooded. When present in the right doses, these are important and useful feelings that serve a valuable purpose by keeping us honest and striving for self-improvement. When overwhelming, these feelings cause people to avoid thinking about their problem areas, and they can even drive self-destructive behavior. Those who haven't fully accepted their ADHD are at greater risk to experience a burst of these painful feelings that is out of proportion to the circumstances—for example, a forgotten appointment elicits a thousand memories of similar failures, cascading into self-hatred. (Remember Al Franken's

Stuart Smalley character from *Saturday Night Live?*) This self-flagellation just makes people feel bad and actually makes them less likely to deal with it more effectively next time. Full acceptance of our weaknesses gives us greater control over our emotions and destinies.

So as you read this book, especially the parts that make you uncomfortable, push yourself to really understand and absorb it. It isn't easy and it definitely isn't fun, but you will be better off for it.

Personal Responsibility: You Can't Control What You Don't Accept

I sometimes get calls from family members of someone with ADHD, looking for advice on helping that person to accept and work on it. Sometimes this person will completely deny it, even when it's pretty obvious and causing serious problems in his life. Other times he will admit to having ADHD, but won't do anything about it. This seems to me to not really be a full admission, so much as it's mostly lip service with the hope of getting his family members to leave him alone. ("OK, so maybe I do have ADHD. Please pass the potatoes.")

I understand that it can be difficult to accept that you have a diagnosable condition. This may be especially true for those who have spent most of their lives trying to hold it all together and hide the full extent of their difficulties. After years of putting on an act, it can be really hard to admit (even to themselves) that something isn't right. It's as if admitting to anything will somehow make things worse, as if it would add insult to the injury of their daily struggles. Of course, it's the obvious struggles that are the real problem, not the label of ADHD. The disorganization and forgetfulness are far more damning and lead to far more criticism than admitting to themselves that they have a treatable condition. The trouble with denial is that it deprives people of some of the most effective ways to actually improve their situation. This would mean that they could give up the act, because they would actually be doing what they need to.

For this reason, accepting that you have ADHD can be quite liberating. It explains a lot, and probably in better ways than the previous explanations you had—like laziness, bad attitude, or ditziness. It can free you from the ghosts of your past failures by offering a more palatable explanation. Perhaps more important, it also offers the promise that the future can be different, that you won't repeat the same mistakes and fall prey to the same tendencies. You don't need to reinvent the wheel and figure out the best strategies all by yourself. You can benefit from what others have figured out and add that to what you already know works for you. However, to do this, you first have to admit that you have ADHD. As in the rest of life, nothing comes for free, but this one should be worth the cost.

This then brings us to the concept of personal responsibility. With this freedom from past struggles comes the responsibility to apply that knowledge for a better future. You don't have to apply that knowledge, but you can't expect others to work harder on overcoming your ADHD than you do. If you have the ability to influence your fate, then you can choose to do so or choose not to. If you want a bigger, fuller life, then you will need to work for it by mastering your ADHD. If you're satisfied with the way that things are, then perhaps you don't need to do anything about it, at least until your circumstances change and you're expected to perform at a higher level.

Rewrite History: Understand Your Past (and Yourself) in a Different Way

Adults with undiagnosed ADHD know all too well the price they've paid and continue to pay for their struggles. They may not know *why* they struggle so much, but they know full well *how* they struggle. Until the day they received a diagnosis, though, they'd found various other explanations for the behaviors that had caused their difficulties. Most of these explanations tended to be pretty negative. Therefore, it's important to learn about the many ways that ADHD affects your life so that you can replace those old explanations with more accurate ones.

It's not just that it helps you feel better about yourself, as in, "I'm not a bad or selfish person, I just have this brain thing that makes me do these things." It also offers some hope that the future can be different if you address your ADHD in more targeted and effective ways. This will probably make you more likely to work hard on changing these habits since they may actually lead to positive changes. Before being diagnosed, it can be easy to give up after trying a thousand new surefire strategies that turned out to be duds. It's therefore crucial to see getting diagnosed as a fundamental transformation in your life, a break that separates the past from the future. Without this, there's no reason to try anything different or expect any better results.

I'll sometimes use the following joke with clients or during presentations to make the point that it's easy to come up with the wrong explanations for why certain things happen. This then influences what we do, even if our assumptions are wrong.

> Johnny and Sally decide that they are now old enough to be allowed to curse. They decide that they will each curse at breakfast and see what Mom does. As they walk into the kitchen, Mom asks, "What do you guys want for breakfast?" Johnny is the first to speak, saying, "What the hell, I'll have pancakes." Mom whacks his butt and sends him up to his room. She then turns to Sally and asks, "OK, what do

you want for breakfast?" Sally looks Mom in the eye and says, "I don't know, but it sure as hell won't be pancakes."

What makes this funny is the mistaken assumption—Sally assumes that Mom was upset about being asked to make pancakes, rather than the cursing. Similarly, those with undiagnosed ADHD (and their family members) attribute their struggles and failures to various character flaws, rather than to an untreated neurological condition. Therefore, learning that you have ADHD puts you in a position of examining all those old assumptions and perhaps replacing a lot of them. All that old stuff now makes sense in a completely different way. It's similar to how a major scientific discovery forces scientists to re-evaluate many other theories. For example, when it was discovered that disease was caused by bacteria rather than spirits, it changed everything about how doctors treated and prevented disease. In the same way, the ripple effects of your personal discovery can travel to the farthest reaches of your past and rewrite your history.

This affects not just the obvious stuff, like why you had such a hard time with homework or why you now forget to send out the bills, but also the less obvious stuff, like why you tend to be pessimistic about things working out well and have struggled with anxiety and depression. Untreated ADHD is a setup for these effects. That's the double-whammy of ADHD—first you suffer in the moment, then you carry that suffering with you as you face future challenges.

You can feel better about yourself and your prospects for a good future by really understanding your ADHD. This means that you do the following:

- *Understand* the many ways that ADHD affects your life, both currently as well as in the past
- *Fully accept,* without shame or defensiveness, that you have ADHD, as well as other strengths and weaknesses
- *Choose* to address the limitations that ADHD brings to your life, even when this means pushing yourself to do things that don't come easily

We can't change the facts and events from our pasts, but we can change our interpretations of what happened and therefore how those old lessons carry forward into the present and future. It's amazing how some optimism for the future will reduce the sting of past troubles.

Is ADHD an Excuse or an Explanation?

ADHD sometimes gets a bad rap because some people see it as excuses for bad performance. Obviously these people don't fully understand what ADHD is and how it affects all aspects of a person's life. I often talk to my clients about using ADHD as an explanation rather than an excuse. There are some really important differences between the two:

- *Excuses* let someone off the hook of his obligations because he is seen as simply not capable. As a result, excuses lower the bar for what is expected of him.
- *Explanations* help the person understand how and why things go badly and, more important, what she can do differently to increase the odds of success.

People who use excuses expect most of the change, flexibility, or accommodations to come from others. This is great when you can get away with it, but even the luckiest person will eventually come across someone who isn't willing to be so forgiving. As I sometimes tell clients, the electric company doesn't care if you have ADHD—they still want their payments on time.

By contrast, using ADHD as an explanation places most of the onus for improvement on you, whether it is to directly improve the situation or to make amends afterward. Explanations assume that we can't easily change the rules for individuals, at least not without paying an unacceptable price. For example, saying, "I have ADHD and therefore can't be expected to be on time," probably won't fly with most employers, friends, and romantic partners. In fact, they may be even angrier about your cavalier attitude than the fact that you were late. Therefore, the better approach is to really work on getting places on time and avoid their anger.

Although no one likes to admit that she blew it or that something is a real weakness, there's real power in that acceptance. If you expect the world to change for you, it means that you are powerless if other people decide to be sticklers. However, by learning about ADHD and how it affects your ability to get things done, you have the power to do things differently and thereby make things better yourself—a much better situation. By owning up to your weaknesses, you can take active steps ahead of time to minimize their negative effect on your life. This may include not putting yourself into no-win situations. You may not be able to change the fact that you have ADHD, but you *can* change what you do about it.

ADHD Is Bigger Than Good Intentions

Everyone has a gap between what they would like to do and what they actually do. Sometimes this means that we don't do enough of some things, like working out. Other times it means that we do too much of others, like eating junk food. For folks with ADHD, this gap between intentions and actions can feel even bigger.

We could say that ADHD is a disorder of actualizing good intentions. Even though their performance may sometimes suggest otherwise, ADHD folks almost always mean well. After all, why would someone bring these kinds of troubles onto herself if she could avoid it?

Living the life we feel we should takes hard work and hard choices. Doing the right thing requires the ability to resist temptation and distraction in the moment. When we don't do the right thing for ourselves, we are seen as self-indulgent. When we don't do the right thing for others, we are seen as selfish. I'm not sure which is better.

Resisting temptation involves sacrificing a small immediate reward for a larger later reward—for example, eating a salad rather than a cheeseburger in order to feel and look better in the long run, or going to the grocery store rather than watching TV. It's this ability to see beyond the temptation of the moment and into the future that allows adults to be successful—and is something that we work hard to train our kids to develop as they get older. This could be as simple as, "Put your jacket on before you go out so you don't get cold," or "You can borrow the car if you get all your homework done first."

Russell Barkley, Ph.D. created the response inhibition theory to explain why people with ADHD have the weaknesses that they do. (See *Response Inhibition* on p. 8 for more on this.) In order to make that better choice that will benefit us in the long run, we need to first resist the more immediate temptation. By inhibiting that immediate response, we have created a moment to think about what is the best course of action. This is where folks with ADHD run into trouble—their brains aren't as good at creating that moment of reflection, so they tend to respond more based on what is right in front of them or whatever pulls harder. Unfortunately, the stimuli that pull hardest on us are usually not as good for us. For example, a cheeseburger will almost always taste better than a healthy salad; watching TV will almost always be more fun than grocery shopping.

So even though ADHD folks mean well and want to do better when it's hypothetical ("I should order a salad at lunch today"), in the heat of the moment, that cheeseburger will pull really hard on their decision-making process. What this means is that, especially for folks with ADHD, it's best to avoid the temptation; it's much easier to do the right thing if you don't have bad things pulling on you. To tilt the odds of doing the right thing, keep these tips in mind:

- *Don't put yourself into situations that require more self-control than you're likely to be able to muster.* For example, when you have other things to do, just don't go to that website that you tend to spend too much time on. It will probably turn out to be for much more than "just a minute."

- *Eliminate distractions that are too likely to pull you off track.* For example, turn off your email alert when working on something more important.
- *Make the better choices loom larger in your decision-making process.* For example, if you're trying to lose weight, tape up a picture of someone in good shape or hang on the wall the outfit that you're trying to get back into. This may make the hypothetical idea of losing weight feel more real so it can compete more effectively with the temptation of unhealthy foods.

Calling All Frauds, Fakes, and Actors

Adults with ADHD tend to be very aware of their weaknesses and foul-ups, but may be less confident about their good qualities and successes. Unfortunately, many have learned over the years to doubt their abilities, since good skills and good intentions don't translate reliably enough into successes. When hard work and maybe a little bit of luck do yield something good, they may still doubt it. At the extreme, ADHD adults may feel like frauds who are just waiting to be found out—*Sure, I may have done a good job on that one project, but it's just a matter of time before I mess things up again.*

Especially after years of undiagnosed and untreated ADHD, it's easy to focus on your weaknesses. The antidote to that is to actively seek treatment for your ADHD, doing your best to improve your weaknesses while also accepting that some of those weaknesses will remain. This is easier to do if you value your strengths, too. Also, remember that everyone has both weaknesses and strengths; it may just be that ADHD weaknesses are more obvious or that you are more aware of your own weaknesses than others'. Nobody is good at everything. Everyone else has to work to achieve success despite their weaknesses; they may just be different weaknesses than those with ADHD struggle with.

It's easier to feel deserving of your successes, and less like a fraud, if you remember the following:

- Your successes are at least partially due to your good efforts and strengths, rather than just random luck. It was your good qualities that made it happen. Don't give your successes away.
- As a result, because your successes come from within you, they are repeatable. Doing the same things can lead to the same results next time. Maybe not every time, but at least sometimes.
- Everybody benefits from a lucky break sometimes, so enjoy them (and don't get too down on yourself when you get dealt a crummy

hand). However, good luck is also created. You can tilt the tides of fortune by laying a solid groundwork for your various activities. For example, the more resumes you send out, the more likely you are to get a good job. Leaving early will make it more likely that you get somewhere on time.

Perhaps the most insidious side effect of ADHD is that it causes people to doubt themselves, thereby stealing their desire to fully apply themselves. This creates a self-fulfilling prophecy. So take back your sense of effectiveness, throw yourself fully into your projects, and find the successes that lie within your grasp!

Is the Problem ADHD or Motivation?

Families and friends of ADHD people often struggle with this question—and so do the people with ADHD. The trouble is, ADHD can look like a motivation problem —*If only you cared more, then you would do better; If only you tried harder, then everything would be fine; If only....* People seem to think that the ADHD person just has to apply himself more. The other person will point out that the ADHD person does great when the activity is interesting, or maybe that he can do well on a task sometimes, but not always, which is confusing.

Most likely, the difficulties that the ADHD person is having are due to *both* ADHD and motivation, especially before the diagnosis is made and effective treatment implemented. Just like anyone, she doesn't enjoy doing things that hit her weaknesses or that too often work out badly, so she doesn't fully apply herself. Ta-da! Motivation problem. When she does fire herself up and try some new plan and program, she may do well for a little while when everyone is excited, but then real life crashes back in and all those new good habits go down the drain.

With every additional failure, she gets a little less excited for the next new system, since she's learned that not much changes, at least not for long. It takes guts to try something new, especially after repeated failures. Nobody wants to be disappointed again. Sometimes it feels less bad to fail by not trying than it does to try something and fail. The key is to believe it enough to, at least grudgingly, give it a shot. Try it enough to see if there is something to it.

Things Can Be Different

The way out of this pessimism is to work it from both sides, by addressing the neurology of ADHD and also digging deep for some motivation:

- *Learn as much as you can about ADHD.* This will give you a better chance of finding strategies that are more likely to be successful.

- *Actively seek treatment for your ADHD.* Medication, therapy, and coaching can all help you get more done.
- *Review strategies you've tried in the past.* What helped you perform at your best? Is there anything you can do differently this time to be more successful with it?
- *Accept that some things will be more difficult for you.* You're going to have to work a little harder on these things, just as others have to work harder on other things.
- *Maybe change your expectations.* Perhaps by lowering your goals you may be more motivated to work for a middle goal, rather than risk falling short of a more ambitious goal.

Keep the Momentum Rolling

Of course there are always ups and downs, but as successes begin to mount, it's easier to muster the motivation to apply the strategies that will help you get on top of your ADHD. The trick then is to keep that motivation strong when the inevitable backslides occur. Rarely is success a straight line. Expect the slips and recover as quickly as possible to avoid undoing the hard-fought progress. Eventually the progress will begin to top out and things won't change quickly anymore. Rather than getting disheartened, this may be the time to celebrate successes while also accepting that there may be a limit to how much progress can be made. Sometimes happiness is achieved by changing your expectations.

Just Do It

Woody Allen once said that 90 percent of success in life is just showing up. This is especially true when it comes to all the mundane tasks of life, such as paying bills, organizing, and cleaning. These are the sorts of tasks that we all need to do on a regular basis, even though we would rather be doing more interesting things. These tasks are not especially hard, but can cause big problems if they aren't done.

Unfortunately, people with ADHD tend to have great difficulty with consistently completing these sorts of activities. They may do them sometimes, but not often enough; they start them, but don't finish everything; or they do them, but too late. After a lifetime of these struggles, many of these ADHD adults add a layer of dread and avoidance to these tasks, so they are even less likely to work on them.

As a result, I often work with clients to make these tasks into less of a big deal—just show up and do them. No, these chores will never be enjoyable, but they still need to be done. Here are some pointers to help you get going:

- *Commit to do at least ten minutes of the activity.* If you get rolling with it, you can keep going. You're much less likely to start something that will feel like an endless marathon.
- *Build in rewards for completing the boring tasks by allowing yourself to do something more enjoyable.* This reward should be guilt free since you earned it. Don't undercut your successes by knocking yourself for needing these rewards. Instead, give yourself credit for being smart enough to find a strategy that works for you.
- *Designate at least one time per week when you tackle some of these mundane tasks.* Put up a sign to remind yourself, set an alarm, or ask someone to remind you. Do whatever it takes. Then push yourself to follow through.
- *Rotate between a few different boring activities, so the variety helps keep it interesting.* It's still not great, but at least it's a little better.

Do It Anyway: Avoid Avoidance

It seems like I spend a lot of time helping clients do the things that they know they should, but just can't get themselves to tackle. (Yes, I spend a fair bit of time helping them *not* do certain things also.) This is especially true among my ADHD clients. They know they should do certain things in order to be happier, calmer, or more successful, but can't get themselves going reliably enough. As Russell Barkley, Ph.D., has said, ADHD is not a disorder of knowing what to do; it's a disorder of doing what you know.

After a lifetime of struggle, of letting themselves and others down, it's easy to get a feeling of dread at the mere thought of certain types of tasks, so people with ADHD avoid those tasks to make themselves feel better—in the moment, at least. Of course, this psychological avoidance makes sense, in a way. The problem is that avoidance has a tendency of making things worse, creating a self-fulfilling prophecy wherein the undesirable task does become rather awful or works out badly if it's done at the last minute. For example, doing your taxes in a frantic overnight marathon makes it go from bad to worse.

The challenge is to push yourself through that bad feeling and get going on the dreaded task anyway. Yes, you will feel uncomfortable. Yes, you may even hate it—but you'll hate it less. Plus, you'll ideally have some worthwhile product to show for your efforts. When you find that you're trying to talk yourself out of doing something that you know you should do, do it anyway. When you find yourself avoiding something uncomfortable, do it anyway. When you find yourself dreading something, do it anyway.

When England was getting pounded by the Germans in World War II, Winston Churchill supposedly said something along the lines of, "When you're in the middle of hell, there's nothing to do but keep going." Exactly—rather than sit and suffer, keep moving. At those times, any action may be better than avoiding dealing with it. Any action may be more likely to get you out of the situation than doing nothing. At these times, think about approaching your challenges rather than avoiding them.

Change Your Mindset, Change Your Life

A lifetime of undiagnosed and untreated ADHD often leads to a predictable mindset. It colors how you think about yourself and your ability to be successful in the world. These expectations very much make sense, given your experiences, but don't need to be set in stone. Learning about your ADHD and understanding your strengths and weaknesses in a different way may give you some good reason to change your expectations. You may not even be fully aware of these expectations, since they can float under the surface of our thoughts, influencing how we feel about things without making themselves fully seen. It may take seeing a skilled therapist to become aware of how pervasively your mindset colors your expectations and affects your behavior. Whether you see a therapist or not, it's helpful to understand how your beliefs about yourself can play out.

So let's go over the beliefs that adults with ADHD tend to acquire (Rostain and Ramsay, 2006, p. 15):

- **Self-mistrust.** I can't rely on myself to do what I need to do. I let myself down.
- **Failure.** I've always failed and always will fail at what I set out to do.
- **Inadequacy.** I am basically a bad and defective person.
- **Incompetence**. I am too inept to handle life's basic demands.
- **Instability.** My life will always be chaotic and in turmoil.

It's easy to see how a lifetime of undiagnosed and untreated ADHD can lead to these beliefs. People with untreated ADHD often struggle to create the kinds of successes that would disprove these beliefs. Of course, it's also easy to see how these beliefs can create self-fulfilling prophecies. For example, someone who has been unsuccessful at certain tasks in the past probably doesn't have much reason to expect a better outcome this time, so she doesn't really try her best. Ta-da! The predictable poor performance reinforces the initial belief.

Therefore, just as untreated ADHD reinforces these beliefs, treating someone's ADHD may open up the possibility that things can be different, that maybe they don't have to hold onto those beliefs so tightly. It can be a fantastic moment of revelation and relief to realize that your future might, just maybe, be different than your past. As with any habit change, it's easy for us to keep going back to these core beliefs, even when we have experiences that contradict them.

So keep an eye out for them. Catch yourself thinking like this and then hammer at those thoughts with contradictory data—"Yes, I never achieved up to my potential in school, but now that I'm working on my ADHD, I'm better able to do what I need to do. Like how I got my report done with plenty of time before yesterday's meeting." If your mind is going to throw these beliefs at you, then make it prove them—if it says that you're a failure, then make it prove that you're incapable of success. Put the burden of proof on the negative beliefs. Maybe the best you can do is call it a draw—your mind can't prove that you're a failure, but you can't (yet) prove that you can be as successful as you want to be. So collect some more information to break the tie.

Since our habits tend to reinforce our beliefs (and vice versa), you may need to work on those too, so that you have some legitimate successes to throw at the negative beliefs. I talk about this in the next article, *Overcome Unhelpful Coping Strategies, Bad Habits, and Defense Mechanisms.*

Overcome Unhelpful Coping Strategies, Bad Habits, and Defense Mechanisms

As we discussed in the last article, *Change Your Mindset, Change Your Life*, adults with ADHD tend to develop certain mindsets. In this article, we will talk about the coping strategies, habits, and defense mechanisms that tend to reinforce (and be reinforced by) those beliefs.

Even though it can be easy to point out how a particular coping mechanism may bring more problems than solutions, we need to remember that these habits must have worked at one time. Maybe they weren't a perfect solution, but they were probably the best of what was available at the time. If none of your options are great, you go with the one that's the least bad. These habits that now may be really problematic must have done at least a little bit of good. So don't knock yourself if you realize that you use some of these—notice it, then push yourself to replace them with better habits. This involves not only choosing strategies that are more likely to give you successes, but also finding better ways of dealing with your emotions when you do encounter setbacks. Success and happiness requires both.

In *Unhelpful Coping Strategies* (p. 91), I described a number of the habits and defense mechanisms that adults with ADHD tend to use. In this article, we will talk about those same habits and defense mechanisms, but with an eye toward overcoming them.

Rationalization

When we're doing something we know we shouldn't (or not doing something we should) we convince ourselves that it's OK. We don't have to feel so guilty about it then. This convincing underlies all the other problematic coping mechanisms that we use. Therefore, even though it spares us the discomfort in the moment, rationalizing ultimately does us a disservice if it prevents us from using better coping skills or doing the better thing in the moment.

So when you get that guilty itch, when you know you're trying to talk yourself into something, stand firm. Be honest with yourself about what you're doing. You may still make the same choice (no one's perfect), but at least you're not making the situation worse by lying to yourself about it. It takes guts to be honest with ourselves. Even the most civilized among us can have some pretty nasty thoughts and brutal feelings. As long as you don't act on it, no problem. This honest self-acceptance may actually make you less likely to engage in other problematic behavior.

Externalizing

Externalizing involves blaming others or outside events when things work out badly—e.g., "He should've reminded me sooner," or "It would've been ready if the printer hadn't run out of ink right before the meeting." If we can blame someone else or make up convincing excuses, then we don't need to take personal responsibility for the problem. No one likes to admit that he screwed up, but there are times that we have to. If you have ADHD, it may feel like you get more than your fair share of these opportunities.

There are two reasons why it's better to just bite the bullet and own up to it. First, blaming others means that you were powerless over what happened and therefore will probably be powerless the next time something happens. Maybe I'm too much of a control freak, but I don't like the idea of throwing my fate to the winds. Instead, the reward for taking at least some responsibility for what happened is that you may be able to avoid this problem next time. Taking some responsibility doesn't mean that no one else played a part or that things couldn't have worked out better if someone else had done something different. It just means that you're owning up to your part.

The other reason why it's a good idea to own up to your part in things is that defensively denying it tends to really rub people the wrong way. In fact, the denial may aggravate people even more than the original problem. This may make them less likely to work with you collaboratively to solve the problem—or deal with you the next time they have a choice. People tend to be much less forgiving of those who blame others than they are of people who make mistakes.

There may be times when someone looks like he's externalizing, but actually isn't.

More so for people with ADHD, this denial is sometimes driven more by neurology than defensive psychology. For example, if someone isn't paying full attention and therefore doesn't really register what he is being told, then there's some justification for his claims of never being told. He was told, but since it never registered, he doesn't know that. This lack of a memory means that it's neither a lie nor externalizing, even though the person is wrong in what he's saying.

These misses, and similar situations, are a different kind of problem, which then require a different solution. For example, you may want to tell people to make sure they have your complete attention before telling you something. Once you find yourself in one of these situations, it's probably best to avoid a debate over what was or wasn't said and nondefensively admit that it's possible that you were told, but that you don't remember that, then get back to dealing with the situation as it currently stands. Of course, the ability to be gracious about this acceptance requires some strong acceptance of your tendency to miss things. Easier said than done, but worth working on, since it can stop a bad situation from getting worse.

Avoidance and Quitting

ADHD adults have difficulty starting and completing tasks. This is sometimes based in neurology when they can't fire their brains up for an uninspiring task. However, there could also be psychological reasons when they make a conscious choice not to deal with uncomfortable situations or those they fear will lead to failure. In addition to avoiding certain tasks, some people may also avoid social situations that they worry won't go well. Given their rich histories of painful experiences to draw from, it does make sense to avoid previously problematic situations because more of the same usually leads to more of the same. If their skills or circumstances haven't improved, then they would be foolish to expect different outcomes.

They may rationalize their avoidance to feel better about it. For example, they may tell themselves, "I'll wake up early on Saturday and do the grocery shopping when the store is less crowded, rather than doing it right after work today." Of course, the more likely outcome is that they don't go to bed early enough on Friday, setting themselves up to sleep in and get there when the store is even more crowded. However, having a plan in place (a bad one) makes it easier to justify not dealing with it in the moment. So be honest with yourself when your plans are more pipe dream than reality. To put it another way, given your track record, how much money would you be willing to bet on the plan working out?

In some cases, the avoidance is based on an accurate self-assessment that the demands exceed their abilities, causing justified feelings of hopelessness. For example, the person who doesn't have a functional organizational system may have good reasons to justify her avoidance of straightening up her office. It's easier then to simply not think about it, which brings some temporary relief from the stress. Fortunately, there are very few situations where we're completely incapable.

It may be that we're slower than or not as skilled as we wish we were, but we could still make some progress if we pushed ourselves. Or maybe we need to get someone else to help us or teach us the necessary skills. This effort is probably better than feeling forever haunted by these kinds of tasks. I can also say with some fair confidence that addressing your ADHD with an integrative treatment program (education, medication, coaching, and therapy) will make most challenges easier.

Sometimes the person starts the task, but bails out before finishing it. This is usually better than not starting it at all, so give yourself some credit for that. What caused you to lose steam? Did you get bored? Hit a tough spot that you didn't know how to overcome? Get distracted by something else? Run out of time? If you can identify why exactly you got off track, you may be able to prevent it next time.

It's worth pointing out here the concept of *conscious quitting*. This means making a careful assessment of the situation and deciding whether the task is still worth finishing or the goal still worth pursuing. It may be that it isn't. For example, when I was writing my dissertation in grad school, I had thought that I would try to publish it. Once I graduated, I realized that it would take much more work than I had thought. My interests had moved on by that point, too, so it just wasn't worth the effort. I decided that it was better to let it go, without too many regrets. If you make thoughtful decisions about these sorts of things, then there shouldn't be any shame associated with quitting, since sometimes discretion is the better part of valor. This is a situation where you should give yourself credit for being flexible, rather than stubbornly pushing something through to the bitter end. It may be that, in retrospect, you realize that there were things you could have done differently along the way that would have changed the outcome or made you more likely to finish it. Instead of beating yourself up for that, try to use that hindsight as a learning experience.

Procrastination

Most people with ADHD are more than familiar with procrastination (you know, it's that thing you do that your family and boss keep bugging you about). This is basically temporary avoidance, until the pressure of the last minute ignites them into activity. It's often the case that a far-off deadline doesn't have much motivational power, so any work that is done tends to be halfhearted. As the deadline gets closer, the pressure slowly begins to build until it reaches that critical mass that spurs them into motion. It's much easier to focus and apply their full effort at this point. (I call this last-minute pressure "nature's Ritalin.") It's true that the pressure improves performance, but only up to a point. If you wait too long, the stress becomes too much of a good thing and your performance starts to slide. It also leaves you vulnerable to unexpected setbacks, like printer problems, not having everything you need, or things taking longer than you expected. Procrastination also tends to make other people nervous, which tends to make them get on your case. So remind yourself of all this when tempted to put something off "just a little bit longer."

For some people, throwing things together at the last minute serves as a convenient excuse for a subpar work product—"Sure that report was pretty crummy, but I didn't start it until like an hour before the meeting." While there's some logic to this rationale, it also makes it unlikely that a good work product will be created, so the person is forced to settle for good enough (or worse). It's one of those situations of nothing ventured, nothing gained.

It can be helpful to take a few minutes to look at your schedule and to-do list, to see how this one project fits into all the rest. For example, while the project may not take that long, do you have so many other things going on that you won't have the necessary time later? It may take some real effort to make yourself sit down and go through all of your obligations, then plan out your time. Especially if this is a rather new experience, you may not be very good at it. A good coach or therapist may be able to teach you some helpful tricks or you may just want to keep practicing until you get better at it. By being able to see your full schedule, you may be able to see a bottleneck where you're going to have ten hours' worth of obligations but only five hours to do it. Simply being aware of that may not be enough to get you going earlier, but at least then you have the option.

Once you are aware, you may want to break a big project into several smaller pieces and create some intermediate deadlines. These deadlines might get you going sooner if you can hold yourself to them (or agree to have your boss or family member hold you to them). You may also be more likely to work toward one of those mini-deadlines since it isn't a big, hairy undertaking, so you have less reason to avoid it.

Pseudoproductivity

Pseudoproductivity consists of working on low-priority tasks, like checking email, rather than on higher-priority tasks, like writing a book on adult ADHD. Messing around with these somewhat important tasks creates a false sense of productivity that can be used to justify not working on the more important tasks. The person feels busy, but isn't actually using that time well. We all have certain tasks that we tend to use as time fillers when we don't feel inspired to work on what we should really be working on, but can't let ourselves get away with watching TV. The time fillers are either more enjoyable or don't take as much brain power, so they're easy to coast on. The good news about pseudoproductivity is that at least the person is getting *something* done, which in theory frees up time later for the more important tasks. This is a really slippery slope though, because it's easy to talk yourself into an endless flood of these preparatory activities without ever getting to the main act.

Since we all have our favorite time fillers, think about what yours are. What do you tend to do when you don't have the energy to tackle what you really should? What do you do at home and what do you do at work? It's easier to catch yourself sliding into these stall tactics if you identify them first. Then be eagle-eyed about spotting them. When you catch yourself starting one of these activities, be honest with yourself about whether it's really the best use of your time. Sometimes it will be. After all, the reason why we can get away with using these justifications is that there is occasionally some legitimacy to them. If it was never a good use of time, then it would be pretty tough to justify it. That's the slippery nature of pseudoproductivity. For example, there are definitely times that I need to check email, but probably not during my prime writing times. The key is discretion and good choices.

For more strategies, see *How to Be Productive, Not Just Busy* on p. 251.

Abandoning Ship

Abandoning ship involves jumping to new and thereby more interesting projects before completing earlier projects that have lost their shine. As with pseudoproductivity, because the person stays busy, she can justify her actions and feel good about all the progress that she's supposedly making. Unfortunately, most tasks in life don't get partial credit if they aren't finished.

Although it can be helpful to rotate among different tasks if that keeps you interested and energized, at some point you need to circle back and finish some of those projects. When you find yourself jumping around, give yourself some credit for the progress that you are making, but then ask yourself if there's anything that you're avoiding going back to. I know, I know, the new is always more exciting than the old, but the old still needs to be completed. It may also be easier to finish something if you don't have a bunch of other, more exciting projects in view at the time, so you're less likely to be tempted by them. You may also want to ask your obsessive-compulsive friends to explain that feeling of satisfaction that they get from checking things off. Even if you can't relate, it may still be entertaining.

Quasi–Obsessive-Compulsive Behavior

Some adults check things repeatedly (e.g., "Did I turn off the stove?"). This can look a little like obsessive-compulsive disorder, except that it has more of a basis in reality. People with ADHD have a fair likelihood of actually having left the stove on, whereas those with OCD rarely do but still feel compelled to check it. Some adults with ADHD may also stick rigidly with their routines as a way to ensure that things get done right—for example, their keys always have to go in the same place, and they get really angry if anyone moves them. Or they may become hyperorganized because anything less than that too quickly degenerates into total chaos.

If you find yourself doing any of this, remember that it's a fairly reasonable attempt to compensate for ADHD weaknesses. You have good reason for doing what you do, you're just doing too much of it. That is, some checking is a good thing, but too much isn't. Having a routine is good, but being rigid isn't. Dialing it back a click or two may put you right where you need to be. Usually when we push things to extremes, we wind up expending more energy without getting enough back for it, whereas the middle ground tends to give the best returns on our efforts. As you really begin to treat and get on top of your ADHD, you will perhaps find that you don't need the extremes any more.

Controlling or Aggressive Behaviors

In response to the common feeling of powerlessness that many with ADHD experience, some people go to the other extreme and become dictatorial. This often comes from feeling out of control inside, so they try to overcontrol what goes on outside of themselves, in an effort to make things work out better. Although it tends to rub people the wrong way, it comes out of a sincere and understandable desire to feel less overwhelmed. So their intentions are good, even if it comes with a high price tag.

If you find yourself doing this, try to remind yourself that quantity is no substitute for quality. That is, by letting go of some things, you can have more control over others. Be selective about what you try to control. Focus on the things that really count. Pick your battles—and be sure to factor in the collateral damage to relationships and your stress level. You might find it easier to let go once your ADHD is treated and you begin to adopt more effective coping skills and strategies.

After a lifetime of being criticized, punished, and told that they're doing things wrong, many adults with ADHD tend to assume that others have a negative intent as soon as anything happens, so they jump too quickly to the defensive. Or maybe they even jump too quickly to offense. This mindset makes sense given their history, but they may still be seeing more negativity than is really there. The problem is that firing that negativity back at the other person tends to make her negative, even if she didn't start out that way. So it can become a self-fulfilling prophecy. Therefore, especially as you get on top of your ADHD, try to defer judgment until you know for sure that the person is being negative. If she is being negative, then respond to it, but don't create the situation you're trying to avoid.

Learned Helplessness

After a lifetime of things not working out as well as they should, it's easy to expect the worst on your next attempt. As a result, many adults with ADHD won't try their best since it doesn't seem worth the extra effort. As much as this kind of makes sense before realizing that ADHD was the unidentified trip wire, getting diagnosed completely changes the odds of success. By addressing those ADHD deficits explicitly and effectively, you're much more likely to be successful.

There are two lessons in this. First, make understanding and treating your ADHD a part-time job, at least until you mostly get on top of it. Work at it. You owe it to yourself. Second, remember that the better you do with your ADHD, the more likely you are to be successful with your next endeavor. The odds are starting to move in your favor. Maybe some of your prior challenges are worth attempting again. You might even want to stretch yourself and try some things that you never before had the guts to. If you do fall short, look at it as a learning experience, something to learn from and do better the next time. This mindset of getting back on the horse is crucial to progress. See *Failures Lead to Successes (and Better Self-Esteem)* on p. 217 for more on this key component of resiliency.

Impulsively Rushing

Some people with ADHD impulsively rush through boring, difficult, or burdensome tasks in order to get done as quickly as possible to minimize their suffering. Of course, this makes mistakes much more likely and leads to a worse final product. The problem is that these self-fulfilling prophecies undercut any chance of a better life.

No one likes dragging out the suffering, but there may be a balance to strike where you spend at least a little longer in order to increase the chances of getting a better result. You may need to evaluate the situation and decide whether it's worth the extra effort—some are, some aren't. The trick is figuring out which make the cut and then pushing yourself to make the most of them. As with learned helpless, some of these tasks may be less awful and more likely to be successful once your ADHD is treated.

Cavalier Lifestyle

Following a lifetime of inability to function by the "normal" rules of society, some ADHD adults may give up and embrace the chaos in their lives. For example, they may rationalize it with, "Sure, things are always chaotic for me, but that's just the way I like to live my life. I'm not confined by others' rules." Teens are probably even more likely to take this mindset. For many of these folks, this carefree attitude is really a cover for the deep pain and frustration of not being able to live up to others' expectations. This casual disregard often drives other people to try to convince the person with ADHD that he *should* want to live by those rules. To the person with ADHD, this feels like an effort to convince pigs that they should want to fly.

I can certainly appreciate feeling that it isn't worth fighting destiny, but I would question whether your fate is in fact set. There's a difference between adopting a laid-back lifestyle because it's what really works best for you and settling for one because you don't feel as if you have any other options. My hope is that you can see that you do have at least some options and therefore don't have to settle for something less than what you want. So ask yourself whether you really do have to choose this cavalier lifestyle, or whether you might be able to pull off something better. If you really tried, could you do it?

Failures Lead to Successes (and Better Self-Esteem)

There are few challenges in life that can be completed successfully the first time. At least the big ones. We could kind of say that success involves overcoming failure. Too many adults with ADHD have plenty of experience with failure, but not as much as they want with the overcoming part. As a result, they may be prone to abandon ship at the first sign of trouble. This is unfortunate because there's a lot to be learned from failures if we can hold on to our self-esteem and not be flooded with shame. This means staying in the present moment, focusing only on the current setback without dragging out every single stumble over the course of your life. It may be OK to consider some other similar situations if you want to look for a pattern. But there's no character assassination going on here—if it doesn't bear directly on the current situation, then push it out of your mind.

The problem with being too hard on yourself and trotting out all the ghosts of failures past is that it understandably makes you hesitant to take any chances or even get your hopes up. Why would you risk that torture if you didn't have to? This puts a real limit on trying new skills and novel experiences.

The way out of this dilemma is to reframe how you see failure. If it's an indictment of your character ("I'm a loser—I always screw things up") then you'd have to be pretty foolhardy to take any chances. It's like standing in the middle of a minefield—the smartest thing to do is stay right where you are, rather than risk getting blown up. By contrast, if you can see it as a learning experience, then you win either way. If it works out well, then you have something to feel good about. If it doesn't work out well, then you have some homework to do to figure out what happened or what you could do differently next time. Truthfully, even if it worked out well, you probably still have some things you could improve.

When faced with a challenge that you're hesitant about, give yourself permission to fail. You'll be more likely to attempt it that way—and more likely to learn something from the process when you're not flooded with anxiety beforehand and shame afterward. This willingness to take a chance is part of the trial-and-error process, and therefore the only real failures are missed opportunities or setbacks that aren't learned from. Those are the real failures, because they don't move you forward, a little wiser than beforehand. Even a total failure is progress because you've ruled out one way that doesn't work. It may take you some time to figure out what that was exactly. Sometimes, as the weeks and even years go by, we gain a deeper understanding of what happened.

Here's a simple example. My roof was leaking in my kitchen, so up I go with a can of patching compound. I patched all the likely culprits (and a few unlikely ones, just for good measure). Of course, this isn't where the story ends. Next big storm, water starts coming in again (literally while I'm painting the kitchen—seriously). I was totally dumbfounded because I thought I had patched everything. Back up on the roof I go, trying to find something other than the obvious spots I had already fixed. Maybe it had been leaking from them also, so perhaps there was less water afterward, but I clearly hadn't solved the problem completely. So I look and look, including in the less obvious places. That's when I see that there's a rotted-out hole under the roof's edge—exactly the kind of thing that would leak during big storms, but not small ones. Mission accomplished (so far. . .). This is how most complex problems are solved—in stages. We start with the obvious stuff and then move on to less obvious possibilities when we have to. So as long as you're trying new things, you're still moving forward.

If you find yourself hesitant to pursue that daring goal or even just try something different, give yourself permission for that, too. We're not striving for recklessness, but rather for decisions that are thoughtful, rather than emotional and reactive. You may need to mull it over more before you're ready to take the leap. Whatever you attempt is more likely to be successful once your ADHD is being treated. That's often a key missing ingredient beforehand. If you're really feeling hesitant, keep the following advice in mind:

- *Go easy on yourself.* It's normal to feel hesitant.
- *Make this challenge part of your larger goals.* If overcoming this challenge brings you closer to something else that's important to you, then it may be worth taking that chance.
- *Brainstorm new approaches.* If you want the result but aren't sure that your current methods will get you there, see what else you can come up with. Then ask others for suggestions.
- *Bite the bullet.* At some point you just have to jump off the cliff. It's your life, and no one is going to live it for you.

This isn't the empty and annoying optimism reflected in clichés like "All you have to do is put your mind to it." This is about taking reasonable and necessary risks to achieve the things that are important to you. It's about creating a future that's different from your past. Most important, it's about changing your whole mindset so that you are willing to take chances. If you can do that, you'll create a future that's better than your past.

Can I Trust Myself?

When you make a commitment to yourself or others to do something, can you rely on yourself to do it? Will it get done in the way that was promised? And on time? For too many ADHD adults, the answer to these questions is, *I would like to think so, I hope so, but I just don't know, and deep down I suspect the answer is no.* Despite great intentions, many adults with ADHD have learned to doubt themselves.

- *Looking backward.* When they complete something or look back on their day, they may wonder whether they've done everything that they should have. They may say to themselves, "I'm pretty sure I did everything, but I've been burned before when it turned out later that I had forgotten some important things." So it's hard to ever feel really confident that there isn't a ticking time bomb out there somewhere. This makes it really hard to relax.
- *Looking forward.* When they make a commitment to do something, either to themselves or someone else, a voice inside may say, "I hope you can do this. These sorts of things tend to not work out so well. Your batting average should be higher." The lessons of the past carry forward to cause doubt for the future.

The unfortunate reality here is that their skepticism actually has some truth to it—they haven't been able to be as reliable as they would like, so they have some good reason to doubt. But what also often happens is that they take this doubt too far—they generalize it and worry about everything or get really down on themselves, even for the little stuff. The problem is that they don't know when they can legitimately relax because they've taken care of everything or when they just don't know yet that they should be worried. It would be great to be able to tell that difference so that they could actually enjoy themselves sometimes.

So how do you learn to trust yourself more? Actively treating your ADHD will give you more confidence in your judgment. You should also try the following strategies:

- *Really work on incorporating to-do lists and a planner.* I know, I know, you hate these things and they never worked in the past. So find a system that works for you, rather than one that works for your obsessive-compulsive friend. You're more likely to stick with a system that fits your way of thinking and is easier to use. However, you still need to push yourself to stick with it rather than give in to the temptation of thinking you'll remember something without writing it down. You won't.

- *Don't overcommit yourself.* Be honest with yourself about what you can realistically handle so that you don't set yourself up for trouble. Most people prefer to hear a no early, when they still have time to plan accordingly, rather than later when it puts them in a bind. Stop and think for a moment before agreeing to do anything.
- *Accept that sometimes you'll blow it.* Everybody makes mistakes, so don't go overboard with the guilt, since it only makes you less likely to use effective strategies to fix the situation. A little anxiety keeps us all honest, but too much of it causes our brains to shut down so we don't think as clearly. Try to be diligent, but then don't fret over what might be. By relaxing when you can, you'll be better able to deal with situations when they do arise.
- *Learn to fix problems gracefully*. Since you'll never be able to eliminate problems altogether, work on undoing the damage afterward. Face the problem honestly and directly and offer to make amends. Don't take it as an opportunity to knock on yourself for screwing up again. See *The Value of a Good Apology* on p. 318 for more on this.

Take Charge of Your Life

For too many adults with untreated ADHD, life can feel like a runaway train—it keeps barreling along while they hold on as best they can. Therefore, an important goal of treatment (and this book) is to give you a greater feeling of control over your fate. This often involves seeing your ADHD as a challenging fact of life that can be actively managed. By clarifying the beliefs you have about yourself, your ADHD, and how your ADHD affects your interactions with others, you can identify how those beliefs prompt certain behaviors and coping strategies that cause you too much trouble. You can then replace them with better strategies and techniques.

Many ADHD adults suffer from the feeling that they don't have enough control over their lives—including their own thoughts and actions. The solution is to try to increase the amount of control you do have, as well as accept the fact that certain areas are beyond your control or will always be weaknesses. This brings us to an important concept that you might have seen in an intro psych class, if you took one. The concept is *locus of control* (LOC), which basically involves how much control you feel you have over what happens in your life. People with an internal LOC feel that they are the ones primarily driving their fate, whereas those with an external LOC feel that other people or events are the major cause of what happens to them. Then there are those with a mixed LOC, who feel that they have some control over what happens but recognize that external factors play a role too.

As you might expect, studies have found that a mixed LOC tends to work out best for most people, including those with ADHD (Goldstein, 2006, October). They don't overrely on others to manage their lives, yet neither do they fault themselves for every bad situation. This allows them to actively manage their lives, yet also bounce back when they get a bad break on something. So, when it comes to sorting out how much responsibility we each have for what happens in our lives, I often use this example: if you invited friends over for a barbecue, you can blame yourself for not buying enough hot dog buns, but you shouldn't blame yourself for the rain. It's important to find that middle ground, because going too far toward either extreme can cause problems. Let's talk about that.

Some people blame themselves for every little thing that goes wrong, whether they had anything to do with it or not. They're so used to being responsible for things that go wrong, that they automatically assume they had something to do with each new problem. Their inconsistency makes them easy targets. This can create a situation where others don't take enough responsibility for their contributions to the problem because the person with ADHD is taking too much—for example, the person with ADHD doesn't do something that his girlfriend wanted because she yelled it across the house while running out the door. That's just a setup for trouble, even for someone without ADHD. As a result, putting all the blame onto her ADHD boyfriend's forgetfulness means that she doesn't have to work on communicating more effectively. As long as he takes all the blame, she won't work seriously on her contribution, so the same problems will keep coming up. Therefore, as the person with ADHD does better, it also tends to push these other people to work on things too, which is to everyone's benefit.

At the other end of the spectrum, some people with ADHD don't feel that they're at fault for much of anything. They see the world as unfair and that people are too often angry at them for no good reason. If everyone else would just chill out, everything would be fine. What they don't see is how their ADHD causes them to do things that upset others, like interrupting, forgetting, or running late. So these other people have some good reasons for feeling frustrated, even if they blow their credibility by acting like a lunatic. If the person does see the effect of his actions, he may not have workable solutions to those problems ("I just need to knuckle down and try harder"). Unlike the people with the overly internal LOC, those with too much of an external LOC need to work on taking a more active role in shaping what happens, so they can feel less like a victim of circumstances.

Those who are most successful in life find the middle road and tend to share these characteristics:

- *Success* comes from their own hard work and good qualities, so they can repeat it. Luck may help, but it isn't the main reason.

When necessary, they ask for help appropriately while maintaining responsibility for the outcome.

- *Failure* comes from modifiable factors, like not trying hard enough or weak skills that the person can strengthen. They might be able to do things differently next time and create a better result.
- *Challenges* bring out their best, as they dig deep, try new strategies, and reach out for help or guidance, including treatment. As the challenge increases, they work harder and smarter, without retreating, giving up, or rigidly sticking with failing strategies. If necessary and appropriate, they concede defeat and move on.

It can be helpful to think about where you fall on this LOC spectrum. Since you're reading this book, I'm going to assume that you feel as if you have some hope of making positive changes in your life. (And if you're the family member reading this book, I'm going to hold out hope for the ADHD person in your life and you, too.) This will have a big impact on your willingness to try some new strategies and stick with your treatment program, even when it feels like climbing uphill. If you feel pessimistic, then boost your optimism by starting with something small that has good odds of immediate success. If you tend to look to others to make decisions for you, then push yourself to come up with your own solutions, even if they aren't the best solutions possible. Some adults with ADHD exaggerate how easily others achieve success, which sets an impossible and demotivating standard.

A complete treatment program will help you with finding that middle ground. Medication and coaching help you be more effective, so you can feel that you do have that necessary control. Meanwhile, learning about ADHD and maybe doing some therapy can help you let go of unproductive self-blame. When you get down to it, this LOC stuff is really fundamental to success and happiness, since it determines how you respond to your world and create the situations that you desire.

Is ADHD a Gift?

If ADHD is a gift, then why does my present suck so much?

With laserlike precision and stunning bluntness, a woman with ADHD perfectly captured the problem with the idea that ADHD confers some sort of positive qualities. I will also be so bold as to assume that you wouldn't be wasting your time and money on this book if you were reveling in the joys of untreated ADHD.

Despite these well-documented struggles, there is still this conventional wisdom out there that ADHD has positive qualities—for example, that it gives people greater energy, intelligence, spontaneity, creativity, fun, and artistic abilities. Related to this, some people claim that having ADHD makes a person more successful at certain careers, such as entrepreneurship, sales, military service, computers, arts, or hands-on jobs. Rather, I would say it isn't that they are extra-talented in these areas *because of* their ADHD, so much as that their weaknesses are less problematic or better tolerated in those careers. While I totally agree with the well-meaning motives behind helping ADHD folks feel better about themselves and their various struggles, there are some important problems with this tactic.

The first problem is that it just isn't true. Research has consistently found that ADHD does not give any kind of advantage. The handful of studies that found things like greater intelligence had serious problems in their design, making the results questionable (Goldstein, 2002). By contrast, there are hundreds of studies that document the many and pervasive problems associated with ADHD (if you're reading this book, you don't need to read the studies to know this is true).

Of course, people with ADHD have all sorts of good qualities, but it isn't *because of* their ADHD. This is the key point and where some people draw connections that don't exist. It's like saying that blondes have more fun—some of them do, but some of them don't, and in either case it has nothing to do with the color of their hair. The person with ADHD would have those same positive qualities even if he were born without ADHD, so we shouldn't draw a causal connection between the two.

The second problem with touting ADHD's benefits is that a lot of people have worked really hard to gain legal protections and accommodations in school and at work for folks with ADHD. To talk about the positive qualities gives ammunition to the critics who would like to remove those protections. After all, why should we spend extra money and force teachers and employers to go out of their way for these blessed individuals? It also hurts researchers who are fighting for precious grant funding.

Finally, touting ADHD's positive qualities also undermines the need for treatment—after all, why should we treat something that brings all these benefits? Wouldn't that risk losing the good with the bad?

A Better Way

So, rather than relying on something that is incorrect, it's more helpful to keep in mind that you are more than your ADHD, that you have your own particular mix of strengths and weaknesses and your own personality. We all face the challenge of making the most of what we have to achieve what we want. Therefore, since you have all those good qualities anyway, it isn't necessary to assume that they came from your ADHD. If you're creative, then run with it. If you have above-average intelligence, then use it to your advantage.

I'll go into this in more detail in the remainder of this chapter, but in short, you can work on valuing your strengths while accepting your weaknesses with the following advice in mind:

- *Build your weaknesses as best you can, whether they are ADHD based or not.* We don't get to choose our weaknesses, but we do have some choice over what we do about them.
- *Use your strengths to work around the weaknesses that you can't improve.* Don't feel as if you have to do things the way other people do if it doesn't work for you. Use your strengths creatively to make up for skills that you're weak in. It's better to do it differently than not do it at all.
- *Be smart about the situations that you put yourself in.* There's no pride in stubbornly putting yourself into no-win situations. For example, if it's really hard for you to get to work on time, then maybe find one that is more flexible about that. If you can't change your abilities, then change the demands that are placed on you.

Build Healthy Self-Esteem

I'm all in favor of helping people to feel good about themselves, but it's easier said than done. Understanding this process can help you not only explain your past, but also guide your efforts in the present to help you feel better about yourself.

We get our self-esteem and sense of who we are from two related places:

- *What we actually do.* Obviously, we feel good about the things we do well and tend to feel badly about the things we do poorly. Those with ADHD or another learning disability may have a lower ratio of the two than they want. Over a lifetime, this can affect how they feel about themselves.
- *What we make of those experiences.* We aren't robots who automatically click our self-esteem up a notch for every success and down one for every failure. Instead, we interpret our experiences and try to figure out what they mean. We also rely on others' reactions to our actions to help us determine whether something was good or bad and whether it was a big deal. (Think of the different reactions your teen friends had to some of your actions compared to your parents and teachers.)

So what this means is that we have two ways to improve self-esteem—actually perform better (this is where medication and coaching often come in) and change how we interpret what we do (this is where learning about ADHD and therapy come in). As you might imagine, the best outcomes are achieved by working it from both sides.

Although we should be supportive of each other, simply telling someone nice things doesn't ultimately amount to much if they don't have some good experiences to base those comments on. The problem with relying on the nice comments is that it can be too easily undone by someone who says not-so-nice things.

This brings us to the concept of *earned self-esteem* that is based on actual successes in meeting life's challenges. Because it's based on positive experiences, it's hard won and develops slowly, but is stable and long lasting. Facing challenges and sometimes falling short creates a temporary blow to self-esteem, but can actually lead to greater self-esteem if the person rises up and overcomes the challenge. (If at first you don't succeed. . .) Life is obstacles, so it's important to have faith in your ability to survive hitting a brick wall and to figure out a way around it next time—there are always more challenges and they tend to get bigger as we get older. Luckily, we also tend to get wiser.

Earned self-esteem is based on realistic accomplishment. Each success creates a step up the ladder of future success as the person sharpens her skills by really pushing herself and also builds confidence that she can handle the next challenge. This is as true of training for a marathon as it is of moving your way up at work or raising children. Unfortunately, too many folks with ADHD don't have enough of this successful progression from smaller to greater challenges. They have some successes, but then also have a bunch of sometimes inexplicable failures ("That was so easy—how could I possibly have screwed it up?"). There is a momentum to both success and failure and to a person's subsequent willingness to take realistic chances. This inconsistent performance can make someone with ADHD uncertain about what they can reliably handle, so she may then be leery of taking much on.

What this means is that simply telling someone that he can do anything he puts his mind to is actually a disservice if it sets him up to take on more than he can handle. The likely failure will do far more harm than the cheerleading words did good (it also tends to blow the cheerleader's credibility). After hearing too many of these kind words from people with good intentions but insufficient knowledge of ADHD, it can be easy to be skeptical about any encouraging words. The key then is to figure out which encouraging words you can believe and which are just wishful thinking—or, to put it another way, which challenges you can overcome and how you can adjust your strategies to make that happen.

For everyone, self-knowledge sets the foundation for success because they can make informed choices about which challenges to take on and under what circumstances. This means being honest with yourself not only about the situations to *not* take on, but also about how you work best and what it takes for you to get the job done. Give yourself credit for what you do well, without diminishing it with what you do badly. As I talk about throughout this book, there are lots of ways to bolster the areas that you're weak in, so the harder that you work at it, the more progress you will make. At the end of the day, though, you also need to accept the fact that you won't be good at everything and that some weaknesses will remain that you need to find workarounds for.

Related to this, give yourself credit for the ways that you have found to get things done, even if they're really different from the ways that others function. Every single client I've seen has figured out some good ways to get things done, even if they didn't fully understand why these were good strategies for them or how they took their ADHD into account. For example, I had a client who never found himself without a necessary schoolbook when doing homework because he always brought home every single book, even if he didn't think he needed them all. This simple solution saved him a lot of heartache. Rather than beat yourself up about having to be different or take it as some sort of proof of your inferiority, give yourself credit for being smart enough to figure out an effective strategy. The less self-conscious you feel about it, the more likely you are to use it and the more likely you are to get the job done—which is really what counts.

Adversity Makes You Stronger (Hopefully)

It's been said that whatever doesn't kill you makes you stronger, which is true, but only sometimes. I would change it to say that it *might* make you stronger. Whether it does or doesn't depends on what you make of it. Some people allow adversity to make them angry, bitter, pessimistic, or defeated, whereas for other people it brings out their best. Adversity can take many forms—ADHD is one, but it could also be a difficult family situation, unexpected job loss, or health difficulties. We all have our struggles, but if ADHD is one of yours, it's easy to see that more clearly than other people's or to feel that no one else has the kinds of problems that you do. Of course, since about 4 percent of adults have ADHD, we know you have plenty of company, but even beyond that, it may just be that others' struggles aren't so visible. For example, I have a client with severe fibromyalgia that really limits her life, yet you would never know it by looking at her. So don't assume other people's lives are all roses and sunshine.

Living with and at least partially overcoming your ADHD definitely brings its challenges. The research very clearly demonstrates that. But it may also give you something to feel good about as you put together a good life for yourself despite your difficulties. In fact, some might even say that we gain wisdom and peace not despite our struggles, but because of them. We may not have much choice about which crummy cards we're dealt in life, but we do have some choice regarding what we do about them and what kind of an effect we let them have on us. Being angry about them doesn't make them go away. So, given what your life has looked like until now, what do you want it to look like from this point forward?

Is Life a Journey or a Destination?

Is life a journey or a destination? And does the answer matter for adults with ADHD? The answers are that life is both, and yes. Some activities are more about enjoying the journey, such as spending time with family and friends, watching a movie, or clicking around the Net. It's more about enjoying the process, regardless of where you wind up. Other things are more about the destination and having a finished product, such as completing a report for work, going grocery shopping, and getting the bills into the mail.

ADHD folks can be very good at enjoying the journey, but often have difficulty consistently reaching their intended destinations and bringing things to completion—the report isn't quite finished, the groceries are still sitting on the counter, and the bills don't quite make it into the mailbox. These sorts of tasks have an important destination, but the journey isn't particularly enjoyable, so it's hard for the ADHD adult to stick with it—they wind up on other journeys instead. Unfortunately, many of these tasks don't get much partial credit if they aren't finished, so the ADHD adult is judged and criticized.

Other than hiring a personal assistant to take care of all the boring details of life, what is the ADHD adult to do?

- *Recognize that these destination tasks have a boring journey.* Accept it. You will have to work much harder to keep going on these—and keep going you must. Fighting against it just gets you worked up and makes the journey worse.
- *Balance destination activities with journey activities.* It's easier to gut it out on the boring stuff if you have some enjoyable activities mixed into your day, too. (But not too many.)
- *Try to make destination activities more enjoyable.* For example, put on music or TV while folding laundry. Just be sure the fun thing doesn't take over getting to your destination.
- *Farm out the destination activities that you are weakest at or hate the most.* Either hire someone or make a deal with your romantic partner, family member, friend, or neighbor to do it for you, in exchange for something you will do for them. It has to be a fair trade or it won't last.

If you can manage the destination activities effectively, then you can enjoy your other journeys guilt free, without a nagging voice in your head (or in the living room) telling you what you should be doing instead.

Roll Back Anxiety and Depression

Adults with ADHD are more likely to feel anxious or depressed than people without it. Some of them have mild or transient symptoms, whereas others are suffering enough to officially qualify for a second (or third) diagnosis. I usually find that my clients' untreated ADHD is driving at least some of that anxiety and depression. It makes sense—untreated ADHD gives you plenty to worry and feel bad about, since things tend to not work out the way you might hope or expect. I will sometimes tell clients that they have good reasons to be anxious and depressed—given their life history, they'd have to be kind of clueless to not feel bad. (Of course, they wouldn't be sitting in my office if they didn't feel bad.) I'm blunt like this because I don't want them to feel bad about feeling bad or feel as if they have too many diagnoses. These things are all connected.

At the risk of seriously oversimplifying, anxiety comes from feeling as if our demands exceed our abilities, and depression comes from feeling powerless to improve our situation and hopeless that it will get better. These should be rather familiar feelings for those with untreated ADHD.

Fortunately, just as untreated ADHD drove these other conditions, so too does improvement in ADHD symptoms lead to other gains. They justifiably feel more on top of their demands and more optimistic that things can work out well. I make a point of telling my newly diagnosed clients this. It also gives them even more reason to work on their ADHD. My hope is that you will get a two-for-one in a positive way, just as you got it in a negative way. That is, just as untreated ADHD made you feel worse, perhaps treating the ADHD will make you feel better—even if you don't explicitly work on that.

Unfortunately, both anxiety and depression rob us of motivation to try something new or fully apply ourselves. This can create a dilemma where the person needs some improvements in order to feel better, but she has trouble getting going until she has those improvements. If you can't gut it out and make yourself get going, you may need to work on the anxiety and depression directly. This can mean reading one of the many good books on the topic, seeing a therapist, or even taking medication. My hope would be that this would enable you to get over the hump so that you have a fighting chance of dealing with your ADHD. As your mood improves, you should be better able to work on your ADHD.

Since most books on anxiety and depression don't discuss how ADHD can contribute to these conditions, you will need to add that part in yourself. That means learning about your ADHD. The same goes for a therapist that you might see—aim to find one who understands ADHD in adults and can help you work on everything, but you may need to be the ADHD expert in the room and educate your therapist about how it contributes to how you feel. This isn't ideal, but sometimes you have to make the best of what's available.

Manage Excessive Substance Use and Other Addictive Behavior

Perhaps because of their greater need to self-medicate, or perhaps because they tend to be more impulsive, adults with ADHD are more likely to abuse substances or have trouble with other addictive behaviors than those without ADHD. This includes people who drink too much but wouldn't be called alcoholics, as well as people who have tendencies toward compulsive behaviors like overspending, overeating, overusing sex, and gambling. I can understand the desire to feel better and that a few drinks or whatever may help some people to do that. Unfortunately, this solution can become its own problem if it becomes excessive. So if you have more than two drinks a night, use other drugs, or engage in other addictive behaviors, you need to be honest with yourself about the effect that it's having on you. Keep in mind who your comparison group is. For example, you may not feel that you drink much since many of your friends drink the same amount. However, that may not be a good measure, since we tend to choose friends who are similar to us—if you drink too much, they probably also drink too much.

Potential warning signs of excessive substance use can be as follows:

- You do things that you wouldn't do sober, such as spending money, arguing or fighting, engaging in sexual activities, or other high-risk behaviors.
- You get into arguments about your drinking or drug use.
- You spend too much money or time on it.
- You're not as sharp the next day.

If you feel that too many of these apply to you, you may want to think seriously about cutting back or stopping the use altogether. My basic recommendation is that it's OK to cut back but still use sometimes—as long as you're able to keep that use within acceptable limits. I won't say it's good for you, but we all have our vices.

If you feel that you don't have a true addiction, but that you would be better off if you used less, you may be able to kill two birds with one stone by treating your

ADHD. I've found that many of my clients simply have less desire to overuse once they get some control over their ADHD and life. Without even really thinking about it, they just don't engage in that problematic behavior as much. It makes sense—as they feel more on top of their lives and their overall mood improves, the escape offered by drinking too much, or whatever, may become less necessary or appealing.

If you aren't able to keep it reined in and you wind up getting into trouble again, then you may want to think about stopping completely. If you can do this on your own, then that's great. If you can't, you may want to consider getting some help with it. It's hard to make progress on your ADHD, or much of anything else, if your addictive behavior is making a mess of things. In this case, you may need to get that under control first by seeking treatment for the addictive behavior.

Unfortunately, many prescribers are hesitant to prescribe stimulants, the most effective medication for ADHD, to people with a strong history of addiction. This is especially unfortunate because untreated ADHD can make it harder for some people to stay clean. Therefore, you may need to settle for one of the nonstimulants, at least until you get enough clean time under your belt that the prescriber feels more comfortable. Meanwhile, you can work with a therapist on other ways of coping with the urge to use.

Some people find AA, NA (Narcotics Anonymous), or other twelve-step groups helpful, whereas others find them kind of culty. Some people are also turned off by the religious overtones. It depends a lot on the specific group that you attend and also on what you make of it. If you don't like the first group you attend, then try another one and see if the chemistry is better there. As with many things in life, you may need to ignore the negatives and focus on the positives if there are some helpful things about attending.

However, if you're taking medication, especially one of the stimulants, you may find that there are some attendees who will take issue with that. They may see it as cheating on your sobriety and no different than taking street drugs, even though you have a valid prescription and legitimate reason for it. Although presumably well intentioned, this rigid attitude is usually counterproductive and underinformed. These people probably don't understand ADHD and how it can affect your sobriety when untreated, and that there is no high from normally prescribed doses. So you may want to think about whether you want to disclose at meetings that you're taking medication. If you do disclose, you may want to have some prepared thoughts about how to respond to these comments. You certainly don't have to justify yourself to anyone, but it may minimize a conversation that you don't want to get into.

Anger Management: Lengthen That Fuse

It's easy to get angry. For some people, much too easy. Of course, the problem isn't that someone is angry, the problem is what that person does with that anger. This is the part that usually gets people into trouble.

I've had family members of my ADHD clients complain about the person's strong emotional reactions—not just anger, but everything else too. This can be exciting, but also disconcerting if the family members are surprised by the intensity of the reaction. Equally disconcerting is the sudden evaporation of that strong feeling, since they're still processing what happened. So, even if you feel done with the situation, you may need to tolerate that others bounce back more slowly and may need to talk about what happened.

Adults with ADHD may be more likely to struggle with anger problems, and perhaps strong emotional reactions in general, for two reasons:

- *Neurology.* Brain-based impulsivity can lead to strong and sudden emotional reactions, so they're more likely to fly off the handle. (And then feel bad about it afterwards.) I talk about this in more detail in *Emotional Self-Control* on p. 13.
- *Psychology.* A lifetime of bad experiences can create the self-fulfilling expectation that whatever can go badly will go badly, so they're primed to get upset. In addition, the stress of feeling constantly behind the eight ball can make ADHD adults more reactive, as it would anybody.

I have a saying that angry is in the eye of the beholder. That is, someone else may see you as more angry than you actually feel and will base her reactions on what she sees. So, if you don't want to be misinterpreted, make it easier for the other person to see more clearly how you really feel. You may have very good reasons for being angry, but can blow a good message with a bad delivery. If the other person sees you as overreacting, she will focus on that, rather than hearing what you're actually saying. Therefore, the more control you have over how you express your anger, the more options you will have to improve the situation that is bothering you in the first place.

The simplest (but probably the hardest) way to lengthen your fuse is to work on your general stress and frustration level. The more on top of your life you feel, the less reactive you will be. You may have a quick fuse under the best of circumstances, but stress will only make you react quicker and bigger. So in other words, working on all the stuff in the rest of this book should help your temper, too. Furthermore, since part of the anger response is neurologically based, ADHD medications should also help by giving you a moment to think before reacting, as well as reducing your overall stress level by enabling you to function better.

In addition, dealing directly with the things that are nagging at you will also make you less reactive. This is especially true about the gripes that develop in relationships and get bigger and bigger the more we replay them in our minds. So, talking that out and trying to resolve it with the person may be more productive. You may also find that the problem was smaller than it felt inside your head. This may be especially worth working on if you're someone who prefers to jump into action, rather than talk about things. Although there is a time and place for decisive action, there are also situations that call for just talking.

Some adults with ADHD struggle with asserting themselves. They may feel pessimistic about this working out well, even if they do try. Or maybe they feel self-conscious and not worthy to ask for things, since they probably messed some things up along the way. Or perhaps they have this idea in their heads that they should be able to do everything themselves, so they never ask for help. Regardless of the reasons, this then is a setup for them to feel stressed out by a bad situation or resentful when the other person unknowingly doesn't meet their needs. So, speaking up at the right times and in the right ways can spare you a lot of heartache. At the other end of the spectrum, some people may have a lot of experience getting others to do things for them and thus will be angry when someone isn't willing to pitch in. This overexpectation is also a setup for the other person to feel taken advantage of and angry.

It's usually easier to handle a situation well if you know beforehand that it might get tense, so you can prepare yourself mentally. You can plan ways to stay calm or not take the other person's comments personally, then (try to) remind yourself of this when you feel yourself getting heated.

Self-esteem can play a role here too. The better you feel about yourself, the less need you may have to react to others. That is, if you feel good about yourself, you may not feel as if you have to justify yourself to others or prove someone wrong. You don't need to respond to every perceived challenge in order to prove yourself. You may also be able to see that someone else's bad behavior may say more about who they are or how they're doing than it says about you. Therefore, you don't need to react to it. This is a nice situation to be in, because life is a lot simpler.

If things do escalate, you may want to just walk away and clear your head. By paying attention to how you're feeling (easier said than done), you will realize when you're not in the best mindset to deal with a confrontation productively. I had a colleague who used to say that the best arguments are like boxing matches—fought in rounds with breaks in between. That is, taking a break to cool off makes for a more productive discussion. The other person may not want to take a break at that point, so you may need to be firm and promise that you will talk further, but that it won't end well now if you're forced to keep talking. Of course, then you actually need to follow through with that. If you develop a reputation for not coming back, the other person has no incentive to let you go. When you do return to the discussion, you may need to apologize for overreacting, if that is your tendency. It doesn't mean that you didn't have good points, but that your delivery was stronger than you had intended.

With family members or friends, it can be worth talking about how to handle disagreements. This may mean explaining why it's so helpful for you to take a break to calm down when you feel angry or to sort through your thoughts when you feel overwhelmed. Sharing this self-knowledge makes it easier for the other person to understand how to get the best out of you, just as your knowing about others' quirks and tendencies makes it easier for you to get the best out of them. This is what makes relationships get better with time.

Perfectionism: Almost Always Overrated

Counterintuitive as it may sound, some people compensate for the imperfect performance of ADHD by seeking perfection, at least in some parts of their life. The rationale is often based on the idea that they can prove themselves worthy, competent, or whatever if they do a good enough job on something. So even if the rest of their life is in chaos, doing an absolutely amazing job on the report at work will take that all away and make them feel better (at least for the moment). It can be easier to take firm control of one little part of their lives that is easier, more fun, or safer, while avoiding the larger chaos that has no quick and easy solutions. Or maybe they get hyperfocused on something and don't realize when they've gotten it to be good enough. Or maybe inspiration ran away with them.

While I am certainly in favor of a job well done, in perfectionism it goes beyond the point of diminishing returns. That is, the person continues to work on something past the point where it's worth it. Even if someone else could notice the results of the extra effort, they may not care. Unfortunately, those with perfectionistic tendencies often feel driven to continue, even if they do realize that their efforts could be better spent elsewhere. This need to continue can be a tip-off that they are doing it for reasons other than those that are immediately obvious. For example, the person who knocks himself out on tiny little tweaks to a report may not be trying to impress his boss, so much as he is trying to prove something to himself.

The price paid is the loss of time for other pursuits. Every additional minute spent perfecting one project is a minute not available for other projects. There's often an inverse relationship between quality and quantity—you can have either one, but you can't have both. When I have a client who has perfectionstic tendencies, I will sometimes talk about Rolls Royces and Fords. Rolls Royces are definitely very high quality, but you don't see a lot of them around. Fords aren't quite the handmade masterpieces, but there are plenty of them on the road. So, the question then becomes whether the client's project deserves to be a Rolls Royce or whether a Ford is good enough. Most things in life are Fords and a few things are Rolls Royces. The trick becomes telling the difference and not working too hard (or too little) on something that doesn't deserve it. The goal should be flexibility, not perfection.

Related to this, the need to do something perfectly also makes it harder to change gears if something else comes up. I had a client who was asked to build a set of shelves at work. Everyone agreed this was a worthy project, since they needed them. When he was finally done, it was a great set of shelves, all the way down to the fine-grit sanding job. Unfortunately, he spent so long perfecting the shelves that he wasn't available to help out in other ways, and his coworkers resented his otherwise good work. Had he lowered his standards a little, he could have helped out with the other work that needed to be done, so the shelves hurt him more than helped him with his coworkers.

Finally, doing one thing perfectly means that the person is probably ignoring other parts of his life. He then gets further behind, and it all becomes that much more overwhelming. It can be tempting at that point to find another sacred project to focus on and ignore the rest. So the cycle keeps repeating itself.

Rather than limiting your life by seeking perfection, strive for something a little bit lower. Aim to do many things well, rather than a few things great. Don't limit your life by pursuing perfection. Think about what deserves more of your labor and what deserves less—some things in life are Rolls Royces, but most of them are Fords. The trouble is, if you try to make too many Rolls Royces, you will wind up walking a lot.

ADHD, Eating Disorders, and Weight Management

There's some new and interesting research coming out about ADHD and eating disorders, including obesity. However, even if most people with ADHD don't have a formal eating disorder, it's pretty safe to say that ADHD can affect what, how, and when you eat. Maybe even why.

To eat a pretty healthy diet requires some fair consistency in the rest of your life. This is much easier said than done. So adults with ADHD may wind up frequently eating on the run or eating quick meals at home that tend to be less healthy. They may also not eat enough over the course of the day, leaving them prone to overeating when they do get a chance because they're ravenous. In addition, they may also have difficulty resisting tempting foods (mmm, donuts…) and eat them more often and to excess, rather than healthier but less-exciting alternatives. When they do eat, they're more likely to be doing something else at the time and thereby not really attending to what they're eating. This makes it more likely that they will eat on autopilot and not feel the body signals that tell them when to stop. They may also be more likely to eat out of boredom or frustration after a tough day.

As hard as it is to have generally decent eating habits, it gets even harder when someone needs to step it up in order to lose weight. It's slow, boring and doesn't show results quickly—the perfect formula for bailing out early by impatient folks with ADHD. By contrast, ridiculous claims of instant results made by fad diets look awfully tempting, even when good judgment tries to rain on the parade.

If you have a full-blown eating disorder, such as anorexia or bulimia, or are severely overweight, it's worth talking to professionals who really understand how to best treat those conditions—and ideally understand your ADHD, too.

However, probably the larger percentage of readers don't have anything official, but don't eat well and could stand to lose a few pounds. If this is you, it's probably worth thinking about how you got here in the first place. Obviously, more calories came in than went out, but how exactly did that happen? Do you have trouble resisting the vending machine at work? Do you reward yourself with oversized portions of unhealthy food as a way to tame the stress and hard work of keeping all the balls in the air all day? For these reasons (and all sorts of others), it's worth really doing your best to get on top of your ADHD and create a less stressful and more satisfying lifestyle. This should only help your eating habits, even without your consciously trying to. Just as untreated ADHD contributed to bad habits, treated ADHD should contribute to good ones.

What about your past attempts at losing weight? How did they end up? If you're like most people, you probably start well, but have trouble maintaining it. Understanding how your ADHD plays into this will make it more likely that you can pick weight loss strategies that you can stick with. For example, you may find that you get bored with the same workout routine but feel compelled to keep doing it. As one of my clients figured out, you're probably better off finding something else at the point that your initial motivation starts burning out. The added bonus here is that the regular exercise will give you more energy and concentration, reducing some of the impact of your ADHD. Maintaining a solid exercise routine means that there are times that you're going to have to say no to other people and activities that conflict with your workout time. You also have to learn to say no to yourself when you try to talk yourself out of it (just this one time). Taping up a picture of you at your goal weight, or some other tangible reminder, can make it feel much more real and motivating.

When it comes to losing weight, healthy eating, and regular exercise, slow and steady wins the race. There are no quick fixes here, just as in so much of the rest of your life. Being able to do a good job on this stuff is both the outcome of doing a good job on your ADHD, as well as part of the means of getting there.

CHAPTER 9

MEMORY MANAGEMENT: WHAT WAS THAT AGAIN?

There's a lot to remember in our busy lives. Sometimes it's new skills to be learned, like how to operate your new cell phone. Sometimes it's passing obligations, like taking your child to a dentist appointment tomorrow. Untreated ADHD makes it harder to grab onto these bits of information and file them away, causing all sorts of problems later.

In this chapter, we discuss the basics of memory and how to make the most of yours if you have ADHD. This will make the events of your days more predictable and less stressful.

This chapter contains the following articles:

The Fundamentals of Memory: In and Out

Long-term memory has two parts—*encoding* (writing information to the hard drive) and *retrieval* (pulling that information off the hard drive). Both need to function correctly if we are to remember something. As a result, memory problems can be based in either or both—and so can the solutions.

Sometimes the problem is that we never really caught the information in the first place—like when someone tells us something but we're not really paying attention, so there isn't much there to stick in our memory. We may be able to dig up some pieces of it if we're cued ("Remember, you were sitting at the kitchen table when I told you"). These encoding failures aren't really memory problems, since the real culprit is a blink in attention—not much got into memory in the first place, so there isn't much to be forgotten. People with ADHD are vulnerable to being distracted at the moment that something happens or is said, so they may wind up recording only part of it into their memories. This can also be called a working memory problem (see the next article, *Make Your Working Memory Work for You,* for more on this).

Obviously, the more intense and meaningful an experience is, the better it gets ingrained and the more likely we will be able to pull it up later. This has three important related implications:

- *You should make a point of paying attention.* You will be more likely to remember something if you actively pay attention to it and try to remember it, rather than passively allowing the information to float past your ears. This also means reducing the competition for your attention, such as by turning off the TV.
- *Others will make assumptions about your forgetting.* People without ADHD will assume that at least some of your forgetting is based in not caring about the forgotten items. In their eyes, you seem to remember what's important to you but not what's important to them, so the forgetting appears to be intentional, even if it's neurological. People with ADHD require greater effort to remember these less-meaningful items.
- *Others can help you remember.* Fortunately, these other people can make you more likely to remember the things that are important to them by making a bigger deal about them and a lesser deal about the things that aren't as important. This works better than just assuming that you will remember everything, and it tends to make everyone happier.

Once a piece of information is written into our memories, we need to be able to pull it up when necessary. Distraction can play a role here, too; if you're preoccupied with something else or there is too much going on at the time, your search function is less effective. Nerves can also interfere with your recall if you start getting psyched out and your mind goes blank (of course, it pops into your head later when the pressure is off). For people with ADHD, weak encoding tends to be a bigger problem than inefficient retrieval. Nonetheless, you can increase the odds of remembering that slippery piece of information by thinking about the circumstances when you learned it or asking for some information from someone else who was there—these bits of information may give your brain more to work with and enable you to pull the rest of the information out of some back corner somewhere.

Make Your Working Memory Work for You

As we discussed in *Working Memory* on p. 9, we use our working memories to hold information that we are currently processing, the way a computer's RAM does. Our working memories remember what has just happened, pull information out of our long-term memories, manipulate all this information, and remember what we want to do until it's time to do it. So there's a lot going on in our working memories. Because we live in a complicated world and there's usually quite a bit coming at our working memories, this is the place where lots of things get forgotten, whether it's something you're reading or something your romantic partner tells you—it gets bumped out before getting transferred into long-term memory, in the same way that you lose everything when the power goes out if you haven't saved it to your computer's hard drive.

Just as with your computer, the key to not losing information is to not overload your working memory and to record the information regularly. If you know that your working memory is kind of blinky, then don't ask it to do more than it can. Here are some strategies to help your working memory work at its best:

- *Minimize distractions.* The less that's going on around you, the fewer intrusions that the important information needs to compete with. For example, you're more likely to remember being told something if you're not also watching TV at the same time.
- *Write things down.* Rather than keeping everything in your head, put some of it down on paper or on the computer. This could be as simple as writing a quick note on your to-do list, but is equally helpful when working on a big or complex project. That way you don't need to remember as many things at once as you think about a particular situation. For example, if considering a big purchase, scribble out a quick list of your upcoming expenses to make it less likely that you will forget something. Trying to mentally juggle all these bits of data is a setup for forgetting a few and thereby making a bad choice.

- *Make passive tasks more active.* The more thoroughly and actively you process a piece of information, the more likely it is to get transferred into your long-term memory. When talking with someone, practice active listening, such as by paraphrasing back what was said. When told something to remember, repeat it mentally several times and think about how it relates to what you already know. When reading, pause occasionally to think about how what you just read relates back to earlier paragraphs, or highlight important passages and write notes in the margins.
- *Take your medication.* If you have a prescription, use it. Among other things, ADHD medication increases your working memory. It's like a RAM upgrade.

Most ADHD memory troubles result from an unreliable working memory. It may never be perfect, but these strategies can help it work at its best. In addition, there is also a company that offers working memory training, a new treatment that seems to offer some solid promise for treating many aspects of ADHD. You can read more about it in *Computer-Based Training Programs* on p. 182.

Learn New Things More Effectively

In order to learn something, our attention has to hold onto it long enough to process the new information and put it into long-term memory. This working memory, as it is called, is similar to the RAM in a computer—when the RAM gets overloaded, programs start crashing and information gets lost before it's written to the hard drive. If you haven't already, you may want to read the previous article, *Make Your Working Memory Work for You.*

In order to make it more likely that the relevant information makes it into your long-term memory, you may want use one or more of these active learning techniques:

- *Repeat the information either out loud or mentally.* If you say it out loud, you experience the act of saying it as well as hearing it again.
- *Relate the new information to what you already know.* The more connections a piece of information has, the easier it is to remember. Random bits of information floating out there on their own tend to be forgotten. For example, if you find out about a new Web browser, think about how it's similar to or different from other browsers you've used.

- *Think about how the information will be retrieved later*. When, where, and how will this information be used again? Remind yourself to remember it then. Picture yourself in that situation.
- *Process the information further.* For example, when meeting someone new, repeat the person's name mentally while carefully studying her appearance. Or when you're told that you need to scuff up glossy paint with sandpaper before repainting it, think about why that is (the little scratches give more surface area and nooks and crannies for the new paint to penetrate and grab onto).
- *Do it yourself.* Doing the activity yourself may make it stick better, rather than just hearing or reading about it. As you're doing it, talk yourself through it, to give your brain one more channel of information.

Effective learners tend to use these strategies automatically, but we could all do better by using them intentionally at times when we really want to remember something. In addition to these general principles, here are some more specific suggestions:

- *Use flash cards and repetition.* If you have information that you need to cram into your head, you will remember more after several shorter sessions than one long one. It's also less boring.
- *Reduce external distractions.* This will make the relevant information stand out more. However, you may find that dead silence is actually worse, so music or television can help to quiet internal distractions and keep you focused. Do whatever works for you.
- *Study at your best time of day.* If you have the ability, schedule your most intense learning sessions based on the times of day that you have the best mental sharpness or medication coverage.
- *Use a highlighter.* If you have to study written material, use a highlighter to mark up the main points. This will not only keep you more involved while reading, but also make it easier to go back and just focus on the highlighted parts, rather than the whole thing. See *Read More Effectively* on p. 352 for other techniques.

Remember What You Were Told

Lots of little situations come up as we go through our day. Folks with ADHD can have trouble reliably remembering everything that happens or is said in these moments, making for embarrassment or frustration when they remember it differently from other people (or don't really remember it at all). This difference in memory may only come up later when the person is cued; for example, seeing extra place settings at the dining room table reminds him that his girlfriend told him something about having the neighbors over for dinner. Or, perhaps he doesn't remember at all even then, despite his girlfriend's vehement claims that she did tell him (and he was supposed to bring home a bottle of wine).

The solution is to grab onto those moments a little tighter so that they stick better in your memory. Things that flit by tend to not stick well for anyone, but especially for people with ADHD. The basic concept here is to use active learning techniques, rather than passive ones. This is the old trick of repeating someone's name after meeting at a party or paraphrasing what you were told to make it stick in memory better. If you haven't already, you may also want to read about active learning techniques in the previous article, *Learn New Things More Effectively*, since many of the same principles apply.

- *No more yelling across the house.* It's tempting to yell information to people in another room or when running out the door, rather than walk over and tell them, especially when we're busy (or feeling lazy). This is a setup for forgetting. If it's worth remembering, then it's worth taking ten seconds to be sure that the message is received the way it was intended. This is one of those solutions that the non-ADHD person probably needs to work on, too.
- *Ask for reminders.* If you know you'll have trouble remembering, then ask for a gentle reminder if you think the person will be amenable and it will help. For example, have your romantic partner call you at work to remind you to call the bank rather than just saying it at breakfast. After all, you'll be calling the bank from work, not from the breakfast table.
- *Write notes.* Always carry around a pen and note cards or sticky notes. Stash them around in various places at home, at work, and in the car. This way you're always prepared to write yourself a note, if necessary. Index cards are great because they fit easily in a pocket, but are also stiff enough that you can write on them easily.
- *Use a digital voice recorder.* They're great for capturing important information and idle thoughts on the fly. (See *Digital Voice Recorders* on p. 282 for more on this.)
- *Use a memory notebook.* Use this to record important details and take notes, so it's all in one place. Something small enough to keep in a pocket (and therefore always have with you) is usually best.

- *Ask the speaker to slow down or repeat himself.* Adults with ADHD often feel self-conscious about asking this, and instead pretend they heard and understood it all. Unfortunately, you can't remember what you never got in the first place, so it's better to ask for something to be repeated than prove later that you never heard it.
- *Don't put words in the speaker's mouth.* It's tempting to assume that you know where the speaker is going before she finishes her thoughts and then to start formulating your response. The trouble is, you may guess wrong and wind up thinking you heard something that you really didn't.
- *Check in afterward.* After a meeting or conversation, briefly review what was decided, what will be done next, and who will do what, to make sure everyone is on the same page. This can be done verbally right at the end of the conversation or later by email. This not only ensures that you heard things correctly, but also makes it more likely that you'll remember it because you've processed it more deeply. Most people will appreciate this, because everybody benefits from this kind of clarity (as well as getting things done right).

Remember to Remember: Prospective Memory

A lot of success in adulthood depends on our ability to remember to do the right things at the right times. This ability to remember to remember is known as prospective memory: that is, memory that goes forward. This is the place where many good intentions go to die, for many people with ADHD (and everybody else, too): the thought of what you intend to do gets knocked out by some new thought or external distraction. For example, forgetting to put the bills in the mailbox before getting into your car because you're thinking about work already. Or forgetting that your kids need cupcakes for school tomorrow because you get caught up talking to the neighbor.

Prospective memory is essentially our ability to remind ourselves, to set a mental alarm to go off at a particular time. It's somewhat similar to the way that multiple-choice tests are easier than short-answer questions—in multiple-choice tests, seeing the right answer sparks our recognition, whereas in short-answer questions we need to cue ourselves because there are no external reminders. In a related fashion, this is why it's easy to remember in a general sense that you should bring lunch to work, yet forget it at the moment that you're walking out the door. If your wife asked you at the door whether you were forgetting anything, you could probably remember it. This place and time is sometimes called the *point of performance*—the specific moment when something is supposed to happen and the only moment that really matters. Remembering lunch while brushing your teeth and remembering while driving down the road don't really count for much. It's all about timing.

Therefore, if you have trouble reliably remembering the right thing at the right time, you have two general options:

- *Keep it at the top of your mind.* Mentally repeat the desired task *(bills in mailbox, bills in mailbox...)* and actively resist attending to any other distractions *(I'll pick up the newspaper after)* until you do what you're supposed to do. This really only works for things that need to happen within a few minutes, and even then it can be a gamble, especially if you have ringing phones or persistent children.
- *Create external reminders.* At a moment that it's on your mind, put it in your schedule, write yourself a note, set an alarm, or leave yourself a voicemail so that you will be reminded at the relevant moment. If you remember that something needs to be done, but you're not at the point of performance, then capture that thought so that you're more likely to be cued at that relevant moment. This is a much better bet than relying on your memory. It's exactly why schedule books and electronic organizers were invented!

It's basically a matter of taking that remembered thought and moving it forward through time so that you remember again at the point of performance. This ability of prospective memory comes out of our working memory, which was described in *Working Memory* on p. 9 and in *Remembering to Remember* on p. 12.

In addition to these general principles, you may also want to try these more specific suggestions. The theme that runs through them all is that it delegates the remembering away from something glitchy (your memory) to something more reliable. This also make for a lot less effort on your part. Better reliability, less work—that's a good deal.

- *Reduce distractions.* The less stuff you have competing for your attention, the easier it will be to notice the important reminders. This could be objects like paper and clothes, or things like a constant flood of emails from an overactive listserv.
- *Place objects where they will serve as their own cues.* For example, put items to be returned to the store right in front of the door so you can't help but see them. The corollary to "out of sight, out of mind" is "in sight, in mind."

- *Respond to alarms immediately.* Either do what the alarm is telling you or snooze it so it goes off again. Don't believe yourself when you say, "I'll do that in a minute, as soon as I finish this." If you know that your batting average on these sorts of promises is just too low, then don't set yourself up for trouble.
- *Use a family calendar.* Families these days tend to have a lot going on. If this is you, then get a big calendar and put it up somewhere easily seen without having to pull it out of a drawer (never happen). It may also be helpful to meet occasionally (and briefly) to clarify the scribbles.
- *Use sticky notes, whiteboards, and pads of paper as reminders.* Sprinkle them all over your house and workplace. Then when you've done the task (or decided it won't get done), get rid of the note so you don't lose new notes amidst all the old ones.
- *Leave yourself a voicemail or email at the point of performance.* For example, send an email from home to your work email to remind yourself to call the bank tomorrow during business hours. This way you don't need to carry the reminder with you from home to work.
- *Develop routines.* If you make a habit of doing the same things in the same order on the same schedule, you're more likely not to skip any steps.

CHAPTER 10

TIME MANAGEMENT: WHAT SHOULD I BE DOING NOW?

Time management involves using time effectively and staying on track through the day—something that is far easier said than done, but certainly a worthy goal to strive for. This means resisting not only external distractions like ringing phones, but also internal distractions like remembering a website you wanted to look up. As a result, it can be just as difficult to navigate your way through a chaotic, hectic day as it is through a quiet day where you have certain goals in mind. These two scenarios have different challenges and therefore require different solutions. This chapter covers all aspects of time management to help you stay on top of your obligations better and have some time left over for the good stuff. It contains the following articles:

Break the Lock: Dissolve Hyperfocus (p. 257) Hyperfocusing on something enjoyable can throw your schedule out of whack, so these strategies can help you make more conscious choices about where your time goes.

Get Places on Time: It Can Actually Happen! (p. 258) People tend to get grumpy when forced to wait for someone, so you may want to use these strategies to improve your odds of running on time.

Make Your Deadlines (and Impress Your Friends) (p. 259) Deadlines are a fact of life, both at work and at home. You will pay a price for running over them, so you may want to try these strategies to get more control over those deadlines.

Escape the Web: Manage Your Online Time (p. 261) The Internet is a great resource, but it's also a slippery slope for anyone who has trouble with time management. These strategies can help you get more control over how much time you spend online.

Time Management for the Time-Blind

Adults are expected to manage their time effectively. This is much easier said than done for those with ADHD, because time can be a very slippery concept for them. In fact, Russell Barkley, Ph.D., has said that people with ADHD suffer from *time blindness*—that is, they just don't see time and future consequences clearly. So they do their best, but even with good diligence, they still hit snags. (I talk about this more in *Sense of Time* on p. 11.) It's kind of like how someone who is colorblind will have trouble with coordinating his outfits—he understands it in theory, but has trouble pulling it off.

If this is you, there are several tricks you can use to make yourself more aware of time so you don't need to rely as much on your fuzzy internal clock:

- *Hang up a bunch of clocks.* There is still no guarantee that you will actually look at the clocks, but it does increase the odds that you'll know what time it is. Put them where they will be seen easily.
- *Wear a watch with a chime.* Set your watch to beep every fifteen minutes to make you aware of the passage of time. It also creates a small break in the action where you can ask yourself whether you're doing what you're supposed to be doing.
- *Set an alarm to remind you that it's time to do something else.* This could be cheap little kitchen timers, a PDA, or software on your computer—the most important thing is that it's quick and easy to set, or you won't go to the trouble. When the alarm goes off, you may still choose to continue doing what you're doing, but at least then it's a conscious choice and not due to lack of awareness.

- *Time how long some common activities take.* Then write it down so you can use it for future planning. Then avoid the temptation to convince yourself that you will do it faster this time so you can continue doing whatever you're doing.
- *Build in some extra time.* Nothing goes exactly according to plan, so factor in some cushion. Then add a little more.
- *Create a schedule for common events.* For example, for getting out the door on work days, if you know you need to be out the door by 8:00, then you should be in the kitchen by 7:40, in the bathroom by 7:20, and the alarm should go off at 7:10 (you get one snooze). Then tape up those times in each room (e.g., 7:40 out of bathroom) so that you can immediately tell whether you're ahead of or behind schedule.
- *Review your schedule with someone else.* Just as someone who is colorblind may have a friend assemble outfits for him, it may be helpful to regularly check in with a friend, family member, or coworker to go over your schedule. She may be able to see problems that you can't—for example, that you've underestimated the time for a task or forgotten drive time.

The Complexity of Lateness

ADHD folks tend to have a hard time getting places on time. Some people may become judgmental about this, assuming that they just don't care enough to be punctual. If only it were that simple.

I can think of at least eight reasons why people with ADHD tend to run late. Let's go through them, since it may help you feel less bad about it and be more punctual.

The Neurological Reasons

1. *Poor sense of time.* Research is showing that people with ADHD are weak in several executive functions, the skills that we use to manage and balance the multiple demands of our lives. One of these executive functions involves the sense of time (see *Sense of Time* p. 11, as well as the previous article). This is our internal clock that tells us how long we have been doing an activity and warns us when we are coming close to a deadline, such as when it's time to start getting ready to leave. For many ADHD people, time is too fluid and slips away easily without notice, especially if they're doing something enjoyable. It's therefore much harder to hit specific deadlines. Related to this, many ADHD folks aren't great at predicting how long something will take, so they don't plan their time well, often running late.

2. *Distraction.* Even if they do plan well, they may get distracted by other tasks which put them behind schedule.

The Psychological Reasons

3. *Giving up.* After years of struggle and failure, some ADHD folks will simply give up trying to better manage their time, figuring that it won't work out well anyway. Of course, giving up like this only makes things worse, even though it is somewhat understandable.

4. *Avoidance.* Related to this, lateness may bring up so many bad memories of being criticized that they may just avoid thinking about it and avoid even trying to plan in order to minimize those feelings. They may avoid putting themselves into situations that require them to be somewhere on time, even though that means sacrificing otherwise good opportunities.

5. *Feeling overwhelmed.* Alternatively, the ADHD person may feel so overwhelmed getting everything done that she tries to use every last second, doing "just one more thing" that puts her past the time to leave. This leaves her feeling as if she is constantly running right in front of the avalanche.

6. *Dread of boredom.* Still others may dread the boredom or wasted time that occurs from getting somewhere early and needing to wait, so they try to minimize that time by cutting it too close. Of course, this too often puts them on the wrong side of that line.

The Interpersonal Reasons

7. *Retaliation.* Relationships are complex, and one person's actions will affect the other's. Sometimes the ADHD person will intentionally show up late to keep someone waiting if he is angry with that person. Of course, these passive-aggressive tactics aren't the most productive way of dealing with those perhaps justified feelings.

8. *Entitlement.* And finally, let's admit it, there are some ADHD folks who actually do feel a sense of entitlement and therefore expect others to wait for them. They may be unaware of the impact that this has on the relationship and the price that they pay for it.

The more you know about why you do what you do, the better able you are to change it, if you choose to. So think about these various causes of lateness and see if any of them apply to you. If so, work on them directly.

How to Be Productive, Not Just Busy

Everybody's busy these days, but are you productive? ADHD adults in particular are vulnerable to doing a lot, but not really getting a lot done. Or the stuff that they do get done isn't really the best use of their time at that moment, since other more important tasks have fallen by the wayside (other people tend to not be much impressed by what you do accomplish if you haven't done what they wanted you to). Unfortunately, because they're staying active and working on things, they can convince themselves that they're being productive, but busy and productive aren't the same. *Productive* means making progress on the right obligations and eventually bringing them to a conclusion. I talked about this pseudoproductivity in *Unhelpful Coping Strategies* on p. 91 and *Overcome Unhelpful Coping Strategies, Bad Habits, and Defense Mechanisms* on p. 209.

Let's now talk about some specific strategies to avoid this trap. Try to keep the following in mind:

- *Be hard on yourself.* When you remember to, ask yourself, "Is this really the best use of my time?" Be brutally honest. It's easy to justify borderline activities, so don't let yourself get away with that smooth talking. Maybe even tape up a sign to remind yourself. Get creative on what the sign says and change it occasionally so that you don't stop seeing it.

- *Set an alarm.* If you have trouble remembering to ask yourself, get a watch with a repeating alarm that will go off every fifteen minutes to serve as a small break to step back and look at what you're doing. Many watches have a beep, but some also have a vibrate function (see *It's About Time* on p. 281). If you find that you're working on something less than ideal, then bite the bullet and push yourself to get back on track.

- *Plan your time.* It's harder to make the best use of your time if you don't know what you're supposed to do with the time in the first place. Take ten minutes every night or morning to plan out your day and write it down. Tape up a note with the three most important things you need to work on, so you're more likely to stay on track.

- *Reduce distractions.* The fewer of these lower-priority tasks that are pulling at your attention, the less effort it will take to resist them. When appropriate, turn off phones and email alerts or go work where there isn't as much stuff to get sucked into.

- *Start things, then finish them.* The two most common places to let yourself slip into other activities is when feeling overwhelmed with starting something or when you can't make yourself finish it. Acknowledge that these times are harder and then make yourself do it anyway.

Use Time More Efficiently

Folks with ADHD often feel like they just don't get enough done in a given stretch of time, despite their best intentions. Family members, coworkers, and bosses may complain even more about this. Sometimes it's big things that suck the time away; sometimes it's a series of small detours. These techniques will help you get more done.

- *Get organized.* It's easy to waste a lot of time looking for things (and get off on tangents) if you're disorganized. This can really add up over the course of a day or week. If this is the case for you, you may need to invest a chunk of time getting your stuff organized and getting rid of clutter—an investment that will pay back. Of course, you will need to maintain it, too, so look at these as installment payments.
- *Reduce distractions.* It's easier to stay on track if you have fewer temptations. So pick your workplace well. For example, you may find that you get sucked in when folding laundry in front of the TV and get more done if listening to music.
- *Have a plan.* Set priorities and schedule your time accordingly. Write it down and put it somewhere that you can easily see it so it can serve as a constant reminder. Refer to your schedule regularly to see if you're making the progress you expected.
- *Take on less.* There are lots of interesting things out there—probably enough for a hundred lifetimes. But in this one lifetime, we need to make choices. Limit how much you take on, since you can't do everything well. Try to focus more on quality than quantity.
- *Use an alarm.* A beeping or vibrating alarm can alert you regularly to the passage of time and also remind you to consider whether what you're currently doing is what you should be.
- *Use social pressure positively.* Make a commitment to someone else to get a certain number of things done in a given time period. Knowing that they will ask about your progress may tip the balance when you're tempted to drift off.

- *Work next to someone else.* Many people with ADHD find that they get more done if there is someone else in the room, even if she isn't directly involved in the task. She may be reading the paper or clicking through emails next to you. My theory is that the other person serves as a constant visual reminder to stay on task.

Focus In: Fight Distractibility

People with ADHD wind up losing a lot of time by getting distracted by side projects and then don't have enough time to do the things that they were supposed to get done. Sometimes it's big chunks of wasted time, like when they get lost online for a couple of hours, but it can also leak away in a hundred small bits over the course of the day, like by taking a minute to skim over an article in the paper that they saw when walking past.

When it comes to fighting distractibility, the best results usually come from setting things up beforehand to eliminate the distraction before it occurs, rather than on trying to resist the distraction in the heat of the moment. So try to set things up correctly ahead of time, rather than counting on yourself to do the right thing in the moment. Once you're distracted, it's usually too late.

- *Use reminders to keep yourself on task.* This could be small taped-up notes or a large whiteboard with the day's goals written in big letters.
- *Set a repeating alarm.* This creates a small break in the flow of events so that you can notice what you are doing and then make a conscious choice as to whether it's the best use of your time. If you find yourself off task, then you can jump back on again.
- *Reduce the distractions.* To the extent that you can control it, try to work in a quieter and less visually stimulating place so there's less competing for your attention. If you can't move where you're working, you can use a white noise machine or fan to provide background noise or to block other sounds. You can also buy noise-canceling headphones relatively inexpensively these days. Foam earplugs cost virtually nothing, but may block too much sound. Since some people actually find dead silence more distracting, you can turn on the TV or music, as long as it does more good than harm.
- *Reduce clutter.* Try to keep your workspace free of extra stuff. If you notice that you have too many things getting in your way, it may be better to push it all aside and organize it later, rather than

getting sidetracked on cleaning up. Make a commitment to yourself to circle back and actually deal with that new pile.

- *Go back to the original task.* When you find yourself on a tangent, go back to the original task and finish that before moving on to the next.
- *Use hyperfocus positively.* The ability to hyperfocus can be a mixed blessing, depending on when you fall into it. You may be able to set things up so that you're more likely to hyperfocus on a project and really get a lot done. Gather all the necessary supplies, reduce distractions, and pump yourself up for the task at hand. See *Break the Lock* on p. 257 for more information on ways to prevent the negative potential of hyperfocus.
- *Create shorter work sessions for better energy.* No one can focus consistently for long stretches, so know your limits. You will probably get more done over several shorter work sessions with breaks in between than in one marathon session. You may want to set an alarm to tell you when the breaks should end to make sure that the breaks don't become longer than the working time.
- *Use active processing techniques.* It's easier to drift off during passive tasks than active ones. For example, when reading, make it more active by scribbling on the page and talking to yourself about the main points of what you're reading.
- *Work with a partner.* Sometimes just having someone else present can help keep you on track, even if you're each working on different things. It can be even better to work together, but only if you choose the right person, preferably someone who is organized enough to structure the time well, but not so anal-retentive that he'll blow a capillary when you get off topic.
- *Designate high brain-power times.* Some tasks require a good chunk of time to really get immersed in, whereas others can be done more on the fly. In order to make it more likely that you will make good progress on those more intense projects, schedule blocks of time when you won't be interrupted. You may need to ask coworkers or family members for their cooperation in giving you this time by explaining that you won't be able to complete these tasks without it. Then turn off other distractions so you won't interrupt yourself.

- *Capture loose thoughts.* If a new idea for an unrelated project keeps kicking around inside your head, then take a second to jot it down. This way it's captured and you don't need to worry about losing it, but you can get back to your main task with less distraction.

Resist Impulsive Time Wasters

It's an interesting world we live in. Fortunately and unfortunately, technology has given us constant and immediate access to all sorts of fun distractions. (Some of them are even worthwhile.) The challenge for everyone these days is to be more intentional about where we put our time, rather than getting sucked into activities that aren't really worth our time. For people with ADHD, this challenge is especially difficult, which is one reason why there seems to be more ADHD now than there used to be—it isn't any more common, it just stands out more.

Try using the following strategies to stand out a little less. Generally speaking, for all people, impulsivity is best managed by avoiding the tempting situation in the first place, rather than trying to resist it.

- *Reduce temptations.* The fewer temptations, the fewer you need to resist. Eliminate potentially exciting impulse stimuli before they occur, such as by unsubscribing from email alerts, canceling magazine subscriptions that you don't read, avoiding stores where you spend too much time and money, etc.
- *Give the devil his due.* We need a certain amount of downtime each day—some days more than others. Build that time in intentionally so that it doesn't happen unintentionally at less convenient times. You can only run at a breakneck pace for so long before crashing, so remember that slow and steady wins the race.
- *Create visual reminders.* These can remind you of your priorities and keep them at the front of your mind when the impulse strikes. For example, post a picture of the vacation spot that you're saving money for.
- *Use self-talk.* Tell yourself things like, "Write report first, check email second," when you're tempted to jump ship. Granted, the problem is usually that you've jumped into your email before even thinking about it, so there won't be any time to tell yourself anything, but you can at least use this technique when you think about it. Every little bit helps.

- *Get out of the situation.* If you find yourself doing something that you know isn't the best use of your time, just jump back to what you should be doing instead. No knocking yourself, no giving up hope—just do it.

Get Going: Beat Procrastination and Avoidance

Procrastination is a hallmark of people with ADHD—leading to the corresponding hallmark of their family members, nagging. Some of these difficulties may be based in the neurology and primary symptoms of ADHD, such as getting distracted by other tasks or forgetting about a project. The avoided tasks may also be too boring to inspire you into action, or the pressure isn't great enough yet if the deadline is still too far away (i.e., not right now). However, you may also avoid or put off tasks that you feel probably won't work out well or that stress you out. (See *Do It Anyway* on p. 207.) If this is the case, it may be worth seeing a therapist to work on developing a more active approach to tackling these kinds of demands with less interference from negative thoughts and feelings. Meanwhile, these other pointers might help.

- *Remind yourself of the price paid.* Waiting until the last minute may help you get fired up for something, but it also carries the price tag of stress, chaos, and vulnerability to unexpected problems. Remind yourself of this (think of some of your more regrettable moments) when you're justifying to yourself that it's OK to wait a little longer.

- *Build the necessary skills.* Sometimes people procrastinate on tasks that they don't feel competent at. If this is the problem, then seek out the training you need to make the task easier.

- *Break big projects into smaller pieces.* It's easy to avoid starting big projects because they feel insurmountable. This can feel psychologically easier if you break them into several smaller pieces. You may find that you need to work with someone else to visualize how the whole breaks into several parts. If so, then find someone to help you. Then give yourself small rewards for meeting these middle deadlines.

- *Use social pressure.* Tell someone else of your plans to start or finish the dreaded project. It may be easier to get motivated to start it knowing that someone else is going to ask about your progress.

- *Mix it up.* Jumping between several tasks, some of which are better than others, may be more appealing than a straight run of only one activity. Just make sure you actually finish everything.
- *Make a small commitment.* If the thought of a marathon session on the avoided activity is too much to bear, then make a commitment to do only ten minutes and see how it goes. If it's going well (or tolerably), then agree to another ten minutes. Often these activities are not so awful once you actually start them. It's getting over the initial hump that's the hardest.
- *Face motivated distractibility.* There are times when we allow ourselves to get distracted because we don't want to deal with whatever else we should be doing instead. Be honest with yourself about this and focus on why you don't want to do the dreaded task. You may still decide that you don't want to do it yet, but it's always better to be honest with yourself about these sorts of things.
- *Rethink things.* Severe procrastination may be telling you that you need to find a new way to get this task done. We don't always have this option, but it may be a possibility more often than you think. It's just a matter of what you're willing to pay to not have to do it. There are obvious examples, like paying a cleaning service, but you can also barter with family and friends to unload some of your most hated chores.

Break the Lock: Dissolve Hyperfocus

It's well known that people with ADHD have trouble with wandering attention, but excessive attention can also be a problem when you get locked onto something for longer than you realize or intend. The trouble with this hyperfocus is that you don't really know when you're doing it, so that makes it really hard to choose not to do it at that point. Therefore, the best point of intervention is usually ahead of time.

- *Set an alarm.* If you know that you tend to get locked in on certain activities, like watching TV or surfing the Web, then set an alarm before you start. This will provide a break in the action and give you a chance to make a choice whether you want to continue.
- *Ask for help.* It may be appropriate sometimes to enlist others to serve as your reminder, if they are willing to do it. For example, by telling a coworker, "I get really focused on my work, so do me a favor and swing by my cubicle to pick me up on the way to the meeting."

- *Give the devil his due.* You may find that you need a certain amount of time per day or week to just go where your fancy takes you. If you allow yourself some designated times, you may find yourself less tempted to stray when you're supposed to be productive.
- *Get back on track.* If you notice that you hyperfocused on something for too long, then take a moment to reassess and see what the best course of action is. Don't follow hyperfocus with impulsively jumping into something else that may not be the best use of your time under the new circumstances. It's better to take a couple minutes and make a good decision.

Get Places on Time: It Can Actually Happen!

Many ADHD folks have difficulty with running late. Other people tend to notice these sorts of things, especially bosses. Even though they will probably jump to the wrong conclusions, people will make assumptions about you if this becomes a habit, so it's often worth working on.

- *Create a schedule ahead of time.* If you have trouble getting out the door on time in the morning, then figure out what time each transition needs to take place. For example, to leave by 8:00 you need to be in the kitchen by 7:40 and in the bathroom by 7:20.
- *Count time backward.* Starting at the time that you need to arrive, count backward until you get to when you need to leave. For example, "To get to the restaurant by 7:00, I need to park by 6:50, leave home by 6:30, and start getting ready by 6:00." People with ADHD often don't think through everything that needs to happen along the way and then run late when things crop up (like driving there).
- *Avoid best-case scenario planning.* People with ADHD tend to be overly optimistic with their estimations for how long things will take. If you know this is you, then pad your estimates in case something unexpected pops up, which it always does. Then add a little extra if it's something really worth being on time for.
- *Time how long things take.* If you find that you're consistently undershooting in your estimates, it may be worth timing these activities a few times and write it down so you can refer back to it later.
- *Set an alarm for when you need to start getting ready.* This way you won't pass that time without realizing it.

- *Get into bed on time.* Many morning problems are really night problems, so that's where the solution is too. If you find that you oversleep or have trouble getting out of bed on time, it may be because you're getting into bed too late and not getting enough sleep. Also keep the morning routine as simple as possible and do what you can the night before.
- *Minimize distractions.* Getting ready with the television or radio on may cause you to stop and listen too much. Having a newspaper out may catch your eye. All of these side trips delay your getting on your way.
- *Just say no.* Avoid starting engrossing activities when it's getting close to time to leave.
- *Build in extra time.* It's pretty much a given that something will come up every day, even if you often can't predict what exactly that will be. So don't pack your schedule to the gills or you're asking to run over or be forced to adjust on the fly.
- *Bring something to fill the time.* Many people with ADHD don't like arriving early because of the boredom of waiting around. So bring something to work on or entertain yourself with, including by sitting in your car in the parking lot.
- *Nothing takes only a minute.* It's tempting to knock off a couple of those quick little tasks before heading out the door. Most of these don't take long, but they can easily add up, especially if you get sidetracked by yet another activity. If you're getting ready to leave, it's best to limit yourself strictly to what it takes to get you out the door.

Make Your Deadlines (and Impress Your Friends)

Even with the risk of exaggeration, it's fair to say that many ADHD people alternate between feeling haunted by deadlines and being oblivious to them. Of course, each extreme tends to feed the other—the dread of an impending deadline makes it tempting to just not think about it, but this also sets you up to have good reason to worry later.

Our lives are full of deadlines, most of which have consequences for missing them. Obviously, there are deadlines at work, but also at home, such as paying bills or calling a friend back about weekend plans. They are a necessary evil, so you need to find a way to at least manage them well enough that you don't bring yourself unnecessary heartache (and your family members and coworkers unnecessary headaches).

- *Create interim deadlines.* Break large projects into several parts, each with its own deadline. If you can make them feel real, this can give you that sense of urgency several times along the way, so you will get more done and not have to do it all at the end (and perhaps overshoot the final deadline). Put these mini-deadlines into your schedule and plan accordingly.

- *Avoid overcommitment.* No amount of creative time management will fit twenty-eight hours into twenty-four, so don't take on more than you can realistically handle. There are lots of interesting and worthy activities to get involved in, but you can't do them all. Most people would much rather hear a no right up front than have you fail to deliver it later when they can't make alternative arrangements. So be selective about what you take on.

- *Remember the price paid for missing a deadline.* Waiting until the last minute may fire your brain into activity, but it also leaves you vulnerable to unexpected roadblocks. What is the price, both financial and social, for overshooting this deadline?

- *Check your schedule before committing to anything.* Carry your schedule everywhere you might need it and make a habit of never committing to anything before seeing if you have the time. When adding a new task, put it into your schedule or, at a minimum, on your to-do list. This forces you to see what else you need to do and therefore whether there will be time. If you don't have your schedule available or if you aren't sure whether you can squeeze it in, then tell the person that you will get back to them.

- *Learn or strengthen the necessary skills.* You may benefit from some additional training to enable you to get a particular task done more quickly. For example, finding out exactly what does and doesn't need to be kept for taxes will save you time both during the year as well as when you need to do your return.

- *Set up regular meetings with your boss.* Use these meetings to review your progress on various projects and prevent last-minute surprises. Do the same at home with your romantic partner to discuss what needs to be done at home (see *Family Meetings* on p. 302). It's usually better to get input early in the process, rather than later. Plus, the regular meetings may get you going earlier on those long-range projects, since you know you'll be asked about them.

Escape the Web: Manage Your Online Time

People with ADHD often have difficulty setting their own limits on enjoyable activities. Sometimes it's simply that they lose track of time, and sometimes it's that they don't want to stop since they're still having fun. This tendency makes the Internet especially problematic—it's endless and therefore not self-limiting. Unlike a newspaper or TV show, which eventually reaches an end, the Internet just keeps going seamlessly on forever, with links leading to links. Because the Internet lacks these end points, there are fewer built-in opportunities to stop and think about whether you should keep going or switch to something else. Because there are no breaks in the action online, it's easy to get hyperfocused, which deprives you of the opportunity to make a conscious choice about what you're doing.

- *Set your home page to be blank.* It's tempting to set your home page to one of your favorite sites, but this is a setup to get lost as soon as you open your browser. So set it either to blank or to some work-related site that you're less likely to wander off on.
- *Eat your vegetables first.* If you have both productive things to do online as well as fun things, get the productive things out of the way first. Resist the urge to "just check the headlines real quick," since we all know where that tends to lead.
- *Set a timer before starting.* If you know you have a certain time when you need to stop your online travels, then set an alarm before you even open up your browser. Once you start surfing, it's too easy to get lost and forget about the timer. You can use an alarm clock, a kitchen timer, or download a program onto your computer (search for "timer programs").
- *Sometimes it's better to just not start.* If you don't really have time, then don't even start. Be honest with yourself about how likely it is that you won't tear yourself away in time to do whatever you need to do next.
- *There's always more to see.* No matter how much time you spend online, there will always be more links to tempt you. Accept it. You will have to find a way to live your life without checking them all out. When it's time to go on to something else, it's time—no matter how many more links you want to explore.

CHAPTER 11

GET ORGANIZED, STAY ORGANIZED: WRESTLE THE AVALANCHE

Where did all this stuff come from? It seems as if we need to move into a tent deep in the woods to escape the constant flow of things that fill our houses, workplaces, and cars. When it comes to staying organized, we can say two things:

- *Rule 1: The act of living attracts belongings.* Some of these belongings are important and useful, so we seek them out, whereas others just seem to show up on their own. Since things keep coming in, it means that things also need to keep going out—preferably at about the same rate.
- *Rule 2: The act of living creates chaos.* Even if you manage to get rid of things as fast as they come in, you still need to put back what got taken out, clean occasionally, and replace what gets used up. This is a perpetual process.

If you're someone who has trouble managing either one of these, you will stand out much more now than in any prior period in history. If you're reading this book, staying organized (or your inability to) probably makes you crazy—and may even be one of the big reasons why you're reading this book. What's worse, for all the effort that you put in, you probably don't feel like you wind up with enough results. This chapter presents strategies to enable you to manage stuff at least a little more effectively.

Let's talk about the point of being organized, about why it matters. Contrary to what a self-righteous minority may say, it isn't to prove your moral superiority. Being organized means being able to find the right thing at the right time. This is a very functional goal, which means that you don't want to spend more time getting organized than you save by being organized (i.e., no obsessive-compulsiveness here). There are a lot of ways to achieve that goal, so remember to keep your eye on the desired result as you weigh your options.

This chapter contains the following articles:

Why Is It So Hard to Get (and Stay) Organized? (p. 264) I counted eight reasons why adults with ADHD tend to have more trouble with keeping their belongings organized. These eight reasons suggest eight solutions.

Less Is More (Organized): Get Rid of Your Extra Stuff (p. 267) The less you have, the easier it is to keep it organized. Therefore, you may want to lighten the load before even attempting to organize what's left.

Get Organized Enough: Better Than Chaos, Less Than Perfect (p. 268) The main goal of being organized is to have a more functional existence. The secondary goal is that it looks better. You're more likely to be successful at both if you strive to be just organized enough.

The Right Things at the Right Times (p. 270) One of the benefits of being generally organized is that it makes it easier to find what you need. Related to this, you can try these strategies to improve your odds of having all the right items on hand when you need them.

Why Is It So Hard to Get (and Stay) Organized?

If you have any doubt that staying organized isn't a universal struggle these days, you've clearly never let your eyes wander across the magazine covers at the supermarket checkout, where you would see several magazines with articles about decluttering, organizing, or simplifying. Unfortunately, none of them have a headline that says, "Start now by not adding this magazine to your existing mess!" So as a general rule, you're in good company. It may just be a matter of degree—some of your neighbors' houses may be pretty bad, but yours is a disaster. Adults with ADHD have additional challenges when it comes to staying organized. Let's go over the problems and potential solutions.

Weaknesses in Executive Functioning

As discussed in chapter 1, people with ADHD are often weak in certain executive functions and are thereby less efficient and effective at managing the various details of their lives. This is especially true for organizing their stuff. When you get down to it, creating and maintaining an organizational system are actually pretty complex processes. First, you need to keep in mind everything that you need to organize and then mentally manipulate those objects to find good homes for them all. This system should take into account how often you need each item so that the most frequently used are most accessible. This takes a lot of working memory. Without it, things get stuck in places that don't really work.

Once you've conceptualized your grand organizational system, you need to kick yourself into gear (self-activation) to put things away and then follow it through to the end, even when you're tired of it (persistence). Of course, then you need to maintain this system, which means remembering where things are supposed to go as well as managing your time well enough that you have a little extra to clean up as you go. All in all, there's a lot going on here, both when people with ADHD struggle as well as when they succeed.

Lack of Time

For people with ADHD, tasks take longer because they waste time scrambling around trying to find the necessary items. This then leaves them with less time to put things back in their place. When they finish the task, they don't circle back to put everything away, setting them up for trouble next time. So the cycle continues.

Unfortunately, life creates chaos, so a regular input of energy is required to re-create order. This means that we need to spend time every day or week putting things back where they belong, getting rid of what we no longer need, and replacing what we've used up. Or at least someone needs to spend that time. If you can work a deal with your family members or hire a cleaning person, then I suppose you don't have to do it all, but it still needs to be done. The simpler you make your organizational system and the less stuff you have, the less time and effort it will take to restore order.

Impulsive Purchases

The more stuff you bring into your house, the more easily it will slip into chaos. This is especially true if you're much better at bringing things in than moving things out. So, when faced with a tempting purchase, try to remind yourself that something will need to go if this comes. Either that or you will have to move into a bigger house (and you know how horrible moving always is).

Lack of a Good Organizational System

Some people with ADHD are disorganized because they just don't have an easy and effective organizational system. Things get put away somewhat haphazardly, which makes them much harder to find later. These are the people who could get locked into their house for a thousand years and it still wouldn't be especially organized.

Having a good organizational system does two things for you. First, it tells you where things should go when you're putting them away. Second, it makes it easy to find things because you know where to look.

If you can recognize that part of your problem is that you don't have a good organizational system, then get some help with it. You may need help with just one room or one type of belonging (like paperwork). Ask a friend or family member for their opinion or hire a professional organizer (see *Professional Organizers* on p. 170). Just make sure that their suggestions fit your way of doing things and therefore can be maintained in the long run.

Hopelessness

After a lifetime of partial (and short-lived) successes at getting organized, many adults with ADHD don't have much hope that the future will be much better. As a result, they give only the minimum effort required or whip things into shape only when forced to (for example, when expecting company). Of course, applying an integrative treatment program (see section II, *Start with Effective Treatment*) plus the strategies in this chapter may give you some good reason to be optimistic, or at least partially willing to give it a try.

Saving Things Just in Case

After being caught emptyhanded so often, many adults with ADHD get into the habit of saving too many things, just in case they might need them later. Since they have trouble deciding what to keep and what to toss, they play it safe and keep too many things. To some extent this is an information-processing issue, as discussed in the section on executive functions. They reason that everything has at least some value and some possibility of being needed later, so therefore they should keep it all. But that's only half the story. The question isn't whether the item has any value at all but whether it has enough value relative to their other belongings. That is, when figuring an item's value, you also need to factor in that keeping too much will make it harder to find the important things when you actually need them. For example, keeping all those old outfits will make it harder to see and find the outfits that you still wear. This ultimately does more harm than good, even if it started out as a good plan. Ironically, getting rid of these marginal items will actually make you more likely to have on hand the things that you really need.

So when you're holding on to some item of borderline value, remember to ask yourself the second question: *How valuable is this relative to the rest of my stuff?* Is it worth the price paid in terms of not finding other, more important items? It's usually better to pay a smaller price upfront by getting rid of the item than paying a bigger price later when you can't find what you need.

Some people feel bad getting rid of things that still have some good life left. To the extent you can, try to sell, give away, donate, or recycle them, if this makes it easier to let go. Unfortunately, though, it's an imperfect world we live in and sometimes we need to send things to an early grave. There comes a point where it's just not worth your time trying to find a loving home for all those orphans.

Extremes Beget Extremes

Many ADHD adults have an all-or-nothing relationship with keeping their stuff organized—their stuff is either pretty close to disaster or they're in the midst of a frenzied organizing spree. (This second one is less common.) While I give them a lot of credit for these heroic efforts to whip their stuff into shape, it often doesn't get everything put away most effectively. Everything is taken off the floor and desktops but is put away somewhat haphazardly. Because they don't take the time to create a more logical and easily maintained organizational system, it's only a matter of time before they're back in the same spot. This obviously makes the organizing marathon feel like a waste, so they're not too thrilled to do it again. Of course, the longer they wait, the worse it becomes, so each extreme drives the other.

The solution, then, is to push yourself to tackle the mess before your family members threaten to call the health department. It won't be nearly as bad then.

It Keeps Coming

Even if you manage to get so organized that your obsessive-compulsive friends are impressed, you then need to maintain it. This means not only putting back what you already own but also dealing with the constant influx of new things. You either need to find a good place for them or send them quickly on their way. So you'll have less work if you restrict how much new stuff comes into your life. Remember that not everything deserves a place in your home or your life.

Less Is More (Organized): Get Rid of Your Extra Stuff

Whenever I'm talking to someone who's disorganized, my first suggestion is always to lighten the load—get rid of as much as you can before you even try to organize what's left. It's exponentially more difficult to get organized when you're packed to the rafters. So the first step is to make a sweep through it all and make some hard choices to get rid of what you don't really need (see "Saving Things Just in Case" in the previous article). You'll thank yourself for it.

Each time you're tempted to keep something, ask yourself these questions:

- Would you pay movers to move it?
- Would you pack it up and then carry it out to a moving truck on a scorching August day?
- The moving truck is almost full and some choices have to be made. Does it make the cut?
- Imagine yourself frantically digging through all your stuff to find something really important—like your passport or your grandmother's wedding ring. Would you be happy to have all this other stuff then?

Some things will make the cut; others won't. The key is to make smart choices. You may have to make several passes through it all, getting rid of a little more each time. You may find yourself stuck, unable to decide which of several items to get rid of. This is probably an indication that the items all have about the same value. They may be different, but their total value is about the same, so it's really hard to decide which one is slightly less desirable. In these cases, pick just one, even if you have to flip a coin to do it. Ironically, if you can't decide, it may be telling you that it doesn't matter what you decide.

It may also be helpful to set a tangible goal of how much to get rid of—six inches of paper, two bags of clothes, twenty CDs, whatever. Or maybe your goal is something more functional, like being able to close your closet doors. It may not matter that much what specifically goes, so long as you hit your goal. You can't organize ten gallons of water into a five-gallon bucket, so one way or the other you need to get rid of five gallons—any five.

Get Organized Enough: Better Than Chaos, Less Than Perfect

Staying organized is a continual process, not a one-time event. It's a necessary evil that we have to set aside a certain amount of time every day or week to keep the chaos at bay. Just living life tends to create chaos, so it requires a regular input of energy to re-create order. The less stuff you have and the simpler your organizational system, the less effort it will take.

Of course, we're not striving here for a *Better Homes & Gardens* photo shoot—quite the contrary. Just good enough. This means functional first (yes, I'm a guy). That is, focus first on what will make your day run more smoothly and with less stress. Once you've accomplished that, then work on making things look pretty. Your organizational system may be different from your friends'. Don't knock yourself for that—as long as it works for you. This means finding your own personal comfort level when it comes to neatness.

I often have clients who feel bad about their inability to meet others' standards of neatness. I will often tell them that if I offered to give them a million dollars, they could probably pull off anal-retentive perfection, but it isn't realistic on a day-to-day basis. It's a matter of priorities. It probably isn't worth missing other important activities, like time with family or other pursuits. Neatness is a preference and a choice that, like any other choice, involves both rewards and costs. We each need to find our optimal balance.

To the extent that it's worth it to you to get more organized, try these strategies:

- *Bar the door.* Actively restrict the flow of new objects into your world, such as mail, email, magazines, newspapers, and things you buy. Some of this stuff comes in all by itself, so you need to actually expend energy to keep it out. It's like bailing an old, leaky boat—you try your best to plug the holes, but there will always be some bailing to do. But the less that comes in, the less you have to deal with.

- *Outflow = inflow.* You need to get rid of at least as much as comes in. No way around it.

- *Find a convenient home for everything.* Often things don't get put away because they don't have a designated place. Sometimes they do have a place but it's out of the way or not easily accessible. You may need to find a good home for each of these objects. Creating a better, easier organizational system will make it more likely that things will actually get put away.

- *Things should be put away based on how often they will be retrieved.* If it's unlikely that you will need to track down a particular item, then it's probably not worth spending the time to keep it super-organized. These are the sorts of things that should be thrown into a marked box. If it's paper, put the older items generally toward the back and newer items toward the front. Don't spend more time organizing than you save by being organized.

- *It counts only if you can find it.* Remember that keeping something "just in case I need it" isn't really all that helpful if you can't find it when it would actually be helpful to have it. Stumbling across it before or after that time doesn't accomplish much except to aggravate you. So when you're considering keeping something, ask yourself whether you will be likely to find it at the right time. (See "Saving Things Just in Case" in the previous article.)

- *File papers based on how you will find them later.* Sometimes ADHD adults have trouble finding filed papers because they don't remember how they were filed away. It may be better to file first by category (such as financial, taxes, personal, and medical) and then have subfolders within each of those. Don't make it overly complicated and create more subfolders than you really need. You need to make your filing system memorable, which is more likely if it's your own, rather than borrow someone else's system.

- *Work with a partner.* If you know that you're likely to bail out prematurely when cleaning up and putting things away, then get a friend or family member to keep you company. Even if they only occasionally provide some input, it can help to have someone else there. Remember that you will probably need to return the favor in one way or another to keep the relationship balanced.

- *Tackle only a corner.* If you have a lot that needs to get organized, pick one small part of the mess and start there. This will make your progress more obvious than if you were to skim across the surface of a larger area. Seeing some tangible results might motivate you to go on to the next.
- *Take pictures occasionally to track your progress.* If you have a giant backlog to dig out from under, it can seem as if an entire day's effort doesn't make much of a dent. This can be pretty discouraging, so it can help to take some before pictures so that you can see how much you've actually accomplished.

The Right Things at the Right Times

Owning things is nice. Finding them at the right times is even nicer. Knowing that the desired item is hiding somewhere within your four walls isn't much consolation when you can't find it. To have the right things at the right times, you have to have a good organizational system so that you know where to look, but you also need to spend the time to put things back occasionally.

Beyond general organization, many adults with ADHD also struggle with bringing the right items from one place to another, like from home to work. This can be incredibly frustrating and bring up flashbacks of lost homework assignments.

- *Place things where you can't help but see them.* For example, lean them against the door or put them right next to your keys. This way you don't need to actively remember to bring the item with you. Since you'll be less likely to remember those things when dashing out the door, it's best to do this immediately when you think of it.
- *Create a transfer station near the door.* This should be a place that's easy to see when leaving. Anything that needs to leave with you should be put there. Make it even more likely that you'll check it by also putting your keys, wallet, or purse there. Nothing else goes there, no matter what.
- *Get rid of clutter.* The more stuff you have lying around, the more hiding places it creates for the objects that you want to see when leaving.
- *Write reminders on a whiteboard.* This should be directly on your path out of the house so you see it without having to go looking for it. Each note will grab your attention better if you limit how much you put up there and erase the old ones. Use different colors to keep everything from blending together and disappearing.

- ***Have duplicates of important but easily lost items.*** If you just don't want to deal with the hassle of forgetting, then get multiples of things like keys, glasses, and pens.
- ***Build in some time to get ready and leave.*** You're much more likely to forget something when you fly out the door in a frenzy.

CHAPTER 12

USING TOOLS AND TECHNOLOGY TO STAY ON TOP OF YOUR LIFE: GIZMOS

I'm all in favor of using technology, except when I'm not. That is, there are times when a high-powered piece of technology is just the thing to get the job done, but there are also times when something simpler is faster and easier. If you have ADHD and aren't able to keep on top of all your demands by just doing everything inside your head, then you need to transfer some of that work to a tool that will do it better. The trick is to find the right tool for the job. In this chapter, I discuss a bunch of options, from simple wall calendars to complex PDAs. In all cases, though, I take into account how people with ADHD tend to process information—what they do well and where they tend to get tripped up. This will, I hope, make this chapter more helpful to you than a lot of the generic advice that you're gotten in the past.

Which tool will work best for you depends on both your existing strengths and weaknesses, as well as on what your life looks like and what you need to accomplish. This will change over the course of your life. Not only do your skills and abilities change over time, but so do your demands—for example, as you move from being a student to being an employee, from living single to raising kids. So it may be time to find some new strategies to help you cope with your current situation.

This chapter contains the following articles:

Use Your To-Do List Effectively: #1. Make a To-Do List (p. 278) If you have more than three things to do, you probably need a to-do list. Whether it's scribbled on the back of an envelope or color-coded and cross-referenced in a complex software program, there are some important tricks to making the most of your list.

It's About Time: Use Clocks and Alarms to Stay on Track (p. 281) Time keeps flowing whether we notice it or not. Using the right clocks, watches, and alarms can help you be more aware of how much time has gone by and how much is left.

Digital Voice Recorders: Catch Thoughts on the Fly (p. 282) Digital voice recorders are cool little pieces of technology that can be great for recording brief notes or long diatribes.

Tools and Technology: General Concepts

ADHD is an information-processing disorder. Therefore, if your brain has trouble reliably doing certain things, you would benefit from using various tools to do those things for you. Of course, this is what all tools are for—to do things that we can't. For example, I can't push a nail into a board by hand, so I use a hammer. I can't remember all my client appointments, so I use a schedule book. We use tools to live bigger and easier lives. If you have ADHD (especially in this busy, crazy world we live in), you'll function much better with the right combination of tools. There are lots of possibilities, and we'll cover some of them here. The trick is to match the tool to the job, see how it works, and adjust as necessary.

The tools that work well for your friends who don't have ADHD may not work well for you. Of course, when I say tools, I could mean something as simple as a sticky note stuck on your bathroom mirror. It pretty much means anything that isn't your brain cells.

Some adults with ADHD are hesitant to use any tools for fear that it will make them stand out more, as if it casts a spotlight on their difficulties. I can understand the desire to want to blend in, but you need to ask yourself what will make you stand out more—using a PDA religiously or missing meetings? The first might get you a little gentle ribbing; the second will get you fired. Of course, this also assumes that you will remember to use these tools and not lose them. These are very real concerns, so it's a matter of finding the right tools and creating a habit so that you're more likely to stick with them.

The tools presented in this chapter are only the tip of the iceberg. There are lots of other options out there. Feel free to get creative. The only thing that matters is that it works for you.

Sometimes a Simple Calendar Is Enough

I'm all about using the simplest tool to get the job done. I'll talk about paper planners and complicated electronic organizers later, but sometimes a plain ol' wall calendar is enough. If you don't have too many meetings and deadlines to keep track of and you don't need something portable, a wall calendar may do the trick. You may need or want one at home and another one at work.

The most important first step in using a calendar is to put it in a good place, somewhere that you will see it without having to go looking for it. It should also be close to the action so you don't have to walk across the house to check or write on it. Keep these other points in mind:

- *Create a family calendar.* If you or your kids have complicated schedules of after-school activities, it may be especially important to keep it all in one place. See The Family Calendar on p. 304 for more on this.
- *Use different colors for each person or type of activity.* This makes it easier to read quickly and accurately.
- *Meet regularly to review the calendar.* For example, Sunday evenings can be a good time to go over who's going where and when so that there are fewer surprises.
- *Nothing is official until it's written down.* You can eliminate debates about who said (or didn't say) what to whom by requiring that everything be written down. You may also want to include your older children in this.

How to Use Your Planner Well

Most ADHD adults have a love/hate (mostly hate) relationship with planners. They know they need one to keep track of everything, but they haven't had enough success with planners to justify continuing to try to use one. The problem with planners is the same problem as everything else in the person's life—it requires consistently remembering to use it, not once or twice, but forever. This means not only putting events into it but also checking the darn thing to see what's coming (preferably before the event happens). This brings up images of those spy movies where the guy has the briefcase handcuffed to his wrist.

For many adults with ADHD, the first problem is that they've chosen the wrong planner (or were the unhappy recipient of it). Because they weren't quite right, these planners were quickly lost or ignored—and became yet another failure experience. It can be a relief to jettison what feels like an albatross on your neck, but it's harder to escape the feeling that you should be able to use it like everyone else. So let's talk about how to find the right planner. Consider your answers to these questions:

- What kinds of events do you need to keep track of?
- How many events?
- How often will you need to check the planner?
- How many details will you need to record with the entry, and how much space will you need?
- How portable does it have to be?
- What other information will you need—phone numbers, email addresses, and so on?
- Will a daily, weekly, or monthly view work best?
- Do you need it to remind you of appointments and deadlines?

All sorts of planners are available, and it's easy to get overwhelmed at the store. The answers to these questions will help you narrow down which planners would work best for you. You may also want to ask (or spy on) friends and coworkers to see what they use and perhaps ask them how it works for them. I talk about the pros and cons of paper and electronic planners in *Planners* next, but some of the basics of how you use a planner are the same.

You may find that you're more attached to your new planner if you take the time to enter phone numbers, upcoming events, regular meetings, various reminders, and other useful information into it. If nothing else, you don't want all that effort to go to waste if you stop using the planner.

Regardless of what kind of planner you buy, the key to using it effectively is to use it frequently. There is a momentum effect here, in that the more you use it, the more valuable it becomes and the more likely you are to use it again. This means writing down upcoming events as well as occasionally checking it to see if anything is coming up. Of course, the act of writing also provides some incidental checking, since you will see what's coming up. As a practicing psychologist, I look at my planner pretty much hourly as I schedule each client, so I have dozens of opportunities each week to see what's coming up. As a result, I'm rarely surprised, even without trying. If you're not frequently writing in your planner, then you need to make a habit of checking it regularly—at least a couple times a day. You may need to put up a sign to remind yourself of this until it becomes automatic. Even if you're not perfect about it, even partial success can be a big improvement in your life.

If you tend to overcommit yourself, then it's important to make sure that the planner is always present whenever you commit to an activity—and to make an ironclad rule for yourself that you never agree to anything without checking your planner first. Remember also that you will probably have some things that you need to do that go beyond the scheduled meetings and appointments, so you probably shouldn't schedule every moment of the day.

Planners: Paper or Plastic?

It seems that a million kinds of paper planners are available, and the techies keep cranking out more and more electronic ones. Some people prefer paper planners, whereas others swear by electronic ones (other people mostly swear at them). Which one is right for you? Let's talk about the relative merits of each.

Paper Planners

Paper planners come in all shapes and sizes with everything from a basic schedule to various to-do list options, goal-planning sheets, phone number lists, and informational inserts. Some of these bonus features seem kind of worthless to me, but maybe someone uses them. Regardless, they tend to be pretty straightforward to use—you flip to the right page and write events into it. Because it's quick and easy, you're more likely to do it. By contrast, some of the electronic planners can be slow and cumbersome as well as frightening for technophobes. I use a paper schedule book because I like being able to see all my clients for the entire week, something that would be hard to do on a small screen.

The big problem with paper planners is that, if you lose it, all your information is gone. There are no computer backups, and it can be a real bear to re-create all that data. One way to protect yourself is to write your contact information in big letters on the cover or first page and to write that there's a reward if it's found and returned. (I would gladly pay the $250 promised on the inside of my schedule book. Seriously.)

Personal Digital Assistants (PDAs)

If you had any doubt that everyone is struggling to stay on top of their schedules these days, just look at how many PDAs are being sold—it's not as if it's only the folks with ADHD who are buying them. They do offer some features that gadgety adults with ADHD will find really helpful. Perhaps most important, PDAs can be set to beep to remind you of various things, which is great for people who have trouble reminding themselves of things.

The other advantage that PDAs have over paper planners is that the data can be backed up, even if the hardware disappears. This can be a lifesaver. Most of these devices will automatically synchronize when plugged into a computer, creating an identical backup on the hard drive. (Assuming you remember to plug it in, but at least you will lose only the changes made since the last synchronization.) However, some more advanced versions can be set to synchronize on their own by calling in to a server somewhere. This is best if it's an option.

The new PDAs have tons of features, but be honest with yourself about what you're really likely to use. Just because a PDA does something doesn't mean that it does it well. For example, you might be able to view word-processing documents on your PDA, but unless you're on the road a lot, why wouldn't you just do it on your regular computer rather than squint at a dinky little screen? You don't want to pay for features that you won't use, but you also don't want to set yourself up with an endless series of distractions as you mess around with its settings. So try to get a sense of what you're looking for before you go to the store and the glitzy displays beckon you.

Some people like to get a combination cell phone and PDA, which means one less thing to remember, but you may lose out on functionality or ease of use. Speaking of cell phones, pretty much every cell phone these days has a calendar function with an alarm that can be set to go off a designated amount of time beforehand. They may be clunky to use, but they get the job done, so it's probably best for people who don't have a lot of events on their schedule and can deal with the slow data entry.

Use Your To-Do List Effectively: #1. Make a To-Do List

Admit it—you groaned a little bit when you saw the words *to-do list.* Most of us these days cringe when we think of our to-do lists, secretly wishing that someone would sneak in and cross off a bunch of things. As much as a to-do list is a simple thing (it's just a list, right?), there are some little tricks you can use to make best use of one, whether it's on paper or electronic.

- *Put things on your list.* OK, so this seems pretty obvious, but it's worth saying. It isn't a failure of the to-do list if it never got written down. Don't trick yourself into thinking that you'll remember it—it didn't work when you were in school, and it won't work any better now that your life is more complicated.
- *But not too many things.* A to-do list works only when it's the right size. If you have too many things on it, you'll probably feel overwhelmed and almost certainly will miss seeing the tasks that really matter. So make those choices up front and don't write down the tasks that you don't think you'll actually be able to get to.

- *Cross off the things you'll never get to.* Sometimes plans change, and what seemed reasonable when we wrote it down just won't happen. Rather than fret over it forever, just cross it off and focus on the more relevant tasks. This kind of conscious decision making is a sign of wisdom; it's failure only when you don't plan well and circumstances decide for you.
- *Write a new list occasionally.* Sometimes a well-used list gets too messy or chaotic, so it can be helpful to rewrite it and tweak it as you go.
- *Write a new list every day.* Some people find it helpful to write a new list at the beginning or end of each day because it helps them focus on what's most important.
- *Create a master list and a daily list.* Some people keep a master list with all the projects they're working on, then pull from that their more immediate list of items. This keeps them focused on what's most urgent without getting lost in the longer list.
- *Prioritize what's on your list.* You may find it helpful to put your list in some sort of order to keep you focused on what's most important. You can put things in a simple rank order, or classify them as 1 for do today, 2 for do this week, and 3 for do eventually. Alternatively, you may have three different sections on your list. Obviously, some things will change over time—the task that was to be done eventually will need to be done this week and then today.
- *Assess whether you have everything you need.* When putting items on your to-do list, you may want to include a little note about things that you'll need (like a new printer cartridge) or time restrictions (like needing to call before noon).

Whenever a client tells me that he's having trouble getting things done, I always want to know why—down to the nitty-gritty. I want to know where the process breaks down, so I ask these kinds of questions:

- Did he put everything he needed to do on his to-do list?
- If so, did he prioritize appropriately?
- If so, did he follow those priorities?
- If so, was there simply more to do than time allotted to do it, given predictable interruptions and inefficiencies?

If you're having trouble, look for a pattern. That may help you best focus your efforts.

To-Do List Software

All sorts of programs are available to help you manage your to-do list. (My Google search yielded 94,300,000 pages.) Many are free, whereas some have a nominal cost, and others have a cost that's not at all nominal. Search online for "to-do list software" to find one that fits your needs. If you have a PDA or smart phone, it will undoubtedly come with software that synchronizes with a to-do list on your computer, but you may find that you don't like the factory-loaded program and want to find something better.

My best advice is to limit yourself to the simplest program that will work for you. The more complicated something is, the less likely you are to use it consistently and over the long run. You'll simply get tired of wrangling it to do what you want.

Depending on your needs and how you would use the two types of list, a software-based to-do list has several advantages over paper ones, including the following:

- *Tasks are easily sorted and reprioritized.* Your priorities likely change over the course of a day or week, so it may be useful to be able to shift around the items on your to-do list to reflect that.
- *Different types of tasks can be broken into distinct categories.* You may want to have several types of lists, perhaps to reflect different projects or types of activities. A click or two will show you only those items that you want to currently see so that you don't need to visually sort through unrelated items.
- *Completed items are hidden.* Once a task is completed (or at least checked off), it drops off your list. This is cleaner and easier to read than a partially scratched-out paper list. This allows fewer places for your important tasks to hide.
- *Old items are preserved and searchable.* It can sometimes be helpful to go back to an old item to find out when you completed it, look up a phone number, and so on. If you can remember something unique enough to be searchable, you can find the desired information quickly.
- *Electronic lists are more easily backed up.* Unlike a paper-based system that is probably gone forever if it's lost, a computer-based one can be retrieved from a backup. (You back up your computer, right?)

Keep It Simple

Let me share my own to-do list system, adapted from a former supervisor. I make no claims that it will work for everyone, but it will for some. I use a small spiral notebook to write down names and phone numbers off the answering machine and scribble down things to do, letters to write, calls to make, and so on. I write these, one per line, on the right side of the notebook. I leave the left side open for jotting down quick notes that don't qualify as official to-do list items, but that I need somewhere better than the back of an envelope to write it down. I check off items as I complete them, so it's easy to scan down the page and see what's left. I then tear off the lower-right corner of the page once everything on it is completed so that I know that I don't need to go back to it. I put the date that I start a page at the top.

What's nice about this notebook system is that I can easily flip back through the pages to find an old phone number or other note. Because the pages are dated, I can find what I need pretty quickly, give or take.

This system is easy to manage and gets the job done. I will put certain far-off items in my schedule book—for example, handouts for a presentation that are due several months later. You may have more complicated tasks to manage than I do, in which case this system may not work for you. But if your demands are pretty straightforward, then the simpler the better.

It's About Time: Use Clocks and Alarms to Stay on Track

Time is a slippery thing (I know I had some around here somewhere...). If your internal clock doesn't tick loudly enough, then you need to make up for it with external clocks. This could be the simple solution of scattering a bunch of clocks around your home and work so that you're more likely to be aware of the passage of time. This is still a pretty passive solution, though, and depends on your cueing yourself that it's getting close to time to do something.

A more active solution (which requires less activity from you) is to set an alarm to do the reminding. The key is to set the alarm as soon as you think about it rather than count on yourself to remember to set it later (more time to forget). Alarms come in many shapes and sizes, and since most of them are pretty cheap, you don't need to limit yourself to just one. When considering which kinds of alarms might work best for you, ask yourself these questions:

- *Where and when do you tend to lose track of time?* For example, in the kitchen or at the computer.
- *Would a stationary or portable alarm be better?* It depends how much you move around.
- *Would a beeping or vibrating alarm be better?* A vibrating alarm may be better in the workplace, since it tends to elicit fewer

questions. A beeping alarm may be better at home because it also alerts family members who can give you a polite nudge if you ignore it.

- *Where should you put the alarm so you remember to set it?* It can help to have a highly visible designated place for it. Then don't put anything on top of it.

You may find that a cheap digital watch does the trick for you. Less than twenty bucks will get you a watch with multiple alarms, including programmable alarms, countdown alarms, stopwatches, and repeating alarms. You won't see these watches on any best-dressed lists, but showing up late tends to look worse.

If you're looking for something with more options, you can buy one of the several specialty watches on the market. These offer more alarms, as well as vibrating rather than beeping so you don't have to announce your time-management struggles to your whole office. Some of these are worn as wristwatches (WatchMinder and VibraLite) and some are worn like a pager (Invisible Clock). You can get more information at www.watchminder.com, www.globalassistive.com, and www.invisibleclock.com, respectively.

Instead of or in addition to a wristwatch, you may want to use plain old kitchen timers that you can set in a couple seconds. They're cheap enough that you can buy a bunch of them.

Most people use alarm clocks to get out of bed, but you may also want to set an alarm to tell you when it's time to get into bed. Or at least to start getting ready. This may be especially helpful if you tend to get caught up in things and unintentionally miss your bedtime.

Digital Voice Recorders: Catch Thoughts on the Fly

Digital voice recorders are about the size of a cell phone and can record hours and hours of audio as individual entries. They're available at most electronics and office supply stores and just keep getting better and less expensive. They're great for catching thoughts on the fly, like in the car or when running out the door. They can also be used for recording meetings, depending on the microphone's sensitivity and everyone else's willingness.

The more expensive models offer more features, like the ability to sort recordings into multiple folders and flag recordings as high priority. You can also download the recordings onto your computer in various formats and even run them through a voice-recognition program that will translate the audio into text. Pretty cool.

There are two potential problems with these little devices. The first is that they're easy to lose—you're not out a ton of cash, but everything you've recorded is gone.

The second is that you can't remind yourself what you recorded just by looking at it, unlike in written notes. So they're not for everyone, but they can be helpful tools for some people.

CHAPTER 13

ACHIEVE YOUR GOALS: TAKE THE LONG VIEW

I was once talking to a guy who said, "My first goal is to get a goal." That can be easy to relate to. Of course, once we get some goals, we need to work consistently to actually achieve them. This is usually harder.

I think it's safe to say that everything else in this book feeds into your ability to achieve your goals. Therefore, you will benefit from understanding how your ADHD trips you up and applying all the various strategies throughout the rest of the book. However, I offer you some more specific strategies in this chapter.

This chapter contains the following articles:

The Chain of Success: Awareness + Skills + Desire = Success

The pursuit of success is like a chain—it's only as good as its weakest link. To be successful, all the links need to be strong enough, whereas failure requires only one link to be weak. So when you do fail at something, the trick is to figure out which of those links is responsible. This is especially important for folks with ADHD, since it may not initially be clear which links gave way. So let's identify the three links of success:

- *Awareness.* The first link is simply being aware of the desired task. Obviously, if you forget about a project, you can't work on it. Sometimes the problem is remembering something at the wrong moments. For example, it doesn't help much to remember while at work that you need to pay the bills at home. These timing issues are big ones for ADHD folks.
- *Skills.* If you remember a task at the right time and place, you then need to have the ability to do what is required. This is usually not the problem for ADHD folks, since they instead tend to run into trouble with not reliably doing what they know.
- *Desire.* No amount of awareness and skill is enough if you don't put forth the necessary effort. Other people often assume that ADHD folks lack the desire to do the required tasks—that they are lazy or irresponsible or have a bad attitude. This is especially true before they are diagnosed. Unfortunately, over time, the ADHD person can begin to believe this himself, making him even less likely to give something his best effort, which then becomes a self-fulfilling prophecy. (See *Is the Problem ADHD or Motivation?* on p. 205 for more on this.)

It's helpful to think about these three links, since different strategies will be necessary depending on which link is breaking down. Strategies from one link probably won't help much in the others. So if something didn't work out, take a moment to figure out where things broke down. Depending on which link it is, you may want to try strategies along these lines:

- *Awareness.* If you're not remembering something at the right times or places, then set up something to remind yourself. For example, use a schedule book or calendar to keep track of commitments and deadlines. Use an alarm clock or PDA to remind you that it's time to do something else. Send an email from home to your work address to remind you to do something there. The trick is to set things up when you are thinking about it so that you can remind yourself at the times that you may not be thinking about it. Medication can also help with this.
- *Skills.* If part of the breakdown or avoidance comes out of not knowing how to do something, then seek help in learning how to do it better or faster. It's almost always preferable to ask for help than to show by your failure that you can't do something.
- *Desire.* Your desire to do something is related to the first two links. We all tend to be more aware of those things that we want to do,

but this may be even more true for ADHD folks. We also tend to prefer to do those things that we are good at. Sometimes, though, we need to do things that we don't really want to or aren't good at. Try to remind yourself of the rewards for doing it or the cost for not doing it. If you have ADHD, accept that it may take extra force of will to make yourself do these sorts of things.

Reach Your Short-Term Goals

Short-term goals are ones with a time span of a day or so. These can be easier to manage than longer-term goals because you don't need to stay focused for as long to accomplish them. On the other hand, if a couple of hours slip away, you don't have much time to make up for it. In addition to the strategies in the rest of the book, you may find that these strategies help you to stay focused on those short-term goals:

- *Plan each day.* Take the first or last fifteen minutes of the day to plan your activities and set priorities. Doing this regular check-in will help you stay focused on the most important tasks. At first you will probably have to push yourself pretty hard to make yourself do it, but it will become easier once it becomes a habit. Until that point, write the rule in stone that you will continue to do it, no exceptions.

- *Build in small rewards.* Everyone prefers the carrot to the stick, but for many people with ADHD, too many tasks can feel motivated primarily by avoiding the stick. You're more likely to be inspired by a positive, so create small rewards for yourself for finishing those awful obligations. It could be something as small as putting on your favorite CD or calling a friend.

- *Be honest with yourself when you're off track.* It can be easy to rationalize messing around with low-priority items when you should really be working on higher-priority items. (I talk about this in greater detail in *How to Be Productive, Not Just Busy* on p. 251.) If you catch yourself at this, then shift gears.

- *Tie short-term goals to larger goals.* It's easier to get going on some small thing if you know that it supports a larger goal. Think about the rewards from that bigger accomplishment when you feel tempted to wander off in the moment.

- *Use social pressure.* Make a commitment to someone else about what you will accomplish that day. Thinking about having to explain why you fell short may get you moving again. Just be sure to pick someone who will be decent about his reaction if you fall short and also who won't take this as an open invitation to offer advice.

Reach Your Long-Term Goals

Long-term goals involve anything that goes beyond a day. It could be a week, a year, or a decade, even. These can be especially difficult for most ADHD folks since far-away deadlines tend to disappear in the daily hustle and bustle. It's not that people are unaware of these goals or don't want to accomplish them, but rather that they are continually delayed into the future—*I'll work on that later...tomorrow...next week....* So the challenge is to find ways to keep these future goals in mind in the present.

- *Post a picture of the desired goal to serve as a reminder.* This may make it more real for you and inspire you to take action sooner.
- *Put up a note to yourself as a reminder.* This may be less inspiring, but it serves as a good reminder.
- *Break long projects into smaller pieces.* Set interim deadlines for each part. This brings the future closer into the present and can help you work more consistently along the way. However, you need to push yourself to honor these interim deadlines without rationalizing them as empty and therefore easily pushed back. For really big projects, you may find it helpful to talk to someone else about how to divide up the project and how much time to allot for each step.
- *Track your progress.* Spend some time on a regular basis to take stock of where you're at. This may make your progress more tangible and help you see where you need to do better so that you can make adjustments as necessary. This usually works out better if it's before the last minute.
- *Ask someone to hold you accountable.* Give that person your long-term schedule and ask him to check in with you on your progress. This can be two-minute meetings if you're on track, but it may be longer if you aren't. Just be sure to pick someone who will push you but not be overly critical about it.
- *Maybe get a different job.* If your job involves a lot of long-term projects and you keep running into trouble with them, you may be better off in a job with shorter goals or more frequent check-ins.

It's a sign of wisdom to know your limitations and put yourself into situations that favor your strengths.

Survive Repetitive Tasks, Repetitive Tasks, Repetitive Tasks

Repetitive and boring tasks are the bane of most ADHD folks. Not that anyone really enjoys them, but people with ADHD really hate them. Unfortunately, they're a necessary evil and an inescapable part of most long-term projects and goals. Perhaps these strategies will help you tolerate them a bit better:

- *Set specific deadlines.* This may push you to get going on things rather than procrastinate on them unto eternity. We all have plenty of tasks that need to be done at some point, but not necessarily by any one specific time. Therefore, you need to assign those times yourself.
- *Use last-minute pressure to get energized.* This can be helpful but is also risky if things don't go according to plan and you wind up running over, so you may want to be selective about when you do this.
- *Trade or delegate it away, if possible.* Whether at work or at home, you may be able to strike a bargain with someone else to do it for you in exchange for your doing something for them.
- *Do it in small doses.* If a marathon of this activity is more than you can stomach, then break it into multiple shorter sessions that are more tolerable. You just need to promise yourself that you'll actually come back around to it.
- *Work with someone else.* This can make it more fun and also make you less likely to wander off task or take long breaks. You may want to use a hands-free headset and talk to a friend while doing things around the house that don't require your full attention but need to be done, like folding laundry and loading the washer and dryer.
- *Create variety by rotating through several activities.* Even if none of the tasks are especially interesting, it may be less boring if you mix it up a bit.
- *Crank up the tunes.* Unless it will be too distracting, putting on some upbeat music may keep your energy level up. TV might work, too, but that's probably more likely to absorb your full attention and cause you to get less done.

- *Set up rituals to create consistency.* If you have certain boring tasks that need to be done on a regular basis, you may find that it's easier to create a ritual, like always paying bills on Sunday nights. The more automatic it becomes, the less you need to think about it.
- *Work for a specific amount of time.* Set a timer that will tell you when you can take a break.
- *Remind yourself of the cost of not following through.* When tempted to abandon ship on something, take a moment to think about the potential problems that might cause. Also try to be honest with yourself about how likely you are to actually come back and do it later.

Calm Your Hyperactivity

If you were hyperactive as a kid, odds are that you're much less hyperactive now. You probably won't be vibrating off your seat anymore, but you may feel restless if forced to sit for extended periods, like a long meeting or a movie. So you may still need some safe ways to discharge that excess energy (or at least make it less obvious) so that you can more consistently pursue those goals that involve a lot of sitting around. Try these strategies:

- *Exercise regularly.* This is one of those recommendations that I could make to anyone, but people with ADHD may especially benefit in terms of feeling calmer and also having better focus.
- *Work an active job.* If you have trouble sitting still, then find a job where you don't have to. This means obvious jobs like construction or working a sales floor, but it could also be an office job where you're frequently getting up and interacting with others rather than staring at a computer screen for eight hours.
- *Take breaks when you can.* If your job doesn't naturally offer a lot of opportunities to move around, then make the most of what you can, such as taking the stairs instead of the elevator, parking farther away so you have a longer walk, or taking the long way around the building. You may need to explain this to bosses or coworkers, so tell them that the activity makes you more productive when you are back at your desk.
- *Move during lunch.* You may be able to tolerate a sedentary job if you're able to be active during lunch. This could be a real workout or even just taking a walk, depending on how much activity you need and can squeeze in.

- *If necessary, get a different job.* This is a drastic step, but it may be necessary in some cases. If it's just killing you to be so sedentary, then you may be better off finding something else.

Section IV

IMPROVE SPECIFIC AREAS OF YOUR LIFE

Introduction: These Are the Changes That Count

We've covered a lot of information so far in this book, from what ADHD is to what you can do about it. Those articles have all led up to this section, which covers how to make specific improvements in specific parts of your life—household management, relationships, college, and work. When you get down to it, it's the struggles in these places that drive people to pick up a book like this or seek out professional help. For example, it isn't that they want to manage their time better, it's that they don't like the problems that poor time management leads to. Managing your time poorly at the beach isn't really a big deal, but it is at work. So it's the fallout in these areas of our lives that drive us to seek help. It's when they go from the abstract concept of time management to the practical realities of having to stay later than everyone else that we take notice and want something better. It's the negative outcomes that get our attention and motivate us to seek out better solutions.

So the chapters in this section cover where the rubber meets the road. This is where things really matter. In addition to curiosity and a desire for knowledge, it's the hope of making progress in these areas that probably drove you to read the rest of the book. That investment will pay off well as you read the remaining chapters and are better able to apply the strategies to your life. This is where things really begin to get good.

What This Section Covers

This section contains the following chapters:

14. *Household Management: Stay on Top of the Boring Stuff at Home* (p. 297) There's a lot that needs to happen at home, from getting a good night's sleep to paying the bills, not to mention coordinating everyone's schedule. These strategies can help you handle all of these demands and make home a more relaxing place.

15. *Relationships and Friendships: Strive for Balance* (p. 309) ADHD can affect how you interact with others, from coworkers to friends to loved ones. The better you understand this, the more effectively you can actively manage those relationships and make them satisfying for everyone.

16. *College and Beyond: Teach an Old Dog New Tricks* (p. 341) College can be a difficult place for students with ADHD, especially if they don't know they have it. Fortunately, there is a lot you can do to succeed in college, whether you're eighteen or eighty.

17. *Work: Hopefully More Than Just a Paycheck* (p.355) There are lots of things you can do to make work a more rewarding experience. Sometimes small tweaks are enough to bring out your best. Other times you need bigger changes, like a new job. We'll cover both.

CHAPTER 14

HOUSEHOLD MANAGEMENT: STAY ON TOP OF THE BORING STUFF AT HOME

Running a household is a pretty complicated task, especially if there is more than one person involved (and all the more so if some of those people are under eighteen). There are all sorts of tasks that need to be done on a pretty regular basis, from wiping off the kitchen counters to filing taxes, not to mention coordinating everyone's comings and goings. To do this smoothly requires a certain mental organization that is difficult for many with ADHD to achieve. Fortunately, there are lots of strategies you can use to make the whole process simpler and more streamlined. This is important, because ideally home should be the least stressful place in your life, somewhere you can recharge for the marathons and sprints in the rest of your life.

This chapter contains the following articles:

Stay in the Budget: We Have a Budget? (p. 305) Creating and staying in a budget is no easy task. These strategies can help you be more successful at it.

Stop the Flood: Conquer Information Overload (p. 307) Information is everywhere, and we all need to find a way to stay on top of it all. These tips can help you keep your head above water.

Create a Lifestyle You Can Live With

People with ADHD often find themselves in a lifestyle that worsens their ADHD—chaotic, unstructured, or too extreme. For example, I've had dozens of clients who habitually stayed up too late on various pursuits and then, predictably, struggled to get out of bed on time and felt awful the next day. They all knew this was torpedoing their productivity, but it was a real challenge to break the habit in the moment, partly because a lot of it came out of their ADHD-based planning difficulties. Of course, the lack of sleep and stress from the last-minute scrambles also added to their struggles.

Unfortunately, maintaining a balanced and structured lifestyle requires the ability to plan effectively and then follow through on those plans consistently—not exactly what we'd call ADHD hallmarks. As a result, it may always take extra work for someone with ADHD to achieve the desired balance. It's a matter of finding a way to become less reactive and more proactive. This involves managing the small daily stuff that snowballs into big problems and to get better at seeing crunch times before they hit. This requires some decent proficiency in all the areas I talked about in section III—good time management, effective organizational systems, accurate memories, and some sense that the effort will amount to something. In other words, there's a lot that goes on behind the scenes before someone can live a stable and predictable life.

Realizing how much work it takes and how unsuccessful they've been at it before, some adults with ADHD just give up and live life flying by the seat of their pants. Some even embrace the chaos and claim that they prefer it that way, that they're not as anal-retentive as everyone else. I'm certainly not going to judge them if that's how they really want to live—after all, just because I hate paying late fees doesn't mean that someone else should care about them. The question I always have when I meet someone like this is whether they truly want this lifestyle or are they merely settling for it because they don't feel capable of creating something more stable. If they're settling, then I would encourage them to take another look at it, especially once their ADHD has been diagnosed and treated, to see if a different approach may yield better results. If so, then they truly have a choice. With settling, it's choosing the only option that's available.

Psychologist Kathleen Nadeau (2002) says that an ADHD-friendly lifestyle emphasizes the following:

- Good sleep patterns
- Proper diet
- Frequent exercise
- Controlled substance use
- Tolerable stress levels
- Appropriate stimulation
- Supportive social relationships
- Career choices that cater to strengths without playing on too many weaknesses

I like to call this the New Year's resolution stuff—the changes that we all could do a little better on. Obviously none of these will cure your ADHD, but they will enable you to perform at your best. This doesn't mean that you need to move into a minimalist monastery and give up all pleasures or that you need to turn into a robot and live a perfectly scheduled life. In fact, striving for something too extreme is a quick way to give up on all of it. It's like trying to lose weight using an all-celery diet—in an hour you'll be inhaling an entire chocolate cake. So the goal here is a lifestyle that is good for you but is also maintainable. You will need to stretch for it, but not to the point of breaking.

In order to be more likely to be successful, you need to create habits that take both your ADHD and personal preferences into account. For example, if you are barely better than comatose most mornings, then it's asking for trouble to expect yourself to go to the gym before work. It might be really good for you, but it seems unlikely to happen more than once. When you do get to the gym, if you know that you get bored easily, then you may want to give yourself a lot of options for your workouts so that you're more likely to stick with it.

When you do need to let loose, you should be able to fully enjoy yourself. This means having guilt-free fun, which requires that you don't have any avoided obligations hanging over your head. So when you're having fun, you can really have fun. If you require more active pursuits in order to relax, then seek them out. Take care of yourself by doing what you need to do to recharge your batteries. As long as it's legal and doesn't hurt anyone, go for it.

Actually Get a Good Night's Sleep

A good night's sleep sets the stage for a productive day—and insufficient sleep sets a very different stage. This may be especially true for people with ADHD, since they already struggle with focus and motivation. Being tired only makes that worse. Unfortunately, getting a good night's sleep is much easier said than done. I would go so far as to say that we can measure how well someone is doing with his ADHD by how well he does at consistently getting a good night's sleep. It takes a fair amount of stability and control over one's life to be able to get into bed on time.

Let's talk about some of the reasons that people with ADHD don't get enough sleep:

- *Procrastination* forces them to stay up late to finish everything when they get a late start.
- *Hyperfocus* on an enjoyable activity causes them to not be aware of how late it is getting, so they miss their bedtime.
- *Intentionally staying up too late* with a "consequences be damned" attitude—they know they will pay the price the next day, but don't want to stop what they are doing and go to sleep.
- *An overactive mind* makes it hard to let go and fall asleep, even when they are in bed.
- *Stimulant medication* can make it harder to fall asleep if they have too much still in their systems.
- *A true sleep disorder* can make it harder for them to fall asleep quickly, stay asleep, or sleep deeply enough.

When I hear that a client is waking up late or is having trouble getting out of bed on time, I always ask what happened the night before, since morning problems usually start at night. If we can identify exactly what contributed to the sleep problem, we can then work on ways to make that less likely to happen again. It's worth working on, because getting up late sets a negative tone to the morning that can cascade throughout the whole day, and being tired makes everything that much harder.

- *Get on a schedule.* Sleep experts recommend going to bed and waking up at around the same time every day, including weekends. Over time, this will help to program your sleep rhythm.
- *Limit caffeine after noon.* Having too much caffeine too late in the day can make it harder to fall asleep. Sometimes you may fall asleep but then wake up soon after, which makes it seem as if the

caffeine isn't responsible. If you take stimulant medication, you may especially want to limit your caffeine.

- *Create a prebedtime routine.* This will condition your brain to get ready once the lights go out.
- *Find calming activities to help you wind down before bed.* Experiment to see what works for you.
- *Exercise helps sometimes.* For some people, exercising late in the day keeps them up, but others find that it tires them out. It's probably also affected by the intensity of the exercise, as well as the timing.
- *Set a bedtime alarm.* This tells you when it's time to start getting ready for bed so you don't inadvertently stay up later than planned.

The more you work to actively manage your ADHD through the day, the better shape you will be in as bedtime approaches. So look at it as a process. If you're still having trouble getting a good night's sleep, you may want to talk to your doctor about it and possibly get a sleep study. Although sleeping medication can be helpful, be careful of using it for an extended period.

Manage the Mail and Get the Bills Out on Time

That darn mail just keeps coming. Six days a week. Most of it's junk, but some of it is actually important, and then there's some stuff that is somewhere in between. The challenge is to sort through it all, get rid of the junk, and keep track of and deal with the important items. This requires the kind of consistency that people with ADHD have difficulty mustering, which creates two problems. The first is random bits of mail getting spread around the house and cluttering it all up. This is usually less costly than the second problem, which is that the bills don't go out on time, even though there's plenty of money in the bank account. Therefore the broader goal of managing all the stuff that comes in serves the more specific goal of getting things back out on time.

So let's talk about some ways to stay on top of it all.

- *Put a recycling bin next to the door.* It may not be pretty, but it reduces the clutter in other parts of the house (so they look better). Immediately pitch all the junk that you know you won't look at.
- *Make some good choices.* After you pitch the junk, pitch that marginal stuff that you think you will look at, but probably never will. The sooner it gets tossed, the less it lingers around taunting you, and the sooner you forget about it.

- *Create a designated place for the important items.* This should be as close to the door as possible, so there is less risk of detours. Only important items get put here, such as bills, paperwork to file, or things that you need to respond to. This way, you know where this stuff is and don't need to track it down throughout the house when it comes time to pay the bills.
- *Set up as many bills as possible on automatic payments.* The fewer bills you need to actually handle, the less likely you are to get them out late. This way, you just need to enter them into your check register occasionally. You may not want to put your big bills to debit automatically in case you don't have the funds to cover them, but it may be a good idea for all those little ones.
- *Create a designated time to pay bills.* This could be weekly, like Sunday nights, or on parts of the month, such as at the middle and end. If you're not likely to remember to do it reliably, then you may need to put it in your schedule, set reminder alarms, or ask a family member to remind you.
- *Save only what you must.* It can be tempting to save a lot of the paperwork that we get, but much of it isn't actually necessary, especially because we can get copies of most of it for a small fee. So ask your accountant or a friend who isn't too obsessive-compulsive about what you actually need to save. Pitch everything else.
- *Get overdraft protection.* Depending on how much it costs and how many checks you bounce, it may be worth not having to worry about messing up the timing of money coming in and money going out. Try to not use it as a line of credit to borrow money from since the rates probably aren't a good deal, but it's much better than insufficient-funds fees.
- *Cancel unused subscriptions and catalogs.* There are more interesting things in this world than any of us will have time to explore. So if you keep getting a magazine or catalog that you don't read often enough, then either cancel the subscription or don't renew it. The less that comes in, the less you need to deal with.

Family Meetings: What's Happening This Week?

If you have kids who are involved in after-school activities, it can be especially important to discuss the week ahead with your romantic partner—who's going where, what's happening, what are we running out of, what do we need to do, etc.

Even if you don't have kids, you may still find it helpful to meet and keep everyone in the loop. ADHD households are especially prone to those *I told you/you never told me* arguments. Any active family is vulnerable to this because we're all so busy just keeping up that we don't make the time to coordinate what's happening next.

It can therefore be helpful to create a habit of meeting once a week to review upcoming events and let each other know what needs to happen. This makes for fewer unpleasant surprises later. Obviously, things will change and new things will come up between meetings, but it will minimize the amount of last-minute finagling.

If you have kids, whether little ones or teens, they will probably enjoy having a designated time where they can talk about the family schedule (most of the time, at least). This predictability gives them a sense of safety and of being heard. These meetings can lead to other important discussions about what's going on in your kids' lives and what they're thinking of or worried about. So keep your ears open.

- *Choose a consistent time.* You're more likely to keep the tradition alive if you choose a time that will be consistently available. Too much rescheduling makes it too easy to abandon.
- *Review the family calendar.* If you have one, this meeting is a good time to go over everything for the week, fill in missing pieces, and answer any questions. See the next article, The Family Calendar.
- *Make it quick.* To paraphrase one of my teachers, these meetings should be like a bikini—big enough to cover the topic, but short enough to be interesting. If they drag on too long, the bored participants will look for reasons to avoid the next meeting. Besides, if it takes more than ten minutes to discuss the week's schedule, then maybe you need to cut back on your commitments.
- *Try to focus just on scheduling matters.* Other topics will come up, since everything is related in one way or another, but try to hold off on discussing the tangents until all the scheduling matters are covered.
- *Meet half the time without the kids, half the time with them.* You will probably find it helpful to have part of the meeting be adults only, since some of it won't be relevant or interesting to the little ones.
- *Put up a whiteboard for agenda items.* Since things come up throughout the week, it can be helpful to have a place to scribble notes to be sure everything is covered.

- *Ask about big school projects.* The meeting can also be a good time to figure out where those big projects (including shopping trips) fit in, since that can quickly throw a monkey wrench in the plans.

The Family Calendar: Let's Keep It All in One Place

As we discussed in the preceding article on family meetings, life is easier when everyone in the family knows what's going on. If the number of activities has exceeded the limits of your memory, then you need a backup.

You may use a schedule book or PDA for work obligations and then use another one for commitments at home. However, rather than dividing items based on where they occur, it may be better to think of your work calendar for daytime commitments and the family calendar for evenings and weekends. For example, if you need to take one of your kids to a midday appointment, that should go in your work calendar since it will affect your workday. And a work-related holiday party in the evening would go on the family calendar since that's where you'll have to plan around it.

- *Nothing is official until it's written down.* A family calendar is only as helpful as the information that is put on it. So it's everyone's responsibility to write things down and also to check it occasionally.
- *Put it where everyone can see it.* Put it somewhere easily seen to make it more likely that everyone looks at it.
- *Tie a pen to it.* Having to hunt down a pen is an easy excuse to write something down later (or not).
- *Sometimes you need duplication.* If a home activity affects work, or vice versa, you may want to write on both calendars—for example, if you need to leave work early to go to your child's concert at school. The only potential problem with this kind of redundancy is that if something comes up, you might change it in only one place, so try to stay on top of that. You may want to leave yourself a voicemail at the other place so you remember to change it there as well.
- *Use different colors.* It may be helpful to assign each person or type of activity a color. This makes it easy to scan the calendar quickly and see what you need to.

Whiteboards: Low-Tech Reminders

Whiteboards can be a good way to capture various bits of information, so you may want to put one up in the kitchen, home office, garage, workshop, and anywhere else that you will think of something that you want to remember. It could be items for a shopping list, phone numbers, people to call back, messages for family members, or just something you thought of. A busy life will have plenty of these moments, where something that comes up needs to be saved for later. You can improve your batting average by scribbling those thoughts down on something that won't get lost or thrown away.

- *Write notes to yourself.* Use the whiteboard to record those slippery thoughts that will otherwise get away from you.
- *Write notes to each other.* If you have a busy life, you probably don't get a lot of chances to fill each other in on all the little details. A whiteboard can be the perfect vehicle for this—write it and forget it. (Email also works well.)
- *Use designated colors or places.* You may find it helpful to assign each person or type of task a particular color. Or maybe you assign each person a particular part of the whiteboard. Both of these make it easier to quickly see what you need to.
- *Erase the old stuff immediately.* Our brains filter out whatever has been around for a while, so if you have a bunch of old notes hanging around, you may not notice the new notes. At a certain point, you need to transfer that information to somewhere else.

Stay in the Budget: We Have a Budget?

As we discussed in *Money Management* on p. 81, people with ADHD struggle with managing their money for a lot of different reasons. Sure, they know all about how important it is and why they should do a better job of managing their finances. Yet somehow that general knowledge isn't enough to prevent too much being spent on some expenses, leaving too little left over to spend on others. As in so much of ADHD, the problem is closing the gap between intentions and actions. The problem is that managing money effectively requires certain skills that most ADHD adults can't count as strengths.

Let's go back over the reasons for ADHD adults' money troubles listed in *Money Management*, but this time with an eye toward solutions.

- *Resist impulsive spending.* You probably know the stores, items, or situations that are most tempting for you. You can protect yourself by either avoiding them completely or bringing only cash and leaving the credit cards at home so as to limit how much you can spend. As fun as it can be to let an impulse carry you away, work really hard to not commit to an expense without first thinking about how it fits into your overall budget. If you can't stop yourself from buying it, then save the receipt and try to wait to open it, in case you wind up reconsidering your purchase.
- *Remember all those moving numbers.* It's easy to run into financial trouble by forgetting about upcoming purchases and making what turn out to be unwise choices. Accept that budgeting is a pretty complicated process, and don't expect yourself to be able to wing it all in your head. Write down a monthly and weekly budget. You don't need to get down to the pennies, but try to create a general plan so you have something to compare against—for example, how much do you have allotted for eating lunch out? This way you know if you're above or below the line.
- *Get organized.* You can manage your finances effectively only if you know what they actually are. This means having a balanced checkbook (give or take) and something of a budget. You don't need to be super anal-retentive about it, but you need to have a pretty close idea. Actually, making it too complicated and horrible will make you less likely to stick with it. In addition, you need to have a pretty good idea of what expenses you have coming up so you can prepare for them.
- *Get on top of the other details in your life.* We can use money to make up for getting behind in other ways. For example, paying extra to have something express mailed because we ordered it late, or eating lunch out because we didn't go food shopping over the weekend and had nothing to make lunch with. This is one of those easier-said-than-done kind of things, but the better you do in the rest of your life, the better your finances will look. In fact, we can almost use your financial state as a measure of how the rest of your life is going. (Try to not apply this to our federal government.)
- *Kiss late fees good-bye.* Put as many bills as you can on automatic payments so they get paid without your even needing to think about it. If you feel uncomfortable giving up control like that, then set up electronic payments through your bank so you can log on

and get the payment in that same day. This eliminates the variability of the postal system and also gives you a couple more days to do it.

If you have one, you may want to have your romantic partner manage the finances if it better suits her strengths and interests. Just because you're all grown up doesn't mean that you have to be good at everything. That's why we couple up—so we can unload some of those tasks that we hate or are bad at. So maybe the two of you decide that it's your partner's job to manage the details, set the financial plan for the household, and be nice about keeping you on track. Then it's your job to do your best to stick to the plan and to be gracious about her input. That way everybody wins (and she'll keep doing the boring finances).

Stop the Flood: Conquer Information Overload

ADHD has been described as an information-processing disorder. Since we live in an information age, it brings to mind the great quote from Norm on the TV show *Cheers:* "It's a dog-eat-dog world, and I'm wearing Milk-Bone underwear." You don't have to have ADHD to be able to relate to this, but untreated ADHD will make it that much harder to keep up with everything coming at you. The trick becomes sorting through it all and making good choices about what you give your time to.

This brings up a concept from economics, *opportunity cost*—whenever we spend a dollar (or hour), it isn't available to spend somewhere else. For example, watching some dumb TV show costs us the opportunity to spend that hour watching a much better show or doing something more satisfying or productive with that time. So economists would tell us to maximize the returns on our invested time by choosing the best activities since we can spend each hour only once.

On the other hand, don't fret over minor differences. For example, should you go to this website or that one? Should you watch this show or that movie? Pick one and let the other one go. The important thing is that you're enjoying that moment in time. Don't worry about what you're not getting to, because there will be a million other interesting things created by the time you would come back to it anyway. It's like going to a giant buffet—you won't get to taste everything, but you'll still get a good meal, even if it's different from the meal that someone else selects. So enjoy what you have (and stop eyeing your neighbor's chocolate cake).

- *Accept that you will miss a lot.* There's way too much new stuff coming out every single second of every single day for any of us to have any hope of getting to all the good stuff, or even some small fraction. Your local big bookstore has more books, magazines, DVDs, and CDs at this very moment than any of us will read, watch, or listen to over our entire life. And let's not even talk about 200 cable TV channels and a billion websites.

- *Limit how much comes at you.* Even if you don't do much, information still has a way of finding you, so you need to set up barriers to what you don't really want. For example, resist the impulse to sign up for catalogs, listservs, or email lists, then unsubscribe from them when you get them anyway. Be selective about what you let into your life. The less that comes in, the less you need to deal with. This is especially important if you know that you have trouble resisting things in the moment, so you then should remove that temptation before it even strikes.

- *Make good choices about what you seek out.* The situations that you put yourself in will influence the kinds of choices you need to make. For example, popping into the video store will put tempting movies under your nose that you will need to decide about. Clicking on the link that someone sent you can lead to even more clicking and far more time than you originally planned. This takes time away from more satisfying pursuits.

- *Follow your fancy sometimes.* Give yourself permission sometimes to just go where your heart leads you, even if it brings you to some completely mindless activity. Get done what you need to, then just play.

- *Stop flipping channels.* TV is an easy place to waste a lot of time. There are some great shows on, but also a lot that aren't. Perhaps a better option is to invest in a digital video recorder (Tivo is one brand) so that you can record specific shows and then watch them whenever you want. Not only does this free you from having to plan other activities around the TV schedule, it may also be easier to resist flipping channels before or after you watch your show.

CHAPTER 15

RELATIONSHIPS AND FRIENDSHIPS: STRIVE FOR BALANCE

It's been said that if one person in a relationship has ADHD, then the other person kind of has it, too. The one person's ADHD affects not only how he interacts with his romantic partner, but also his ability to meet his practical obligations in the relationship, like getting to dinner on time and picking up after himself. This can lead to some predictable and interesting dynamics between the two people as they work to find a better way. Every couple faces their own challenges, but a relationship where one person has ADHD will tend to face certain kinds of challenges—and benefit from certain kinds of strategies.

It's important to remember that when it comes to improving your relationships and friendships or reducing the effect that your ADHD has on them, you don't need to strive for perfection. Often, some partial improvements are enough to make things much better and create a situation where your positive qualities outweigh the negative feelings the other person has about your ADHD-based behaviors. Of course, you may also decide that you're tired of trying to be something you aren't and make some choices about who you interact with. Some other people may be much more appreciative of your good qualities and much more tolerant of your negative ones.

I use the word *relationship* broadly to refer to interactions of all kinds: family member, friend, coworker, boss, for example, so it doesn't apply just to romantic relationships. Besides, a lot of the same rules apply to all of these. Usually romantic relationships intensify feelings and thoughts that we can keep simpler in other relationships.

This chapter contains the following articles:

undiagnosed ADHD. This article discusses how to approach that person in a constructive way about seeking an evaluation.

We See Others Through Our Own Lens (p. 315) We understand others' actions based on what we ourselves do. This makes it easy to misinterpret ADHD behaviors, because they look intentional to someone who doesn't have ADHD.

Expectation Management: Promise Only What You Can Deliver (p. 316) Given that ADHD behaviors are so often misunderstood, your relationships will be more satisfying and less stressful if you actively manage what others should and shouldn't expect from you.

The Value of a Good Apology (p. 318) Since everyone blows it sometimes, we could all benefit from knowing how to give a really good apology. It may not change what happened, but it can change how the other person feels about it.

To Tell or Not to Tell? (p. 319) There are no absolute rules about whether you should tell someone about your ADHD, but there are some issues you should consider when making your decision.

Relationship Patterns to Avoid: You Can Do Better (p. 323) People with ADHD tend to fall into certain kinds of relationships. This is understandable, but you may find that you want something different and more satisfying.

Restore Balance in the Relationship (p. 324) Every relationship entails struggling to maintain balance. You can use these techniques to bring a little more balance (and peace and satisfaction) to your relationships.

Fun Stuff in the Bedroom: Improve Your Sex Life (p. 329) A couple's sex life can be affected by many things, including one partner's ADHD. A satisfying sex life is a worthy goal for every romantic relationship.

Work It Out with Some Help: Couples Therapy (p. 330) Sometimes it may be necessary or helpful to call in a couples therapist to enable you to get over a roadblock or make your relationship even better.

Social Skills Training: Helpful or Obvious? (p. 334) Social skills classes are sometimes recommended for adults with ADHD, but they may not be that helpful if you already know what to do. The trick then becomes doing the right things at the right times.

Parenting: Stay Sane While Wrangling the Offspring (p. 336) Children can add a lot to your life, including more complexity. You can use these strategies to make it more satisfying for all concerned.

True Intimacy Means Hearing the Bad News, Too

For better or worse. Ideally, relationships have more good moments than bad, but conflict, anger, frustration, and disappointment are an inherent part of relationships and life. It's only in the movies that we see just the good parts of romance (if we got enough of that in our real lives, we wouldn't have to go to the movies). So the challenge is to find a way to deal with these other emotions in a manner that doesn't interfere too much with enjoying the good parts of the relationship. If you're the one with ADHD, it's easy to focus on the troubles that you contribute to the relationship, but you're still only half of it. Your partner also plays a part and contributes both to the problems and the potential solutions.

If your goal is to have a strong relationship that lasts over time, then you need to be able to be honest with each other. This means not just the good news, compliments, and things that you agree on, but also the bad news, criticisms, and disagreements. Every relationship will have them—even the ones where neither person has ADHD. If one person does have ADHD, then it's easy to make that look like the biggest problem. It's a great smoke screen that hides all the other problems.

Psychologist and relationship expert David Schnarch, Ph.D., has a saying that I use a lot—the sign of a good relationship is that it forces you to become a better person (1997). That is, our partners push us to deal with our issues and bad habits and hopefully rise above them. By contrast, being overly tolerant of our partner's issues is actually a disservice—being an *enabler,* in AA lingo. So being forced to deal with your ADHD is a favor. So is forcing your partner to deal with her reaction to your ADHD. We may not always like what we hear, but that doesn't mean that it isn't good for us to hear it.

Of course, working on your delivery is a way to make it more likely that your message will be received by your partner the way you intend it. This is another place where we can all work on becoming a better person—not just dealing with our own issues, but also in sharing our perceptions about our partners' issues in a constructive way. If there's too much anger behind your delivery, it distracts from the real point and makes it too easy for your partner to justify not hearing what you're saying.

Your or your partner's ADHD may be the thing that starts you really looking at the relationship, but it won't be where it ends. No relationship is so simple that the *only* problem is someone's ADHD. No one is that lucky.

Of course, if we want people to be honest with us, then it's our responsibility to be sure that we handle their honest comments appropriately. Truth is earned—that is, if you want people to continue to be honest with you, then you need to react well when they tell you what you don't want to hear. If you react badly or use the information against them later, they have no reason to be good enough to be honest next time. Everybody loses then. So strive for something better. Work on really hearing what these other people are saying. It doesn't mean that you have to agree with it all (you won't), but you at least should listen. This becomes a matter of integrity—I want to be the kind of person who can handle bad news. I also want to be able to say that I've done my best to make this a better relationship.

No Man Is an Island: How to Get Help When You Need It

ADHD is definitely not an invisible condition. It may not always be obvious *why* someone does the things that she does, but there won't be much doubt about *what* she does. Therefore, part of managing your ADHD involves managing how you relate to other people. This involves making good decisions about how and when to ask for help, striving for balance in the relationship, living up to your obligations without making your problems other people's problems, and not promising more than you can deliver. We'll talk about all of these topics in further detail in the rest of this chapter, so in this article we're going to focus on the basics of effectively getting help from the people in your life.

Many adults with ADHD have mixed feelings about getting help from others. On the one hand, they may be hesitant to reach out for help because they feel that they should be able to manage all these details themselves and that asking for help is therefore a sign that something is wrong with them. On the other hand, some adults with ADHD may rely on others too much to manage the details of their life and keep them on track. It can be even more confusing for all involved when the person vacillates between these two extremes because she hasn't figured out where she really stands and what she really wants the relationship to look like.

As with most things in life, the best path is usually something in between. This means asking for help when it's appropriate. This tends to lead to the best outcomes—things tend to work out better, you get to take credit for your contribution to the successes, and the other person feels both needed and appreciated. This sure beats the alternatives.

In order to be able to manage your relationships effectively, you first need to know yourself and what you want. How much input do you want on what happens in your life? What are your limits? What are you willing to ask for help on, and what would you prefer to figure out for yourself? The answers to these questions evolve over the course of our lives as both our abilities and the demands on us increase. Being diagnosed with ADHD will almost certainly shift your answers as well, in both directions—you may find that you're better able to take on certain responsibilities once you take your ADHD into account, whereas you may find that you're now more willing to let go of other responsibilities.

Once you know what you want, you need to communicate that to the people in your life. You may or may not tell them that you have ADHD (see *To Tell or Not to Tell* on p. 319), but you will need to tell them what you're looking for from them, what you don't want from them, and what you're willing to give. Ask about their expectations and what they are willing to give. Then the negotiation begins! Whether you have ADHD or not, what you ask for from other people is probably different from what they ask of you. You could take it as a sign of weakness that you need to, for example, ask for reminders, but look at this way—isn't it kind of asking for trouble to associate with people who have exactly the same needs as we do? Isn't it better to have people in our lives who have needs and abilities that differ from and complement our own?

When you approach these other people with your requests, you might want to emphasize how they will also benefit from your doing better. For example, if you know that you will probably forget things that are said in passing, it may be better to ask people to leave you a note. Everybody wins—the only solution that lasts.

Overcome Denial: Help Someone Else to Recognize His ADHD

I would wager that a decent percentage of you are family members or romantic partners of adults with diagnosed or suspected ADHD. The reason why other people tend to get involved in politely encouraging (or nagging, depending on your perspective) the person with ADHD to get treatment, is that untreated ADHD tends to affect family members, too. ADHD is hardly unique in this regard.

I often get calls from family members seeking treatment for someone else and am asked at presentations how to get that reluctant person to see someone. Sometimes the situation is complicated by having a child who seems to be struggling with ADHD, but the parent doesn't want to see it. As a guy, I hate to say this, but it's usually we dads who are more reluctant. These fathers justify not getting treatment by minimizing the child's difficulties or saying that he'll grow out of it—just like he himself did (not really). No parent likes to admit that his child is struggling, but this responsibility can be doubly difficult for the parent with ADHD who is reliving his own childhood while watching his child suffer. I understand the desire to avoid this pain. Unfortunately, the pain only gets worse the longer it's avoided.

Whether you're trying to get the adult or the child into treatment, some of the basics are the same. It isn't about pathologizing or casting blame. It's about making our lives easier and better. We do this all the time in all sorts of ways. For example, many of us have air conditioning, even though few of us would die from a hot day—why would we suffer if we don't have to? Is it a moral failing to admit that you don't like swimming in your own sweat?

Talk to the person in a calm way about how his ADHD (or whatever it is, if it hasn't been diagnosed yet) affects him and you. Don't be accusatory; just state the facts as neutrally as you can manage. About how it makes both of your lives harder than they should be. About how it can be hard to admit these things, but that the reward for doing so is that life might get easier. Then tell him what you're willing to do (and perhaps not do) to make things better. This is about collaboration and improving the lives of everyone in the family—*What do we need to do to make our lives better?*

If you get a strong negative reaction, like anger, denial, or finger-pointing, then you obviously hit a nerve. Back off and let it ferment. Wait a few days or weeks, then bring it up again. These sorts of conversations sometimes need a few rounds before anything definitive happens. Of course, it's easier to take the long view if you start this discussion before you get to the end of your rope. By that point, patience is long gone.

If these conversations continue to fall on deaf ears, then it's time to turn up the heat, in a nice way. Let him suffer his own consequences, and be a little less generous about bailing him out of the situations that you mentioned. This doesn't mean giving him the cold shoulder and refusing to do *anything* nice for him—just the ADHD-related stuff that you talked about. For example, you won't be giving him those additional reminders or helping him get out the door on time when he gets distracted. Tell him this ahead of time so there are no nasty surprises, and explain to him that you would be happy to do these things again in the future, but only after he meets with a knowledgeable professional (see *Getting Diagnosed* on p. 41). Explain that you feel that it isn't helping him or the relationship for you to be working harder than he is on these things.

If it's a child that you would like to have evaluated but the other parent is resistant, you may need to approach it a little differently. Explain why you think that it's worth looking at. If you have it, provide backup information, such as emails from teachers, report cards, and comments from coaches, so it doesn't look like this is just your opinion. If the other parent doesn't see the same problems, it may be because he doesn't interact with the child in the same situations. For example, you may be the one who is responsible for getting the child to do his homework, so you see the distraction and fight the battles. If that's the case, then ask the other parent to take over these responsibilities for a time—not just once, because the novelty may mask some of the ADHD symptoms. Let him experience what you experience and see the struggles firsthand.

Most likely, you and the other parent have the same goals for your child, but may disagree about the methods of getting there. You may feel that you need to address his potential ADHD in order for him to be most successful, whereas the other parent may not see this as necessary. Remember to keep these common goals in mind, since that will tend to keep the discussion calmer and more productive. This is especially the case if you and the other parent do not live together.

It may be that the other parent needs to see the gains that a child makes once his ADHD is addressed in order to agree to look at his own difficulties. Of course, the better we are doing in our own lives, the better parents we can be, so his getting on top of his ADHD and feeling more effective and less stressed will only be a good thing.

We See Others Through Our Own Lens

It's a fact of human nature that we try to understand other people's actions by assuming that everyone else has the same motives we do. For example, if someone without ADHD forgot to do something, it may be because she didn't really care that much about it ("If something is important, I remember it"). Therefore, if someone else (perhaps with ADHD) forgets to do something, the first person will assume that it must be because that task wasn't important to her. After all, if it was important to her, she would have made a point of remembering. This makes sense, especially since she seems to remember some things pretty well, at least some of the time, so therefore it must be intentional when she doesn't remember.

Since we can't see inside other people's heads, we have to make the best guesses we can based on what we see. This leaves a lot of room for error, especially when we don't know someone well and don't have enough experience with him to inform our interpretations of his actions.

Undiagnosed and untreated ADHD very much lends itself to this kind of misinterpretation. So rather than seeing it as a neurologically based information-processing problem, it's labeled as a problem of motivation, attitude, or character—none of which is anything to feel proud of. Besides the effects it has on the person's self-esteem and the other person's resentment, it ultimately hurts them both because the strategies that are used to fix bad motivation, attitude, and character don't help someone with ADHD perform better. So everybody gets more frustrated.

It's important to understand how easily this kind of misinterpretation can occur, because it probably explains a lot of the reactions that you've gotten from other people. So it isn't that these other people were intentionally trying to make you feel bad (any more than you were intentionally trying to make them feel bad). They just didn't know what to make of your behavior and how to improve things, so they took their best guess at it. They weren't trying to be critical, make up arbitrary rules, or be controlling, they were just trying to get things to work out better. Your behavior made them feel out of control, so they tried to do what they could to feel less anxious.

If you're the family member or romantic partner, understanding this misinterpretation probably goes a long way toward explaining some of your reactions along the way. Even with good intentions, it's easy to make a situation worse if you don't fully understand what's driving the other person's actions.

So whether you're the person with ADHD or the other person, you probably didn't act in the best way because it wasn't a great situation—you were both trying to figure something out that didn't make any sense, so you made the best sense of it that you could. Now that you know about the ADHD, though, it can be a completely different situation. Now you both have the ability to do things differently and to achieve better outcomes. Don't take the lessons of the past as being set in stone—if you approach other people differently, they may approach you differently.

Expectation Management: Promise Only What You Can Deliver

I'm a big fan of expectation management—that is, actively managing the expectations that other people have of me, telling them what they can expect me to do and what they shouldn't expect of me. By contrast, the times when I don't do that, I wind up feeling stressed out and making myself nuts trying to live up to something I can't easily deliver. Because ADHD affects an adult's ability to consistently do what others expect, expectation management is an especially important skill to develop (see the preceding article, *We See Others Through Our Own Lens*).

For example, if you tend to run late, you may want to tell a new friend, "I'm really bad at getting places on time. I try to, but I still tend to run late a lot more than I would like. So if I'm late getting to the restaurant, just call me and I'll tell you when I'll get there. Better yet, call me before you leave to make sure that I'm not running too far behind. If I'm really late, order an appetizer and it's on me." This way the friend doesn't expect you to be on time and then get resentful when you're not.

This doesn't mean that you get a free pass whenever you tell someone that you're not good at something. Most people probably won't go for that one-sided arrangement. Rather, expectation management has the goal of keeping both people happy, of preventing bad feelings, misinterpretations, and resentment.

Obviously, in an ideal world, we would all be able to do everything perfectly. But in this messy world that we live in, we need to accept shortcomings in ourselves and others. The shortcomings exist whether we accept them or not—by accepting them and actively managing them, they have less of an effect on our happiness.

You may not have any choice about having ADHD, but you can choose what you do about it. For example, you may always be forgetful to some degree, so you may need to tell the people in your life that they shouldn't expect you to have a better memory than you actually do. Nothing personal, you just don't remember things as well as you might wish. It's better to be up front about this than to let other people come to their own conclusions. Of course, to do this effectively, you need to generally feel pretty good about yourself and be able to admit your weaknesses without getting defensive or crumbling into shame.

Expectation management involves five parts, as the lateness example illustrates:

- *Acknowledge your limitations.* Be honest with the other person (and yourself) about what you can probably pull off and what you probably can't. You will quickly be found out if you try to hide it, so it's better to deal with it directly.
- *Explain what the limitations mean (and don't).* As we discussed in *We See Others Through Our Own Lens* on p. 315, it's easy for others to read all sorts of negative intentions and character traits into typical ADHD behavior. It's therefore really important to nip that in the bud so that the other person doesn't assume the worst.
- *Do your best.* Tell and perhaps show the other person how you're trying to compensate for this limitation. Intentions count.
- *Give the other person some options.* Not that he should be limited by your options, but this way he doesn't need to guess about what you will find acceptable. You may also want to give him permission to do certain things (like remind you) that he might not otherwise feel are appropriate.
- *Rebalance the relationship.* Make whatever amends are necessary and that you're willing to make.

We all make our own choices in life. It isn't your job to be perfect for anyone or to make choices for others. However, it is your responsibility to inform those choices that other people make. This means describing what you do and perhaps why you do it. They then get to decide what they want to do. You will encounter some people who just aren't willing or able to make that work. It's unfortunate, but that's the way it is. By the same token, you will encounter some people you aren't interested in making it work with. It takes two to tango, and both people need to do their part, so don't take full responsibility for things not working out. Being too hard on yourself and blaming yourself for things that weren't entirely your fault will only make you less willing to apply yourself to the next situation.

We may not have as much control over our limitations as we would like, but we do have control over how we handle them. Expectation management involves actively managing our interactions with other people so that everyone is happier with the outcome.

The Value of a Good Apology

We all blow it sometimes. If you have untreated ADHD, it probably feels as if you blow it a lot. Treatment can improve your batting average, but you'll still never attain perfection. The ability to give a good apology is a great skill to have, regardless of who you are, so let's talk about it. It isn't as simple as saying you're sorry. In fact, a lousy apology can actually make things worse.

In order to apologize for something, you first need to be aware that you've done something wrong. It's possible that something happened that you weren't aware of. Or perhaps the other person interpreted events differently than you did and feels hurt by it. You may not know what exactly happened, but you may get a sense from the other person's mood or actions that *something* happened. This is the time to show concern and start asking questions—it isn't your responsibility to make the other person tell you, but it is your responsibility to ask. At least if you ask, you can't be faulted for not trying to make the situation better. Of course, if you want to increase the odds that the other person will tell you, you need to be known as someone who handles these sorts of things well, rather than getting defensive, flipping out, or making things worse. (See *True Intimacy Means Hearing the Bad News, Too* on p. 311.)

Once we're aware of what we did, we need to deal with it within ourselves before we can say anything to the other person. It feels bad to make a mistake or realize that we hurt someone. If it feels as if this happens too often or we keep making the same mistakes, it's easy to get down on ourselves and either put up defenses or crumble into embarrassment. At these times, we may be so overwhelmed with our own feelings that we can't possibly deal productively with the other person's feelings. So the first step in an apology is to calm our own reaction so we can see beyond our own needs. It may take some time to do this, so we may need to come back afterward to clean things up—better late than never.

Since ADHD behaviors are so easily misinterpreted by other people, part of the apology may also involve reinterpreting the behavior—"I really do value your time, but it's really hard for me to run on time. It always has been." It's important that the other person not personalize the ADHD behavior—as in, you did this to her because you don't care enough. That just adds fuel to the fire. Others will be much more forgiving if you come across as genuinely concerned and well intentioned. They may still not be thrilled with you all the time, but they won't get as angry about it.

When you do blow it and need to apologize, remember to take the following steps:

1. *Admit what you did wrong.* Be honest and thorough; minimizing it will probably only make things worse.
2. *Recognize the impact on the other person.* Helping the other person feel understood will go a long way.
3. *Say what you will (try to) do differently in the future.* I feel that an apology inherently contains a promise to not repeat the problematic behavior. Otherwise, it can come across as something of a free pass. Of course, you shouldn't promise what you can't deliver, so you may need to acknowledge that it will probably happen again, but you will do your best to minimize it. No one can ask you to do more than that.
4. *Make amends, if necessary.* There are times when it's best if you fix whatever the problem is, such as replacing something you lost. Other times, a token gesture can soothe ruffled feelings, such as doing someone a small favor or buying someone a drink.

There are times when someone else feels hurt but we don't feel that we're responsible for it or we didn't do what she is accusing us of. Generally the best approach to take in these situations is to acknowledge her feelings and say that you're sorry that she feels bad. You shouldn't accept responsibility for something you don't think you did, because that's potentially as problematic as denying what you did do. You might say something along the lines of, "I'm sorry that messed up your day, since that really wasn't my intention. I'm pretty sure that I left you that message, but if I didn't, I'm sorry."

You may not have tons of control over your ability to do all the right things at the right times, but you do have the ability to fix things afterward. Remember that the hallmark of a good relationship is resilience—the ability to rebound from trouble spots. In fact, it's that ability that gives us real confidence in the relationship and the other person. We're judged only partly by our actions, but mostly by our intentions—a good apology may not change the action, but it can reveal the intention.

To Tell or Not to Tell?

I'm often asked by clients and audience members at presentations about whether someone should tell family, friends, coworkers, or bosses about having ADHD.

There are no right or wrong answers, since it depends on the circumstances, the ADHD person's openness, and the other person's trustworthiness. My hope is just that the decision to tell someone is well thought out, rather than impulsive or based in what turn out to be shaky assumptions.

Generally speaking, there are more potential complications from telling someone at work about your ADHD, especially a boss. This is because people at work may jump to conclusions about how your ADHD affects your ability to carry out your job duties. It then creates a self-fulfilling prophecy where they start looking for certain things and predictably start to see them, even though nothing about your performance has changed or is any different from what anyone else is doing. For example, this could lead to being passed over for promotions or plum assignments or even to disciplinary actions. It's highly unlikely that anyone would ever be callous enough to come out and say that it was because you have ADHD, but it may still affect their behavior toward you. You may have a great boss or coworker who would handle this information well and work with you, but otherwise it's generally safer to not disclose at work unless absolutely necessary. See *Formal Accommodations Through the Americans with Disabilities Act* on p. 361 for information on legal rights and seeking accommodations at work, including when it's best (and worst) to disclose.

Although these same kinds of problems are less likely with family and friends, there are three potential reasons to hold back on telling someone you have ADHD (or whatever):

- *You can't get the cat back in the bag.* Once you tell someone, you can't untell them if you change your mind or they handle it badly.
- *Myths and misinformation abound.* Before saying anything, you may want to dig a little to find out what the person thinks about ADHD. If he says something overly negative or dismissive, you may want to seriously consider how likely he is to take a more balanced view of the condition. (More on this education below.)
- *People talk.* If you reveal this personal information with this person, will he respect your privacy, or will he tell others? There's nothing to be ashamed of, but it's your personal information and therefore your request for privacy should be respected. It should be your choice about who gets told what, when, and how.

I don't want to give the impression that you should never tell anyone about your ADHD or that there is anything so sinister about it that you need to keep it to yourself. Rather, it's about making a good decision. As a way of avoiding having to make this weighty decision, I often recommend that people talk symptoms before diagnoses. That is, talk about the specific symptoms that the other person sees, without getting into formal diagnoses. For example, you could say, "I sometimes get really caught up in an idea and stop hearing what someone else is saying, so just give me a poke if it seems like I'm not listening." This addresses the problem of distractibility and offers a potential solution without getting into explanations of why it happens. Spend some time and come up with concise ways of explaining your ADHD symptoms so that you don't need to make them up on the spot. Maybe even practice saying them out loud or run them by someone who knows about your ADHD.

There may be times when talking about symptoms isn't enough or you feel that you want to tell someone about your ADHD. Let's go through the three potential problems just mentioned and consider ways of overcoming them.

Are You Sure You Want to Say It?

Intimacy and connection in relationships are built by sharing personal information. This is then maintained by treating that information respectfully. So you want to make sure that the person you're contemplating telling will be able to hold up her end of the bargain. This means stopping and thinking about it long enough to really make a good choice.

This topic came up often in an adult ADHD support group I ran. One attendee described how he knew that he had a tendency to get caught up in the moment and blurt things out. So he came up with two rules for himself about telling people about his ADHD: "1. Never tell anyone you have ADHD. 2. Even if you forget rule number one, never tell anyone you have ADHD." Obviously, this got a good laugh, perhaps from the recognition that good intentions beforehand sometimes get lost in the moment.

On the other hand, I had a client who had been dating a woman for a few months but hadn't told her about his ADHD. Even though he hadn't said anything about it, his troubles with time management, paying attention, and interrupting her were frequent sources of frustration for her. We discussed whether he should tell her. Ultimately he decided that he needed to, because she was coming to her own conclusions about him on account of his actions. This helped her better understand why he did certain things and gave them less to argue about.

You May Need to Educate the Person

Even though there is a lot more good information available about ADHD in adults, there's still a lot of misunderstanding and misinformation. As a result, you may want to educate the person about ADHD. Probably the best way to do this is to provide the information in your own words and to speak from your own experience, but some stubborn ones may need to see something more official, like an article, website, or book. This may also be helpful if the person is genuinely interested but is asking questions you can't answer.

It can be helpful to create a thirty-second soundbite of how ADHD affects you in the context that you're talking about, such as at work or with friends. Ideally the conversation will go for more than half a minute, but it can be a good way to start things off on the right foot. You may also want to be prepared to answer some common questions or address common myths, such as:

- *ADHD is just an excuse.* ADHD has been the subject of thousands of research studies, including at the National Institutes of Health. People with ADHD often need to work harder to achieve the same successes.
- *Everyone has some ADHD.* Everyone has their moments of distractibility, but people with ADHD have suffered for it, consistently and across all parts of their lives.
- *Adults grow out of their ADHD.* Some people grow out of some of their symptoms, but most adults still have significant troubles.
- *ADHD medication is addictive.* When properly prescribed and taken, the medications are safe and nonaddictive.

Someone may throw you a curveball and ask a question you don't know how to answer. No problem—tell him you will look it up and get back to him.

Truth Is Earned

Some people in your life deserve to be given personal information; others don't. The difference is how comfortable you are about how they will treat that information. Those who treat it with respect, by keeping it confidential and not using it against you later, tend to be told more. Those who misuse your information tend to be told less. So when contemplating telling someone about your ADHD, ask yourself whether that person has earned that information. If so, then go for it.

Of course, someone's response to your disclosure also tells you something about him. There may be times, especially with a new relationship, that you want to find out quickly where someone stands on these matters before investing too much time in the relationship. As an example, I was recently on a panel that was shown online with a young man who had been diagnosed with ADHD. While we were talking beforehand, he told me about friends who told him not to do the panel for fear that a potential employer would find out about it. His feeling was that he didn't care if they did. In a way, any employer that would screen him out on account of his having ADHD is probably not a good place for him to work anyway. Better to find this out before being hired than afterward. The same may go for potential friendships and romantic relationships.

Relationship Patterns to Avoid: You Can Do Better

When someone has ADHD, certain relationship patterns tend to develop, since we all tend to attract certain kinds of partners and create certain kinds of relationships. Generally speaking, these dynamics are more likely to occur in romantic relationships than friendships since relationship dynamics are generally more intense when the heart is involved. The patterns below may not fit your relationships, but it's worth thinking about for a moment. By knowing what to look for, you're less likely to fall into it and more likely to shift the relationship if you do. You may find that more than one pattern fits, particularly across relationships.

These patterns are equally worth knowing for both the person with ADHD and the other person. It takes two to tango, so either person can drive a change to something better.

The person with ADHD is:	*The person with ADHD needs to:*	*The other person needs to:*
The Incompetent (needs to be cared for)	Build skills. Increase self-sufficiency. Take more initiative.	Step back. Let her fail sometimes. Cope with her anxiety.
The Lost Soul (needs to be rescued)	Find his path in life. Do the hard work to get there.	Give him space to discover his path.
The Victim (needs to be protected)	Learn to stand up for herself. Focus more on improving functioning than on gaining accommodations.	Step back to give her space to advocate for herself.
The Easy Target (is to be blamed)	Take responsibility only for what is his doing. Improve overall functioning and thereby reduce easy targets.	Take responsibility for her half of the interactions. Work on her own issues. Meet her own needs directly, without nagging or playing the victim.
The Prince/Princess (needs to be served)	Expect less from others. Increase self-sufficiency. Become more aware of others' needs.	Focus on his own needs. Resist the pull to do too much for her.

It's easy to fall into these kinds of patterns, and each makes sense in its own way. Each one kind of solves certain problems and meets each person's needs.

Nonetheless, I hope that you can find a better way of relating. I definitely don't want to give the impression that I'm advocating a tough love approach—it should be all about the love, without being too tough. Rather the goal is to push yourself and your partner to strive for something better. This goes over much better when it's done supportively, because otherwise your partner can just write you off for acting like a jerk and thereby miss the real point of what you're doing.

If you're already in a relationship, it's an unwritten law that working on your own issues will gradually push your partner to work on his own, since he can't keep doing the same things when you're doing different things. This can make your relationship more satisfying, peaceful, and loving. If you're not in a romantic relationship, then you may find that you attract more grounded partners once you work on your own issues.

Just as important, personal growth in our intimate relationships also tends to translate into improvements in our friend and coworker relationships, so there's a lot to be gained. For example, it gives you more options in terms of the people that you interact with, since you will have a harder time finding someone who wants to play the other half of each of these patterns. The better you're doing, the more satisfying and productive these other relationships will be.

Restore Balance in the Relationship

Relationships work best when they're balanced, but keeping some semblance of balance is also one of the major struggles in most relationships. This is especially true when one of the people has ADHD and isn't able to reliably and consistently turn his intentions into reality. As a result, the other person often feels the need to make up the difference and then winds up feeling as if she is carrying more than her share. This imbalance likely grows as the relationship develops—there isn't much overlap of responsibilities when a couple is dating, but there is much more when they live together and especially once the kids show up. As a result, what was seen as merely quirky or mildly irritating when casually dating becomes justification for homicide when living together. Every couple faces these adjustment challenges, but couples where one person has ADHD will have an extra helping.

One foundation of a stable and satisfying relationship is some sort of balance. This doesn't mean a perfect division of labor, where each person does exactly half of everything ("Honey, I loaded my half of the dishwasher!"). Rather, it means a complementary relationship where each person takes care of his share of the responsibilities and helps out where he can. Ideally tasks are assigned based on abilities and who hates them least. Regardless of how everything is divided up, the key is that both partners feel as if they're on the same team and working together. At some stages of the relationship, one person may do more (like when her husband is writing a book about ADHD), but there's a sense that it will all balance out in the end.

Few relationships achieve perfect balance. Each partner has different abilities and energy levels. Ultimately, one person will probably wind up doing more. You can fight this, but beyond a certain point it probably won't do much to balance the scales, so much as cause frustration and resentment on both of your parts. Rather, it's probably better to accept the realities. Of course, this is easier to achieve if you feel that your partner is doing his best—it may still be less than you want, but intentions and effort should be given a lot of credit.

Talk It Out

Since life is constantly evolving, it's easy to stick with a division of labor that worked before but doesn't really work as well now. Or perhaps one partner has slowly accumulated more than her fair share of tasks or maybe someone is just sick of a particular chore. It can therefore be helpful to sit down occasionally to take stock of who's doing what, what isn't getting done, and perhaps what shouldn't be done anymore. If you're busy, it's very easy to not be fully aware of what your partner is doing. For example, my wife does all sorts of things around the house that I have no idea about and never even think about. (Presumably I do a few things, too.) You know it's time to have one of these conversations when one of you finds yourself grumbling (or yelling) about the other not doing enough.

So find a quiet moment to sit down and review all the various tasks that are required to keep your household and family running smoothly. Discuss who's doing what. Make suggestions about different ways to accomplish those goals. Maybe even let some of those goals go, at least for now.

Different Strokes for Different Folks

We all have our individual preferences. Our partner probably has different preferences. The trick then becomes finding a way to meet both of those sets of needs—at least mostly. It's easy, though, to get moralistic about our own desires and be dismissive about our partner's (only slobs don't wipe off the counters, but no one really cares what the garage looks like). Any time you find yourself talking in absolutes like this, step back and take a look at what you're saying. If it sounds at all dismissive in your own ears, it's probably ringing in your partner's. This is a setup for him to get defensive and not really hear what you're saying: "It makes me nuts when there are crumbs all over the counter. Please wipe them off."

These extreme positions make productive negotiation much harder. So remember that your preferences are merely preferences, not moral indictments of your partner's character. Of course, as in any negotiation, you want to try to get what's important to you, but that often means giving up the things that are less important. You're more likely to get what you want if you approach your partner respectfully and keep in mind what's important to her (especially the stuff that's not important to you).

It's also not helpful to use other people as examples of what your partner should aspire to—for example, "John always loads the dishwasher after dinner." There are two problems with doing this. First, your partner can probably easily cite counterexamples from other couples, so that doesn't move the discussion forward. Second, you don't live in those other houses, so you need to find a way that works for the house that you do live in. There are lots of ways to create a satisfying relationship, so the only thing that matters is that it works for you and your partner, not whether anyone else would be happy about it. By aspiring to do what other couples do, you limit your options and may wind up trying to cram a square peg into a round hole—especially if none of these other relationships have someone with ADHD. Every couple has its own challenges and therefore must find its own solutions.

Reminding Is Better Than Doing It Yourself

The forgetfulness that comes from ADHD is an easy setup for the non-ADHD partner to feel that too many chores fall to her. After too many of her reminders go unheeded, she may take the path of least resistance and just do them herself, rather than expend the energy to chase down her partner. This makes sense, but is also problematic in the long run.

Often the better approach is to stick with the reminders. It's a two-way street, though. The non-ADHD partner agrees to give the reminders with a friendly tone and without nagging (mostly) and the ADHD partner agrees to receive the reminders graciously and do his best to follow through (mostly). Of course, in these arrangements, each person is more likely to stay friendly if the other person does, too. So you're both responsible for that.

You may find that a whiteboard, family calendar, and family meeting are helpful for keeping things on track and therefore require fewer verbal reminders (see articles on these topics in chapter 14).

It may be necessary for the non-ADHD partner to let go of certain situations and let the partner with ADHD face his own consequences—for example, not get on his case about leaving the house late when she isn't involved. This doesn't mean that she needs to be happy about his being late, but she doesn't need to involve herself in it. If it doesn't concern her, she may choose to stay out of it. This is one of those pick-your-battles scenarios—if she gets on him about these low-priority items, she then has less impact when something big comes up. Therefore, for her own sake, she may want to be more selective. Of course, in order to leave it alone, she needs to control her anxiety over what might happen or embarrassment over her partner's behavior. She needs to be able to see this as reflecting on him, but not on her. Otherwise it creates a situation where she cares more about it than he does—and so the power struggle begins.

Finally, there may be some activities that are best delegated away, such as cleaning the house or cutting the grass. It isn't that one member of the couple couldn't do these activities, simply that it too often becomes a problem when it isn't done quickly enough. Therefore, there may come a time when it's better to just pay someone else to do it, if you have the money. It will mean sacrifices elsewhere when that money isn't available for other things, but it may be money well spent.

One Steps Up, One Steps Down

ADHD relationships come in all shapes and sizes. However, there's a stereotype of the scattered adult with ADHD and the superorganized partner. Even if your relationship doesn't fit this extreme, it may still have some of this flavor.

It's easy to get into a pattern where the non-ADHD partner feels resentful for having to take on responsibility for too many of the details in the couple's life, whereas the partner with ADHD feels constantly criticized for not living up to the other person's standards. As with any couple dynamic, this arrangement works in some ways and doesn't work in others. You will feel better about it and have more options for coming to a more satisfying arrangement if you can be honest about both sides of the coin.

The organized non-ADHD partner easily falls into the role of being the responsible one. It fits her strengths, she likes doing it, she likes being needed, and she likes not having to worry about the other person messing things up. What's probably not as acknowledged is that she likes doing things her way, so she benefits from taking on all this responsibility. She may rationalize it as being necessary purely because of her partner's unreliability, but she really likes it. Therefore, if anything is to change in the relationship in this regard, she needs to acknowledge this need of hers, find a way to let go of some of this control, and tolerate her partner's doing things differently.

Meanwhile, the partner with ADHD is more than happy to unload all these burdensome chores, since he never liked doing them in the first place. ("No, I insist that I be allowed to do our taxes!") He may not enjoy the feeling of being beholden, but he's willing to tolerate it as long as it doesn't get held over his head too often. It's probably more obvious what the partner with ADHD gets from this unbalanced relationship. However, in order to buy himself freedom from being seen as the less capable one, he needs to step up and begin doing more of those undesirable chores. He may not need to do them to his partner's highest standards, but he needs to do them at least well enough to prevent his partner from having an anxiety attack and taking them all back.

Therefore, in order to rebalance the burden of responsibilities, both partners need to come toward center and give up part of what they like. That is, the non-ADHD partner can't have everything done her way *and* not be the one to do it all, and the partner with ADHD can't get out of these chores *and* be seen as equally capable.

Each partner needs to compromise, not just with the other partner, but with himself. So if you see yourself in one of these descriptions, then be honest with yourself about both sides of the coin. It's easier to make a satisfying decision if you take all of the information into account, including the stuff you don't really like to admit.

Give Credit Where Credit Is Due

Relationships have momentum—when things are going well, we tend to give our partners the benefit of the doubt. When things are going badly, though, we nail them on every potential infraction. This is especially easy before someone's ADHD is diagnosed and the couple has a different way to understand these behaviors.

It's easy to get into a nag and passive-aggressive cycle in which the non-ADHD partner is seemingly always on the other person for what he did or didn't do. He then feels as if he can never do anything to please her, so he gives up and doesn't really try. He then lies about things in an effort to avoid further criticism, which only drives her to hammer him even harder when she finds out about his cover-ups. This quickly goes from bad to worse. It's easy to see how this pattern can develop—and harder to get out of it.

Therefore, if you find yourself snapping at each other too much, call a truce. Someone needs to, so it may as well be you.

- *Express appreciation for what your partner is already doing.* No matter how frustrated you are with your partner, he must still be doing some things well. Look for them.
- *Do something nice for her.* Change the tone of your interactions by going out of your way to do something that your partner will appreciate. I know, I know, it's probably the last thing you want to do when you feel frustrated, but it may be the best thing you can do.
- *Resist the temptation to criticize.* You will undoubtedly see plenty of things to comment on, but that doesn't mean that you have to. Remember that you also have plenty of opportunities when things are going well, but you often choose to keep those criticisms to yourself, for the sake of peace in the house. This doesn't mean that you shouldn't comment on anything, just that you should try to limit it to the things that really matter.
- *Remember why you like this person.* In the hustle and bustle of daily life, it's easy to focus on chipping away at the pile of chores and forget about the romantic connection or even just enjoying each other's company. Take a moment or two to remind yourself about what you love about your partner.

No matter how much your partner is driving you nuts right now, you are not purely the passive victim of her bad habits and snippy attitude. You have the power to change the tone of your interactions—and thereby change hers. It's much easier to get your partner to change what she does when you both feel like you're on the same team.

Fun Stuff in the Bedroom: Improve Your Sex Life

Sex is an important part of a romantic relationship. As you undoubtedly know, a couple's sex life is vulnerable to interference by all sorts of stressors, some of which are an individual issue (like changing hormone levels or depression), and some of which are a couple issue (like resentment about an unbalanced workload). Not surprisingly, then, just as ADHD can affect every other aspect of a romantic relationship, it can also affect the couple's sex life, for example in the following ways:

- *Pragmatically,* when the inefficiencies resulting from one partner's ADHD means there is simply less time available for sex or romantic intimacy in general. Alternatively, the partner with ADHD may not be available at the right time; for example, if she is frantically cleaning up around the house before company comes over the next day.
- *Neurologically*, when the ADHD interferes with reading the other's signals, responding patiently, and delaying gratification.
- *Psychologically,* when the non-ADHD partner feels resentful about the unbalanced workload and too many misunderstandings, whereas the partner with ADHD feels resentful about being scolded too often.

Although some couples are able to maintain an active sex life despite other difficulties in the relationship, for most couples, a happy relationship is a requirement for sex. This may then be something of a motivator to work on the other parts of the relationship discussed in the rest of this chapter—and also all the other stuff discussed in the rest of the book. This doesn't mean that you should wait until everything else in your life is going great before working on your sex life, because few of us would ever have sex if that was the case. Rather, look at it as a process that will hopefully continue to get better.

As with every other topic that may come up in the relationship, it's likely that you and your partner will have some differences of opinion regarding your sex life. It could be about frequency and timing, as well as other matters. These discussions shouldn't really be any different those you might have about more mundane matters, except that we tend to be sensitive when sex is involved. We feel more vulnerable and might take things more personally than we otherwise would.

Therefore, tread lightly and work really hard to be respectful of your partner's desires and insecurities. Because of this, you may want to be smart about where and when you discuss sex—ideally when there isn't too much going on and neither of you has too much else on your mind. If you take medication for your ADHD, you may want to have these discussions when the medication is working, so that you're better able to listen and hold back eager comments.

Perhaps not surprisingly, an effective medication regimen can improve things in the bedroom, too, by helping the ADHD partner to maintain attention, be more aware of the other's needs, and display an improved capacity to delay gratification. Of course, because the most commonly used medication class, the stimulants, will have mostly worn off by the end of the day, it may be helpful to change the timing of sex to take advantage of this improvement.

The goal is a satisfying sex life—as *both* of you define it. That can mean very different things to each person. The challenge then becomes finding a way to meet in the middle so that both people are mostly happy. It's possible that the person with ADHD will need more variety to prevent getting bored with the same old thing. The other partner may not understand it or may feel threatened by it, as if it implies that she isn't exciting enough. As with everything else related to ADHD, it's important to not take these things personally and to instead focus on how to deal with it productively within the relationship. This means finding a good compromise and perhaps talking specifically about what is acceptable and what isn't. Clear ground rules tend to make everyone more comfortable and prevent problems later.

Work It Out with Some Help: Couples Therapy

There are times when a couple either needs some professional help in order to get their relationship back on track or wants it to make their relationship even better. Some people feel self-conscious about needing to see a couples therapist; I see it as a sign that you care so much about your relationship and partner that you're willing to really work on it. Avoiding something that could make things better at home is more likely to be a sign of a problem.

Of course, by the time most couples get to a therapist's office, things are usually pretty strained. They've tried everything they could think of, probably including some ridiculous but well-intentioned suggestions from friends and magazine articles. Some of this undoubtedly helped, at least a little, but the couple is still left with more conflict and unhappiness than they're willing to settle for.

Some people slip into couples therapy sideways, as the romantic partner joins the adult with ADHD in his individual sessions. This could involve practical matters, such as education about ADHD and how the partner can help the person with

ADHD to more successfully meet both of their expectations. However, it can also take the form of "true" couples therapy, as the couple deals with weightier topics of intimacy, trust, and sex.

Regardless of the focus of the sessions, what will quickly become clear is that both partners play some role in what goes badly and therefore can both play some role in improving the relationship and the running of the household. This may come as a surprise to some partners who would like to keep the focus solely on the ADHD as the primary problem ("I wouldn't complain so much if you weren't so forgetful"). The bad news is that they will need to look at their own part in things; the good news is that they therefore have more control over the ultimate outcome than they realized.

Find a Couples Therapist Who Knows About ADHD

I'm hesitant to even write this section, since many readers will have a hard enough time just finding an individual therapist who understands the many ways that ADHD affects an adult's life. Nonetheless, I'll forge ahead, with the hope that more and more therapists are learning about ADHD in adults. The reason why I think this is important is that ADHD affects all sorts of things in the relationship, so a couples therapist who doesn't understand this will not likely be as helpful as a well-informed one would be.

It may be that you can't find a local couples therapist with a lot of experience with ADHD (by which I mean one who knows about ADHD—I guarantee you they all have clients with ADHD, but many of them may be undiagnosed). If you strike out, then find one who is willing to learn a little and listen to what you have to say on the topic. For example, if the therapist suggests that you each write down a daily log of positive behaviors, I would hope that she would be willing to adapt the assignment so that it isn't a setup to make the ADHD partner look less committed. It may be that you need to be the ADHD expert in the room—not ideal, but workable if you find a therapist who is humble and strong in other ways.

Romantic Partners Need to Learn About ADHD, Too

Even if it was the romantic partner who initially discovered and researched ADHD and pushed her partner to get evaluated, it's still often important for the non-ADHD partner to learn about ADHD. This means more than just, "You get distracted and forget things. Got it." I invariably find that the partners are curious and full of questions. Some of them are eager and dying to learn. Others are skeptical about this whole thing, from the legitimacy of the diagnosis to the potential benefits of treatment.

As the designated expert in the room, the therapist can do several things:

- *Inform the skeptics.* This involves teaching your partner about ADHD, how it's diagnosed, what the research tells us, risks and costs of not treating it, and potential benefits of treatment, as well as answering all the pointed questions. I'm more than happy to talk to a doubtful partner or family member. At least they showed up, so they have at least some sliver of curiosity that I can work with.
- *Fill in where the books and websites leave off.* Ideally your partner has read some of the material that you've passed along, as well as listened to your explanations. Even if he has, though, he may still have some questions either about ADHD in general or how it specifically applies to your life.
- *Serve as an authoritative voice.* It's annoying when our family members give more credence to someone else saying the same thing that we said, but it's a fact of life. Therefore, it may be helpful for your romantic partner to hear some things a second time from the therapist in order for it to really sink in. (Afterward you get to say, "That's what I said!")

What to Expect from Couples Therapy (Give or Take)

As we just discussed, the crucial first step is getting informed about ADHD—for both partners. If the relationship is to have any hope, it's really important that the partner not take the ADHD-based behavior personally or see it as willful—for example, seeing unreliable follow-through as a sign of not caring enough about the partner's happiness. This path leads into a tar pit that is almost impossible to get out of cleanly. By contrast, seeing the ADHD as a fact of life that both partners need to compensate for and work around can shine a ray of hope that things can improve. They both have a stake in the solution as well as the outcome. Often one of the first things that's lost when a couple really starts to struggle is that feeling of being on the same team; learning about ADHD can get them back on the same side. A good therapist can help you connect again.

You can't leave the past in the past if it's still happening in the present. It's really hard for both partners to forget about those old battle scars if the same problematic behaviors are still happening. Therefore, it's easier to let go of that old hurt and resentment if your partner is doing a better job now or at least seems to be working toward it, even if he isn't hitting home runs yet. The couples therapist may help you both with strategies that can reduce the negative effects that the ADHD is having on the relationship, but it may be that this piece of the puzzle actually comes from an individual therapist, coach, or medication. Regardless of the source, this opens the door for you to do better as a couple and work on other things. Meanwhile, the non-ADHD partner will have to work on changing her reactions to the ADHD-based behaviors, since that is also contributing to the conflict.

Generally speaking, we're more likely to work on our issues if we see our partner working on his—remember this when you catch yourself telling yourself that you'll only do your thing if he does his. This is a setup for a stalemate. Therefore, someone needs to be the bigger person and do the right thing so the other person will, too. It shouldn't always be you, but maybe this time it will be. A good therapist will work with you two on this balance so that it doesn't feel as if one person is doing all the work. This is why it's important to find a therapist who understands ADHD; otherwise, she will spend all her time trying to get the ADHD partner in line and mostly repeat the other partner's unsuccessful strategies. In other words, more of the same, except worse because a perceived expert is saying it this time.

The therapist may also help you to clarify what you are each looking for from the relationship and to find common ground. It may not seem like it when you're not getting along, but there's probably more similarity and complementarity than you realize. A skilled therapist can tease out these unifiers and help you negotiate the differences so that you are both happy—the only arrangement that can last.

Along the way, it's probably a safe bet that the therapist will work with the two of you on communication strategies. This is a common technique in couples therapy, but may be especially important when one person has ADHD because a lot of good intentions get lost in the cracks of ineffective communication. To be honest, all of the lessons of good communication for those with ADHD apply to every other couple, too—it's just that the couples where one person has ADHD benefit even more from them. Keep these pointers in mind:

- *Talk when it's quiet.* That is, minimize distractions like TV, kids, or impending deadlines when it's time for the serious conversations. This is the first and most important suggestion. Since these calm moments are probably hard to find, you will need to actively create them—schedule them and turn off the noise.
- *Don't talk right before bed.* For many couples, especially those with young kids, the only time that they get a quiet moment is right before the lights go out. This can be a good time to talk about the day's events and tomorrow's plans, as well as other matters. Try to avoid the big discussions, though, since it's likely that at least one of you is too tired to be at your best at that point. Besides, there are more enjoyable activities you could do when the door's closed.

- *Keep it short.* Long diatribes are fun and all, but they rarely get our main points across. Mostly what they accomplish is to give our partners time to think about what they want to watch on TV afterward. Don't exceed your partner's attention span, and definitely don't repeat yourself more than once. It's easy to feel as if we need to keep talking to make sure our partner gets it, but this just makes the partner shut down. Short and to the point works much better.

- *Stick to one topic at a time.* Topics tend to be related in a relationship, but to the extent that you can, try to focus on just one at a time. It's better to finish one than start three.

- *Repeat what you heard.* Without sounding like an annoying parrot, reflect back what you heard your partner say, but in your own words. Process the information and show you understand it. This doesn't mean that you agree, just that you heard and understood what was said.

- *Ask your partner what he heard.* Related to the prior point, it's fair game to ask your partner to repeat what he heard you say if you're worried that he's drifting while you're talking or that you're not making your point clearly. This isn't about catching your partner so much as keeping you both on the same page, so intentions count for a lot with this one.

- *Talk about how and why, not just what.* Most couples tend to agree about the fundamentals of the relationship, such as mutual happiness, secure finances, satisfying sex life, and peaceful home. Where they tend to disagree is in how to get there or why certain things are important in the pursuit of those goals. So rather than get stuck on the superficial aspects of what each of your preferences might be, talk about why these are important to each of you. If you can understand your partner's position (and maybe even share the ultimate goal), you may be more willing to work with her on how to get there.

Social Skills Training: Helpful or Obvious?

ADHD has a big social impact. It affects how you relate to others and how others see you. I talked about this in detail in *Social Skills and Friendships* on p. 83. So what are you to do about this?

There are some clinicians who offer social skills classes, mostly for kids but also sometimes for adults. These can be helpful for people who don't know how to read social cues or don't understand other people well. However, this doesn't really apply for most people with ADHD, especially adults. They generally know what they should do and even why they should do it, but have trouble translating that knowledge into consistent performance, just as they do in all the rest of their lives. Adults with ADHD may act impulsively and regret it afterward, or may miss social cues because of their inattentiveness. It's kind of like flossing our teeth—we all know that we should do it daily, but few people actually do. Awareness doesn't translate consistently enough into action. (Don't tell my dentist.)

The solution, then, is the same as for those other difficulties. Medication can help close the gap between intentions and performance. You may also want to work on being more mindful about how you relate to others. I know, this is one of those easier-said-than-done kind of things, so I'm not expecting miracles here, but I'm also not willing to say that you're completely powerless over it. Even if it only works sometimes, that's still an improvement. Try to remind yourself to pay attention better. You may also want to make a point of scanning the social scene occasionally to make sure that you're still on the same page as everyone else. For example, do the people that you're talking to still seem interested? Does someone look like she wants to say something? If you have a romantic partner or friend who is often with you, you can arrange a secret sign that this other person can give you when you're crossing lines—then you have to agree to be a good sport about getting this advice.

When you catch yourself doing something that you wish you didn't, offer a quick apology and get the interaction back on track. For example, if you realize that you interrupted someone, you could say something like, "I just realized that I cut you off back there. I'm sorry about that—I get excited sometimes and can't stop myself. So, what were you saying?" You may even want to add something like, "Feel free to stop me if I interrupt you again. I promise I won't take it personally." It isn't the other person's responsibility to keep you on track, but it benefits her happiness if she has permission to more actively manage the conversation.

The same goes when you realize you tuned out for a few seconds and missed what the other person was saying. Many people with ADHD get good at covering up when they feel out of step with the other person. The good news is that it keeps the conversation rolling along. The bad news is that it can lead to some uncomfortable discoveries later and give you something to worry about in the meantime. A better approach may be to own up to the lapse in attention and ask the person to repeat it, which shows that you care about what the other person was saying. For example, "Sorry, I think I lost you for a second there. I sometimes get wrapped up in thinking about what someone said before and then stop hearing what he's saying now. Tell me that last part again, if you could. I don't want to miss anything."

You may also want to think about the kinds of situations that you put yourself in. For example, if you get easily distracted in large groups, then try to choose smaller groups when you have the chance. Or if your attention gets pulled away from the people at your table when eating in a busy restaurant, either pick quieter restaurants or sit facing the wall, rather than out into the room. I had a couple I saw where the wife would feel hurt when the husband kept getting distracted by the young cuties walking by, so we talked about not putting themselves in those kinds of situations.

Some people with ADHD run into trouble because they get bored when things are going well or not enough is happening. To remedy this problem, they may create some otherwise unnecessary drama to spice things up, much to the chagrin of the other people who were enjoying the calm. I had a client whose husband would immediately catch on to the fact that she was stirring the pot and instead would ask what else they could do that would be more fun. If you catch yourself itching to create some excitement, then own up to your boredom—it's OK to feel bored, but it may not be OK to fire up your friends and family members to cure that boredom. Instead, admit that you feel bored (maybe just to yourself) and go find something less problematic to occupy yourself. Maybe you can also give your family members permission to call you on this habit, like my client's husband does, so that they don't react negatively and get sucked into the downward spiral.

Parenting: Stay Sane While Wrangling the Offspring

Most couples settle into a pretty good groove when it's just the two of them. Adding a child to the mix then disrupts many of those patterns and forces them to find a new way to stay on top of all the old demands, plus managing all the new ones—and ideally keeping some of that romantic connection alive. The habits that used to work no longer do—for example, staying up late to get caught up on things at home doesn't work when a child wakes up early, regardless of when you go to sleep. In addition, some things used to be no big deal before having kids, but now really are—for example, not getting around to fixing the door to the basement so that it's lockable. It's easier to overlook things when it's two independent adults living together. Children have much less tolerance for these things.

Parenthood is no easy task and involves a big adjustment. Therefore, it will reveal many weaknesses in the relationship that might have been mostly under the surface beforehand. For example, an adult with undiagnosed ADHD may find that the demands of parenthood make it impossible to cover up for her inefficiencies by working harder, because there just aren't enough hours in the day anymore. Because parenthood requires that people function at their best, it creates an unintended opportunity for each parent to work on her own issues, as well as what she contributes to the relationship's struggles. A child's happiness can be a good motivator to push us to work on what we've been able to avoid up to that point. So take the opportunity to rise to the occasion and see what your best really is.

I'd been doing therapy with a teenager for a few months for the typical sorts of things that teens struggle with these days. His mother pretty clearly had ADHD, but had never been formally diagnosed. As we talked, it became obvious that she was working really hard to manage things at home, but didn't have enough progress to show for all that good effort. She freely admitted that her ADHD slowed her down and contributed to some of the things that her son and I were working on. As we talked about it, she agreed to get her ADHD evaluated so that she could do a better job at home and as a parent. She realized that this would make it easier to work on the other things going on with her son.

As this mom knew all too well, the challenge for parents with ADHD is to do all those good things they know they should do, but can't pull off consistently—just like in the rest of their lives. As a result, moralistic lectures rarely do anything except make them feel bad about themselves. Typical parenting books can be helpful in the sense that we could all do with learning more strategies based in child development and other parents' experiences, but they won't correct the fundamental disconnection between intention and action that hamstrings people with ADHD. In fact, obsessively reading parenting books can just give you more things to feel guilty and inadequate about, so know when to say when with those.

Because of this inconsistency, the other parent may be recruited (or volunteer) to be the one who keeps the family on track. This is an easy arrangement to fall into since it caters to this parent's strengths and reduces her anxiety. The trick is to still maintain some semblance of balance, even if it's a balance that's somewhat off kilter. As long as both parents are happy, it doesn't matter if it's 50/50 or 60/40 or even 70/30. As a related example, I tend to rely on my wife to be the expert on our young son and childrearing in general. She spends more time with him and reads more of those books. This doesn't mean that I do everything her way or always agree with her, but I see no need to reinvent the wheel when she knows the answer. This balance will likely shift the other way as he gets older, but it works for now.

If you're frustrated by your ADHD coparent's inconsistency, then please, please, please do not make it out to be some sort of measure of his love for his children. Not only does love have nothing to do with these matters, but the implication can be extremely damaging to his sense of himself as well as the relationship between the parents and between the parents and children. Only bad things come from these sorts of comments, so do your absolute best to avoid them. Some legitimate debates over parenting techniques will undoubtedly arise, but that's totally different. Every parent wants his children to be happy and healthy, but they may disagree about how best to achieve those common goals. These sorts of debates work out best when they focus more on techniques and less on motives.

It's also worth keeping in mind that the two parents will almost certainly have different approaches to childrearing. Children very quickly learn to expect different reactions from each parent. As long as you don't contradict or undermine each other, this is a good thing, because it increases the range of your children's experiences and makes it more likely that they will receive the kind of parenting moments that work best for them. So rather than put unnecessary pressure on each other to be on the same page in every way, focus on the items that matter most.

Fair, if Not Balanced

Even if one parent winds up taking on more of the responsibility of managing the details of running the household and raising the children, it's important to keep it from sliding to extremes where the parent with ADHD is seen as the fun one and the other parent is seen as the strict one. This gives the parents too much to argue about as the strict parent feels unappreciated for his work and cheated of the opportunity to have some fun sometimes. Therefore, the non-ADHD parent needs to be sure not to treat his partner like another one of the kids, and the parent with ADHD needs to do her best to share the workload. Each parent will naturally gravitate toward his strengths when it comes to raising the children. This is fine, so long as neither parent takes on a role so completely that the other parent gets totally squeezed out.

Often, One of the Kids Has ADHD, Too

Given the strong genetics of ADHD, there's a pretty good chance that at least one of your kids will also have ADHD. If so, that child will likely require and benefit from more hands-on parenting than your other children. This can increase the demands on your time.

For a child with ADHD, it can be both good and bad to have a parent with ADHD. On the one hand, it can be helpful for her to know that one of her parents faced similar challenges, which can help her feel better understood. This can be reinforced by sharing relevant stories from your own childhood or even from that same week. On the other hand, it's that much harder for a parent with ADHD to create the predictability and structure that helps children with ADHD to perform at their best. In addition, an impulsive, stressed-out parent is more likely to blow up when a rowdy child doesn't go along with the plan.

Perhaps more influential, though, is how the parent handles his own ADHD. That is, does he accept it and actively address it or does he deny his continuing struggles? Children take cues from their parents about how they're supposed to feel about themselves and others. If they see a parent clearly struggling but not taking active steps to better manage it, or even outright denying it, that can send a powerful message—this is too big to overcome, so don't even try. This message gets reinforced even further when that parent minimizes those same struggles in the child.

By contrast, a very different message is sent by a parent who strikes an appropriate balance between taking these matters seriously and having a sense of humor about them. That is, he admits it when he blows it and tries to fix the situation, but is also sometimes able to laugh at himself about it—for example, after leaving the milk out on the counter all day, he says something like, "Don't tell the genius award committee about this. It won't win me any prizes." This is said in a lighthearted way that shows that he recognizes it was a knuckleheaded thing to do, but he isn't going to get down on himself because he can see that it's really no big deal. It's important to model self-forgiveness for your children so that they can learn to do it for themselves. A child with ADHD probably needs this more than most, since she will likely feel that she makes more than her fair share of mistakes.

Telling Your Children About Your ADHD

At some point, you will probably want to tell your children about your ADHD. More specifically, you will want to give a label and reason for the behaviors that they are intimately familiar with—it's not as if they didn't notice these things. For younger kids, you may want to avoid diagnoses by talking in general terms, such as, "Mommy sometimes loses things, so you can help her find them." The most important thing to convey to your kids is that you love them and are doing your best, even when you blow it sometimes. An adult may be able to figure this out intuitively, but you may need to come out and say it more often with children so they don't misinterpret the ADHD-based behaviors as somehow indicating that they aren't important enough to you (it doesn't hurt to say it to adults, too).

Your kids will also watch how the other parent reacts to the ADHD behaviors. If the other parent is tolerant and accepting, they will be more likely to be. If the other parent is critical and disrespectful, the kids may either follow suit or feel compelled to protect the attacked parent—neither situation is a good one. So if you find that there is too much of this going on at your house, then work together to find better ways of getting things done and to manage the stress in the relationship. Not only will you both be happier, but your kids will be better off for it, too.

Parenting Under Two Roofs

Creating a unified front can be hard enough when both parents live under the same roof. It can be even harder when those parents are no longer together (and even harder when new romantic partners come on the scene). A parent with ADHD, especially if it's undiagnosed or untreated, is an easy target for the other parent to blame for all sorts of troubles during the relationship and afterward. Of course, both parents contributed to the difficulties in the relationship, so it's too convenient to place so much blame on the other person. I understand that there are hurts and resentments when a relationship ends, but if children are involved, the relationship is never truly over since you'll always be connected through the children. So you need to find a way to live with it.

The first and most important thing I would say here is to keep your issues with your ex between the two of you. Do not put your kids in the middle of this—it's tempting to take cheap shots, but it hurts your kids the most and ultimately does more damage to your relationship with them than it does to their relationship with the other parent.

If the other parent is the one mudslinging, then address it directly when the kids are elsewhere. Focus on the kids' needs and remind the coparent that conflict hurts them most. If this isn't enough, then focus on being the best parent you can be. Work on your ADHD and whatever else interferes with your doing a great job. Answer their questions directly, telling them only as much information as they need to know, even if it's a topic that you wish never came up. Don't lie about or minimize what your kids can plainly see—this only adds insult to injury since they will know that something doesn't add up. Be mindful of where the line is between being honest with your kids and taking an opportunity to trash your ex. Your kids will know where that line is, even when you don't.

Remember that you may not be able to control your ex, but you can control what kind of a parent you are. One imperfect but hard-working parent is infinitely better than two bad ones.

CHAPTER 16

COLLEGE AND BEYOND: TEACH AN OLD DOG NEW TRICKS

College can be a great time of life, filled with personal growth and enriching experiences. Despite all this potential, students with ADHD often struggle with getting the kinds of grades that they and everyone else know they should. This is not only disappointing and painful in the moment, but can also limit their long-term career options if they don't get a degree. Fortunately, knowing about your ADHD and actively managing how you approach your studies can make for a much better outcome, whether you're eighteen or eighty. So let's talk about how to make college or graduate school a more fulfilling experience for you.

This chapter contains the following articles:

Use Available Support Services (Preferably Before Finals) (p. 353) Colleges vary a lot in the kinds of support services they offer, but since you already paid for them, you may as well use whatever might be helpful.

Is College Right for You?

I see a lot of kids and teens with ADHD. This means that I also see a lot of parents who are really concerned about these kids' grades and their ability to get into a good college. This is certainly understandable, but I don't automatically assume that every teen I see is destined for college or even that college is what would be best for all of them. College can be a great experience for many people, but it isn't necessarily the best place for *everyone*.

Therefore, the first question to ask is what you expect the college experience and a degree to do for you. If you can achieve your occupational and financial goals without one, then perhaps it isn't worth the investment of time and money. For example, going to a technical school or getting on-the-job training in a trade may be a better way for you to learn and prepare yourself for a satisfying career. Or perhaps the military is a better fit. Or you could try just getting a job and seeing what appeals to you.

Having said all that, there are other teens I see who hate school or just aren't strong students but want and would be good at the kinds of jobs that require a college degree. These students should get that degree so that they're not limited to jobs that they don't really want. These folks will struggle more with staying on top of their academic demands and getting grades that at least somewhat resemble their abilities. They may be more than smart enough to handle the work, but will struggle with juggling multiple classes and longer assignments when parents and teachers don't hound them about it. These students will have to find a way to suffer through school and get grades that are good enough to get them to the next level and eventually get them a diploma. Better things await once school is done, so they need to keep their eye on that prize.

Whether you decide to go to college or not, I would hope that you make your choice based on the right reasons. By contrast, there are lots of bad reasons to go to college, including these:

- *Someone is making you.* If the main reason that you're going to college is that someone else wants you to be there, then perhaps they should go instead. It's unlikely that you're really going to give it your best effort or get much out of it if you're just going to pacify someone else.

- *You don't know what else to do.* Many graduating high school seniors go to college immediately because they don't feel they have any other options. Considering what college costs these days, you should be there only if that's where you want to be, not just because you don't know what else to do.
- *Everyone else is going to college.* Perhaps that's a good choice for them. But does that mean that it's good for you?
- *It's your ticket out of Dodge.* It's true that going to college out of the area is a great way to flee your hometown at least partly on your parents' dime, but you can probably find another way to get out if you really want to.

If you decide to go to college, I would hope that you go with a clear conscience and are able to make the most of the experience. This means more than just grades and a degree—it means meeting lots of interesting people, getting involved in extracurricular activities, and finding your place in the world. It's hard to pull this off if college isn't the right place for you. Instead, you get an expensive uphill climb. So spend some time and really think about it. Talk to others—some who went to college and some who didn't. Would they do the same thing again? Does their experience apply to your life at all? What are they doing for work? What kind of a lifestyle does that give them (not just financially, but also matters like job stability, work hours, type of work, and flexibility)? Ask what a typical workday looks like. This is a big decision, so you want to gather as much information as you can.

It may be that college will eventually be right for you, but isn't right now. I talk about this further in the next article, *Some Students Do Better in College After Taking Time Off.*

Some Students Do Better in College After Taking Time Off

There can be a lot of pressure for a graduating high school senior to go straight into a four-year college. While this path works for many, some students are not yet ready to handle the academic and social demands of college, even if they're more than smart enough to handle the classwork. This is especially true for students with ADHD who relied heavily on parents, teachers, tutors, and other support staff to get their good grades. For these young adults, a delayed entry can make a world of difference in their performance when they do start college and, ultimately, in their success and happiness in later life.

College success requires two maturities:

- *Intellectual maturity* to be able to handle the academic challenges on one's own without parental guidance. This also involves knowing who, when, and how to ask for help, if necessary.
- *Emotional maturity* to be able to strike an appropriate balance between studying and enjoying the social and recreational aspects of college. This may also involve overcoming the resistance to use available support services on campus, if necessary.

While most parents will have some doubts about how their children rate on these two dimensions, some graduating seniors are truly not yet able to function in a college environment. Packing them off prematurely, simply because that is what many of their classmates are doing, may prove ultimately disastrous. Placing these students in a college environment before they are ready risks a failure experience that will only make them feel bad about both themselves and school. Passing but scraping by doesn't gain a student much as a stepping stone—after all, is the goal to simply get a diploma, or is it to set oneself up to lead a successful and satisfying life? By twenty-five, it won't matter that the student started a year, or even two, later. Students with ADHD or other learning disabilities are especially prone to struggling if they start college before they're ready. Given their increased difficulties with classwork, they are more likely to overdo the recreational aspects of college.

Of course, the decision to delay starting college is not an easy one. It requires that the family make an honest, if perhaps painful, assessment of the student's abilities and likelihood of success. Information from teachers, guidance counselors, and mental health professionals may be helpful. Keep in mind, though, that there usually are no absolute answers—ultimately it's a judgment call. Related to the two maturities, there are two factors to consider in determining whether a student is ready for college:

- *Prior academic performance.* To what extent is the student a self-starter? Was she able to consistently produce work that is at least good enough? College success requires a much greater ability to manage the details of more complicated assignments on one's own, so scraping by in high school is kind of a bad sign.
- *Ability to balance work and play.* The move from home to the dorm room presents almost all college students with much more freedom and a whole lot more temptation. At any given moment, there are at least a dozen activities that are more fun than slogging through a fat textbook, but the textbook still needs to be read. How has this student done in the past when it comes to getting down to work?

Whether you're the student or the parent, you need to be totally honest with yourselves about how the student rates on these two factors. If someone is claiming that college will be different from high school, I would want to know specifically why that is—what is going to be different so that it's reasonable to expect different results? The ultimate goal of this discussion isn't to convince anyone of anything, but rather to make the best decision possible—if a student isn't ready, that will eventually become obvious. Those hard facts will be far more convincing than anything anyone could say. By contrast, if you decide that the student isn't yet ready, then something that would be different is that he is a year or two older (and hopefully wiser) from having done something else before going away to college.

If the decision is made to hold off on starting college, the family needs to find a way to tell friends and extended family and deal with the social pressure of people's reactions. This can be an uncomfortable moment, but often the best approach is to simply state, "We thought about it and decided that he will get more out of college later." The issue here is not what most classmates are doing, but rather what is best for this specific student.

Put the Break to Best Use

Just as college is an investment in one's future, so too can taking time off first be if it enables the student to get more from the college experience. The best way to spend that time will depend on the individual, as well as on circumstances and what's available. There are several options.

- *Attend a local college while living at home.* This gives the student experience with college-level work, while still providing the structure of living at home. Parents are available to help with assignments, as well as to provide guidance on time-management choices, such as the balance between socializing and studying. The goal is to provide a smoother transition to living independently at school. Community colleges offer the most flexibility in terms of how many classes are taken, as well as usually being the least expensive.
- *Get a job.* This could be something personally meaningful, such as working for a nonprofit, or simply something to make a buck. If the parents are willing to foot the bill for living expenses, volunteer work may be more rewarding, as well as look better on a resume. For bright students with poor motivation or little direction, the time spent in the types of clock-punching jobs available to high school graduates with little work experience may provide a concrete example of why a college degree is worthwhile. The new graduate should probably be expected to pay more of his own way than he had to before, such as his cell phone bill or car insurance. This

teaches responsibility and signifies that this is a new phase of the young person's life. Additional chores around the house may also be imposed to give a taste of living independently, especially because some of these chores would have to be done anyway if he lived somewhere else. Of course, additional freedoms may also be appropriate, such as later curfews.

- *Live abroad or in a different part of the country.* Whether through a formal program or with relatives or friends, this can be a fantastic opportunity to gain exposure to other ways of life. During the time away, the young adult may take classes or work, or both. Depending on what type of structure is provided in the living arrangement, this may actually be easier to manage than a busy college campus.
- *Join the military.* The armed forces can be just the thing for some graduating seniors who need a great deal of structure and don't know what they want to do for a career. The military tends to offer perks such as job training and college classes. Nonetheless, this is a decision that should be considered thoroughly in that it is much more difficult to undo.

Going Off to College

Some parents may worry that if their children take a break before going to college, they will never get there. While this is true for some young adults, if the break is well conceived, it will serve its purpose as a solid stepping stone that enables them to make much better use of the college experience. Of course, some people simply do not fit the traditional college mold and would be happier and more successful seeking their fortunes elsewhere—and a break won't change this. Attempting to jam these square pegs into round holes will only lead to failure, resentment, and fruitless struggle.

The college experience involves far more than the academic knowledge gained. It is a time of self-exploration. Exposure to diverse ideas, people, and opportunities provides the raw material for crucial decisions about what each student is looking for in life, both in terms of work as well as in more personal areas. Although the ultimate product of a college degree is often emphasized most, college is really a process by which teens become young adults.

A Smoother Transition into College

Every summer I get calls from the parents of ADHD college students who had a rocky year and are now either on academic probation or a hair away. They may even need to get their grades up in the next semester or be forced to take time off. Most of these students had already been diagnosed with ADHD, but some of them didn't know they had ADHD until we start discussing what gets in the way of getting better grades.

They may be very bright and certainly capable of doing the work, but have trouble managing all the demands of living on their own. All of a sudden, parents and teachers aren't available to keep the student on track, and she needs to make it to class on time (or even just show up), keep track of assignments, and actually finish those assignments. The transition from living at home to living in a dorm can be too much to do all at once, so it can be helpful to break it into smaller, more easily mastered steps and avoid these wobbly starts to a college career.

For example, the student could take some classes at a local college while still living at home and perhaps working part time. Parents are thereby available to assist with the following typical trouble areas:

- *Time management,* such as sleep and wake times, the timing and extent of studying, and other activities
- *Temptation management* regarding the many enjoyable but non.-academic activities available to college students (this means valuable extracurricular activities, as well as the sex, drugs, and rock-and-roll kinds of things)
- *Financial management* to help the student stick to a weekly or monthly budget to prevent going broke halfway through the semester

ADHD students may also need extra help with planning a balanced courseload, including realistic scheduling in terms of avoiding morning classes or several classes in a row without a break, as well as ensuring that prerequisite and required courses are taken in the appropriate order. All of these issues can be better managed with some assistance from parents living under the same roof, rather than several hours away, thereby reducing the likelihood of disastrous end-of-the-semester surprises. Of course, the goal is that the student will gradually take over all of these tasks, but in the meantime it's better to not set them up for what may be too likely to be a failure. The trick for the parents is to strike just the right balance between assisting and infantilizing, a line that's often easier to see after the fact.

It's important to see this middle step of living at home as a place for the student to build skills and prove to everyone that he's ready for the big time. This isn't a punishment for doing poorly in high school. He may feel that it's unnecessary, so the parents may need to weather that storm and insist that he prove himself ready before they're willing to commit a big chunk of tuition. It's usually best to create specific requirements for the student to shoot for, such as a GPA, number of classes attended, number of assignments completed on time, etc., rather than leaving it open and subjective. The goal of going off to a four-year college may still be the same; it's just a question of how and when the student gets there.

Part-Time or Full-Time Student?

"It seems like no matter how many classes I take, there's always one that I don't do well in." This was said by one of my clients, but could have been said by lots of them. For many college students with ADHD, one of the biggest challenges is juggling all the various commitments. Or it may be that because they take more time to get the work done, a full courseload is simply too much. For these reasons and others, it can be better to take a reduced load. It's smarter to do well in fewer classes than worse in more.

Because academics often emphasizes exactly those areas where students with ADHD are weakest, they often need to work twice as hard just to keep up. Therefore, it's even more important that they gather some successes here, to justify that extra effort and maintain their motivation. It may be helpful to see college as a rite of passage, after which they can find a niche in life that caters more closely to their abilities. Meanwhile, to ensure that they actually get to that better situation, they may benefit from a reduced load.

This reduced load could be as simple as taking four classes instead of five, especially if one of those classes is known to be a killer. The missing class could be made up over the summer or an additional year beyond the standard four (which is looking more and more like the standard five these days).

Another option is to take fewer than four classes while also working part time. This can be more complicated to schedule, but can provide enough variety for the student to stay interested, especially if he's ambivalent about college in the first place. It will take longer to earn a degree this way, but at least some progress is being made toward that goal for a student who wouldn't be willing to go full time.

If a student is going full time and really struggling, it may be better to drop down to one of these part-time options—the sooner, the better. If the semester has already begun, it may be better to drop a class or two and focus on doing well on the remaining classes than to do badly in all of them. You can then reevaluate what to do for the coming semester.

There are certain practical matters involved in going to college part time that will need to be explored before any decisions are made. You may need to find out how it affects scholarships and financial aid, since that may preclude doing anything less than full time, at least at that college. A community college may be a more affordable option then, at least for some classes. There is also the issue of health insurance—full-time college students can usually be kept on the parents' health insurance, whereas part-timers can't be. You may be able to buy an inexpensive individual plan through the college or other source, so consider that when calculating costs.

If considering going to college part time, remember that college isn't a race to see who can get a degree fastest. It may be better to take more time but get more out of it.

Strategies for College Success

I jokingly say that I have a subspecialty in wayward college students—the ones that go off to school and then run into trouble for various reasons, forcing them to take some time off. In the interest of helping other students avoid these struggles, let's talk about how to succeed in college if you have ADHD.

Going from high school to college can be a gigantic transition. For most students, the hardest part isn't the work itself (although it does get harder) but rather the sudden need to manage their lives with minimal outside support. The parents and teachers who might have helped keep you on track before aren't around anymore.

Here are my top tips for succeeding in college with ADHD:

- *Create a full-semester calendar.* To avoid discovering at the last minute that you have three tests in two days, write all of your big assignments on one calendar that covers the entire semester. Post it on your wall. Then mark off the days as they pass. This will help you see better what you need to do and when you need to do it.
- *Go to all your classes.* Yes, this is an obvious one, but it works. Don't talk yourself into skipping "just this one class—I'll go to the next one." Once that snowball starts rolling, it picks up speed pretty quickly.
- *Do all your reading.* Ditto.
- *Go to bed on time.* This is another obvious one, but it's much harder to get up on time, pay attention in class, and not fall asleep while studying if you stay up too late. This will mean missing out on some fun, but life is all about making choices.
- *Talk to your professors as soon as you start to struggle.* The deeper the hole, the harder it is to dig out of. Professors are much more willing to work with you if the situation hasn't yet become a total disaster.

- *Keep taking your medication.* It's always amazing to me how many college students stop taking their medication. If it helped you succeed in high school, why would you stop taking it when the demands are that much greater?
- *Find the professors who teach the way that you learn.* Ask your advisor and all your friends about professors' teaching styles so you can find the ones who will be the best fit for you.
- *Choose your living situation wisely.* Living with your slacker friends in the party dorm would be a lot of fun, but won't help you study. Therefore, the less social dorm or off-campus housing may be more conducive to getting good grades—and being there next semester.
- *Find a good mentor.* This could be your faculty advisor, another professor, an administrator or secretary, or even an upperclassman. This is someone of whom you can ask questions and who will give you good advice on the various challenges that you may face. You may want to schedule regular check-ins to have someone to be accountable to. Or maybe it's just an informal sort of thing where you can go and talk when needed.
- *Use the available support services.* Most schools offer at least some sort of support services for students with ADHD and other disabilities—or any student who needs extra help. Find out what they offer and what it takes to qualify for those services, then use what you need. Don't wait until the end of the semester (they hate that). For more on this, see *Use Available Support Services (Preferably Before Finals)* on p. 353.

Older Students: You Can Teach an Old Dog New Tricks

Adults with ADHD may find themselves going to college when they're older than typical college age. They may be returning to finish their studies or starting for the first time.

Some of these students may have struggled through high school with undiagnosed ADHD and never thought of college as a possibility before being treated. Others may have started college but not finished because of their untreated ADHD. In either case, it may be fairly reasonable to expect a better outcome from college once they know about their ADHD and are being treated for it. This isn't merely empty cheerleading, since treating your ADHD can significantly change your odds of success. It's your judgment call to assess how much things have changed and whether they've changed enough for you to be successful this time.

Going to college as an older student can have both advantages as well as disadvantages compared to going at eighteen. Let's run through them. The advantages of going when older include:

- *A greater appreciation for college.* I have a saying that there's nothing like a crummy job to convince someone of the value of an education. It may be that you've grown tired of the jobs that are available to you and want something better. You may not enjoy the classes any better, but you'll have more motivation to get your degree.
- *Greater maturity and self-knowledge.* The experiences from a year or two (or twenty) out of high school might have taught you not only why it's important to get a degree, but also how you work best in pursuing that degree. You may have more self-discipline now than when you were eighteen.
- *Greater appreciation for the cost of college.* If some or all of the cost of tuition is coming out of your pocket, you may be much less willing to skip classes or shortcut assignments.
- *Clearer sense of what you want to study.* You may know a little better what you want to get out of college and can focus on those classes. They may be more interesting when you can see how they build toward a more rewarding career.

Going as an older student also brings some disadvantages, but none of them are insurmountable. Let's talk about them:

- *Rusty academic skills.* You may never have been a spectacular student, and those skills probably didn't get any better over the years away from school. It may be best to start by taking only one or two classes so that you can get up to speed. You may also want to make use of the various support services that are available to all students—see *Use Available Support Services (Preferably Before Finals)* on p. 353 for more information on this. You've paid for all these services whether you use them or not, so take advantage of what's there.
- *More complicated lives and demands.* Most eighteen- to twenty-two-year-olds have fairly simple lives. This may not be as true for you anymore, especially if you're married or have kids. So it may take more juggling to make it all work. If you have one, talk to your romantic partner about how the two of you can work together to survive the semester. If you have a job, talk to your boss about your scheduling needs. Use this additional headache as a motivator to do your best in class so that it will all be worth it.

You may feel self-conscious about being older than the other students and worry that it makes you stand out from the crowd. As I have told many clients in this situation, going to college at eighteen is easy; it's showing up later that really takes guts. Remember this and give yourself credit for getting your degree the hard way. The only thing that matters is that you get your degree, not when. However, if it makes you feel more comfortable, you may want to attend a college that caters more to older or working students so that you aren't the only old guy in a classroom full of kids. You may also want to keep in mind that once you get your degree, most people will simply assume that you got it at age twenty-two, even if you got it at fifty-two.

Read More Effectively

College involves a lot of reading. This is bad news for a lot of students with ADHD because they often complain about having trouble reading. Most people with ADHD don't technically have a reading problem, such as dyslexia, but they do have trouble keeping their attention on the page and remembering what they've read. They may find themselves at the bottom of the page and realize that they have no idea what they've just read. This forces them to either reread it or just skip it. In either case, it's frustrating to put so much time and effort into it and not have enough to show for it, so they may not even bother. Therefore, a college reading load may be daunting and difficult to keep up with.

As I explained in *Working Memory* on p. 9, this is primarily due to a working-memory weakness in that the words that are being read are dropped before being transferred into long-term memory. You can improve this by making reading a more active process.

- *Flip through the chapter before reading it.* Read the summary or key points, if available. Read the subheadings. This can give you an overview of the chapter so that the smaller points that you read along the way make more sense.
- *Use a highlighter.* You probably spent a lot of money for your books. They're yours, so you can do whatever you want to them. Use a highlighter to mark up the main points or things to remember. Scribble notes in the margins. Not only does this keep you more engaged while reading so you get more out of it, but it also helps you narrow down how much material you need to study for the test.
- *Take notes.* Depending on the type of reading, it may be helpful to jot down notes or create an outline. Doing this forces you to process the information more deeply, which will make it stick much better.

- *Find a quiet place to read.* A good spot might be a corner of the library where your friends won't come find you. The less that's going on around you, the less you need to actively screen those distractions out. You may also want to invest in a bunch of cheap foam earplugs.
- *Find a not-so-quiet place to read.* Some people actually do better with a little bit of noise around them because it drowns out the chatter inside their heads. So listening to certain kinds of music or reading in the middle of a bustling coffee shop may actually help you focus better or keep you energized. Go with whatever works.
- *Talk it out afterward.* Find a classmate with whom you can discuss the reading. This will help solidify what you read and enhance your understanding. Of course, this also forces you to finish it before the meeting.
- *Move while reading.* There's no rule that you need to read at an official and uncomfortable wooden desk. Pace around if that helps you feel less restless. Maybe even walk on the treadmill at the gym, but try to go when there are fewer cute distractions walking by, or at least find a quieter corner. Foam earplugs may also be helpful.

Use Available Support Services (Preferably Before Finals)

Colleges these days tend to offer many more support services than they used to. Some schools are much better than others as far as this goes, so you may want to look into that before even applying to a school. Contact the office of services for students with disabilities (ask the college's switchboard operator what they call it there, or look around the school's website) and find out what sorts of services would generally be available for someone in your situation.

Every college offers certain informal support services to every student. This includes things like tutors, academic advisors, a counseling center, a writing center to review your papers, librarians who can show you how to do research, and study skills seminars. Of course, you can also go straight to the source and meet one on one with professors or teaching assistants during their office hours. Many students find that these services plus a good work ethic are enough to enable them to succeed.

Other students require more formal accommodations, such as extended time on tests or assignments, taking tests in a quiet room, or using a note taker. Find out what is required to qualify for accommodations for ADHD and any other potential disabilities. There is a wide variety in what schools require. Some are pretty easy, whereas others require a full psychoeducational evaluation. This is a rather involved process that necessitates almost a full day's worth of testing with a psychologist, followed by another day's work for the psychologist to score everything and write a report. Given how much time it takes, expect to pay at least $1,000, but probably more. Also, don't wait until the last minute—you will probably need at least a month's lead time to get on someone's schedule. You may be able to get your testing done much less expensively through the university counseling center, with students doing the testing and being supervised on the report writing.

Regardless of what kind of support services you use, don't wait until the last minute to use them. First of all, they may no longer be available—for example, tutors' hours get all scheduled up. Second, you don't want to spend the last weeks of the semester digging out of a hole. This is easier to pull off in high school and harder in college where there's much more work, so you can fall much farther behind. Whereas teachers may pursue students in high school, college professors leave it up to the student to come to them and to seek out needed support services. If you know a particular class or semester is going to be challenging, then don't wait for trouble before getting help.

CHAPTER 17

WORK: HOPEFULLY MORE THAN JUST A PAYCHECK

Adults spend a lot of time at work—about a third of the day, if we're lucky, but many of us spend more than that. So it shouldn't be surprising that adults with undiagnosed ADHD often seek treatment because they're not doing as well there as they would like. Because we spend so much time at work, we want it to be an enjoyable and fulfilling experience—maybe not every moment, but overall a satisfying endeavor that gives a sense of contributing to the world, even in a small way. It's hard to feel like that if you're struggling just to keep your head above water or your boss off your back. This then spills into other parts of your life—for example, if you feel so burned out at the end of the workday that you don't have much left for your romantic partner or family.

The good news here is that working on your ADHD in all the ways discussed in the rest of this book will benefit you at work, too. So it isn't completely coincidental that this chapter comes last. Because there are a million and one ways to make a buck in this world, I won't go too much into the specifics of various job possibilities—that's an entire book all by itself. However, I will talk about some of the more general concepts as they apply to an employee with ADHD. I'm going to assume that you have the skills to be successful at work (perhaps in a different job) and that the main problem is that your ADHD is preventing you from showing what you've got. Therefore, using the strategies related to time management, organization, remembering, relationship management, and so on in the rest of the book should take care of whatever is tripping you up on the job. So what's left are things related to finding a job that's a good fit for you and tweaking your job so you can perform your best.

This chapter contains the following articles:

Find a Job and Career That You Can Enjoy (p. 356) It's much easier to be happy at work if you're in the right job. This may involve a small change or a big change.

Career Counselors Can Help You Find the Right Job (p. 357) Some people find themselves in a job or career that isn't a great fit, but don't know what else to do. A career counselor can help you figure out what kinds of positions would better suit your abilities and interests. It's much easier to be happy and effective if you're in the right job.

Informal Accommodations Often Work Best (p. 358) It's pretty likely that your ADHD is affecting your work performance. You may want to approach your boss in an informal and collaborative way with requests that can make you a better employee.

Formal Accommodations Through the Americans with Disabilities Act (p. 361) There are times when you need to invoke your legal rights at work. This is usually best avoided, so you should know what you're getting yourself into.

Sometimes It's Better to Just Find a New Job (p. 364) For all sorts of reasons, you may find yourself in a job that just isn't working out. Therefore, you may be better served looking for something else.

Should You Work for Yourself? (p. 365) Rather than continue to work for someone else, you may find that you're happier starting your own business. This can be a great opportunity for the right people.

Find a Job and Career That You Can Enjoy

Work is a big part of adult life. It pays the bills and feeds the family, but it also takes up a big chunk of our week and can play a role in how we define ourselves. If you have ADHD, your work life is probably harder and less rewarding than it should be. Compared to the relatively few options for school, though, we tend to have many more options in the world of work—if you have trouble sitting still, you can get a job where you don't have to. If you're lucky enough to have a good assistant, then you don't need to worry as much about the boring and devilish details. As a result, many adults who weren't phenomenal students can be quite successful at work if they put themselves into the right situation. On the flip side, as adults we're held to higher standards than we are as kids, so coworkers and bosses may cut you less slack than your teachers did (well, some of them).

Sometimes a Small Change Is Enough

You may find that you enjoy your career and believe that you could be good at it, but that your current job isn't working out as well as you would hope. In these cases, you may just need to change to a different job in the same career. This may be as simple as a transfer to a different job with the same employer. Other times you may need to seek your fortunes elsewhere. For example, you may love the thrill of the chase of working as a salesman, but find that your current job hits too many of your weak points. I had a client who had been successful in sales until he took a job that involved selling giant products to giant companies—the sort of thing where the top sellers close only a handful of deals a year. This requires lots of follow-through and tons of details. Although he had some success with it, he had done better when the sales cycles were shorter so he could jump on a prospective client, make the sale (or not), and move on to the next. This gave him a bunch of sales per year, which inspired him to keep going for the next exciting sale. By contrast, in his current job, those sales were so far apart that he didn't get that adrenaline kick often enough and would spend a lot of time drifting between sales. It wasn't that he didn't have the necessary skills—his previous successes showed that he did—but rather that this particular job wasn't a great fit for his strengths.

Consider Your Options

It may be that you need a bigger change, such as a whole new career. People find themselves in jobs and careers for all sorts of reasons, some of which are pretty random and make for a bad fit. So if you're struggling in your job or career, you may want to think about how you got there and whether it's the best place for you. (Some readers will be pretty darn sure that their current situation definitely isn't.)

If you don't know what you want to do (but maybe know what you don't want to do), then you need to gather more information about what kinds of jobs are out there. My advice is to ask everyone you know about their job: What does a typical day look like? What do you like and hate about it? How did you get it? What are some related types of jobs? Don't be shy about asking—most people are happy to talk about themselves. Also don't worry that they may like different things than you would, because it's still worth hearing their experience. What you're looking to do is just to broaden your range of possibilities and to give yourself more options. This will perhaps give you some leads to explore further. Essentially what you're doing with this is an informal career interest inventory. (See the next article for more information about formal career assessments.)

Career Counselors Can Help You Find the Right Job

Some people are lucky enough to have a clear sense of what they want to do for work. Others aren't so lucky. Even if they have a good idea of what they want to do, adults with ADHD may still have a somewhat haphazard career path. They may not have a clear plan to follow or, even if they do, they may impulsively take a job that is good in some ways, but doesn't fit that plan—or maybe even their strengths and weaknesses. Perhaps more so than some other people, adults with ADHD need to find a job that is a good fit for them, since they are more vulnerable to performing below their abilities. Even if they are in the right career, they may be in the wrong job or working for the wrong boss, so they can't do their best.

If you don't know what you want to be when you grow up, whether you're twenty or fifty, a career counselor can help you narrow your options. This can save you a lot of wasted time, false starts, and dead ends, so it can be money well spent.

A thorough career assessment will help you find those better jobs or careers by evaluating your

- interests,
- strengths and skills,
- temperament and personality type,
- values and needs, and
- how your ADHD affects your work performance.

It's probably not worth going cheap on this, since a quick but superficial evaluation probably won't tell you anything that you don't already know. Worse yet, it may offer suggestions that are not a good fit for you. Most important, a career counselor needs to know how ADHD plays out in the workplace, since that may rule out some possible positions. Beyond potential careers or jobs to pursue, a knowledgeable career counselor can also give you good advice about other job-related factors to consider, such as the extent of self-starting that is required or how much paperwork is entailed. She may also include recommendations for reasonable accommodations to ask of employers, compensatory strategies you can use, and areas where additional training would be helpful.

If you're struggling in your current position, a career counselor may be able to identify precisely how your weaknesses are tripping you up, with the goal of applying that knowledge to help you perform better. It's almost always better to seek accommodations before the situation at work has reached a crisis and you're already halfway out the door. I talk about the legal matters of employment law (including whether to disclose your ADHD) in *Formal Accommodations Through the Americans with Disabilities Act* on p. 361, but you don't need to invoke the Americans with Disabilities Act to ask your boss for help.

Informal Accommodations Often Work Best

Most employees find that they do better at work with some small tweaks. Employees with ADHD may need bigger tweaks than some, but smaller than others. Of course, any employee will do best in a job that is a good match for his strengths, interests, and weaknesses, so finding the right job is kind of like the first and biggest accommodation. If you wind up in the wrong job, no amount of accommodations may be enough to make it a decent situation. (See *Sometimes It's Better to Just Find a New Job* on p. 364.)

Regardless of how much assistance you need, it's usually better if you're the one who seeks it out, rather than having it foisted on you by your boss. My advice is always to try first to seek out accommodations informally with your boss in a constructive and collaborative way, rather than with a sense of entitlement or legally. (I talk about the legal stuff in the next article, *Formal Accommodations Through the Americans with Disabilities Act.*) The sales pitch is that some relatively minor accommodations will enable you to do a better job, which ultimately benefits your boss, too. You might say something like, "I would get a lot more done if I wasn't sitting right next to the copier, since I get interrupted every few minutes when people use it." Of course, for your boss to go for your suggestions, she has to get back more than she gives, or it isn't worth it.

No matter how accommodating an employer may be, ultimately employees need to do most of the work to either improve their performance or find a job that's a better fit. Unless you're brilliant or irreplaceable and therefore have some leverage, you need to keep your requests for accommodations reasonable. This can include things like moving your desk, more frequent check-ins with a supervisor, a white noise machine to block distractions, some additional administrative support, or a PDA to assist with time management. If your employer isn't willing to pay for these accommodations, it may be worth paying for them yourself—if nothing else, it shows your commitment to the job and may spur your boss to do some other things. The Job Accommodations Network website (www.jan.wvu.edu) has a long list of reasonable and effective accommodations for ADHD, so you can get some ideas there.

As long as you're trying to resolve problems at work informally, you may not want to disclose to your boss that you have ADHD, as discussed in *To Tell or Not to Tell?* on p. 319. As I discussed there, I often recommend that people talk symptoms before diagnoses. That is, without saying that you have ADHD, talk about difficulties with time management or forgetfulness. You can always reveal your ADHD later if necessary, but you can't unsay it once it's said.

One potential danger of revealing your ADHD to a boss who isn't so enlightened is that he may then start unintentionally looking for certain behaviors that he hadn't noticed before. For example, if you tell him that you have trouble with distractibility, he may then notice every single time you appear to not be paying attention—even though you're not any more distractible now than you were before. Worse yet, if you are only a little more distractible than your coworkers, he may perceive you as being far more distractible. We tend to see what we look for—like when we buy a new car and notice how many other people are driving that car. There aren't more of them on the road—we just happen to notice them all. Think about how much to disclose, so that you don't inadvertently make the situation worse.

Keep in mind that using ADHD as an excuse after a reprimand for unacceptable performance is the absolute worst way to disclose the diagnosis. That shouldn't be the first time that your boss hears about it. In fact, all of these accommodations are best done when there is still a good working relationship and your boss is most willing to assist you.

Extra Training May Be Necessary

You may need to seek additional training to really be able to do your best at your current job. It may be as simple as a single meeting with your boss or a coworker to teach you a better way of doing something. Or maybe an online course, a book, a seminar, or even a formal college or graduate school class. It may even be in something indirectly related to your career, like a writing class or how to more effectively use a computer program. Your employer may pay for these and allow you to use work time or may feel that it is your responsibility to do on your time and your dime.

If your employer is unwilling to pay for these things, it becomes a question of how much this current job is worth to you and how much you feel that these additional skills will make you more marketable for the next job or a raise. It may be a worthy investment in your career if it allows you to move up to a better position, either in the same company or elsewhere.

Therefore, if you're thinking about using legal means to push your employer to grant you accommodations, it may be more worth your while to invest that time and money in improving your skills so that you can walk away to a new job with your head held high.

You May Want to Bring in a Professional

There may be times that it would be helpful to bring in a professional to talk to your employer, either by phone or in person. This could be a therapist, psychiatrist, or coach (lawyers are discussed next). Sometimes the same words will have more credibility if they come from someone else, especially someone who is seen as having some expertise in these matters. The professional should have not only a good understanding of ADHD in general, but also of your strengths, weaknesses, and job demands in particular. You may consider bringing in a professional when meeting with your boss to explain how ADHD affects your work performance and the rationale for the requested accommodations or change to a different job. Ideally it doesn't come to this, but you may have one of these professionals participate in a disciplinary meeting in an attempt to gain some understanding and leniency from your employer—and perhaps a better plan to prevent the problems from happening again.

If it isn't necessary or possible to get a professional to speak with your employer, she may able to write a letter on your behalf. Alternatively, if you've had psychological testing done, you could share a copy of the report. However, it's likely that the report contains far more information than your boss needs to know—some of it will be purely irrelevant, whereas some you may feel is too personal to share. In this case, the psychologist may be willing to write an abbreviated report containing only the information that is relevant to your job.

Formal Accommodations Through the Americans with Disabilities Act

Some employees find themselves in such a bad situation that it's worth consulting a lawyer. Unless you're looking to sue an employer over past misdeeds, it's hard to keep a job through legal means. Yes, it is possible to sue an employer to provide accommodations through the Americans with Disabilities Act (ADA) and the Rehabilitation Act, but this is by no means a done deal and is often hard to win. State and local laws may also apply, depending on where you live. Unlike school accommodations, which are relatively easy to get for those with a longstanding, documented disability, it's hard to force an employer to do something it won't do voluntarily. Besides, do you really want to work somewhere that had to be forced by a lawyer to create a conducive work environment? It's hard to imagine that the general tone of the workplace would get any better after that. In these cases, if you can't make something happen informally (as described in the preceding article), it may be best to just cut your losses and find another job.

However, if you're determined to fight for accommodations and are willing to go through the time, expense, loss of privacy, and headache of legal action, first take a moment to ask yourself these three questions:

- Is this a job that you really love, except for where your ADHD is interfering?
- Do you feel you could be successful with some minor modifications?
- Is this a job that isn't easily replaced?

If you can answer all three questions with a hearty yes, then it may be worth consulting a lawyer—specifically one who specializes in employment law. Don't let a burning need for justice (a.k.a., vengeance) cloud your judgment, because almost all of these cases are won by the employer, unless the employee was clearly being mistreated. You need to be on really solid ground before ever taking it to court. Some amendments to the ADA were passed in 2008 that may favor the employee more, but it probably still won't be easy. You should also remember that going through legal proceedings can take up a lot of time and mental energy and make public some things that you would prefer to keep private. You may get more traction instead by invoking your rights under ADA and using that to encourage your employer to work *with* you, rather than *against* you by getting lawyers involved.

Nonetheless, telling your employer that you're going to talk to a lawyer should be your absolute last resort—as soon as you let that out of the bag, your boss is likely to get nervous and contact human resources, who will get even more nervous. You then have fewer options for working things out informally because they will feel compelled to do everything by the book to cover their butts in case it goes to court. It's far better to work these things out informally and collaboratively, but sometimes you have no choice.

If you feel that you need some legal muscle to make things better, then it's best to speak with a lawyer early in the process, before things deteriorate too far and while you probably have more options. She may have some suggestions for you that don't involve making things contentious. You should definitely talk to a lawyer before disclosing that you have ADHD, because you can't take that back once you've said it. You should also talk to a lawyer before telling your employer that you're going to talk to a lawyer.

Walk the Tightrope

The ADA and Rehabilitation Acts prevent discrimination against people with disabilities, which includes ADHD. However, if that disability can be remediated through medication or various devices, then it may not count as a disability. If it can't be, the employer is required to provide reasonable accommodations to enable the person to do the job. This could include moving the person's desk to a quieter corner of the office or providing more frequent meetings with a supervisor to ensure that the employee is on track with her projects. Or, as one of my clients discovered after the office was rearranged, she was less distracted when she sat under the heating and cooling vent because it blocked a lot of the extraneous noise, so she asked to be moved back. Providing a PDA may qualify as a reasonable accommodation, whereas hiring an administrative assistant (even part time) might not.

The line to walk is that the person must be disabled but otherwise qualified to do the job. In other words, someone who uses a wheelchair can't be discriminated against for a desk job, but could be denied a job as a firefighter. This creates a very narrow band of people who qualify for legal protection—the disability needs to cause enough impairment to warrant accommodations, but can't cause so much impairment that he can't do the job. So getting the person in the wheelchair a new desk is seen as a reasonable accommodation because the person is otherwise capable of performing the job duties, and a new desk is a relatively minor cost and inconvenience for the employer.

The implications of this band being so narrow is that employers can disqualify employees from both sides. From one side, they can say that the disability isn't sufficient to justify any accommodations at all. From the other, they can say either that the disability is so limiting that the costs of accommodations would be excessive or that the person isn't otherwise capable of performing the basic duties of the job. If you do ask for accommodations, you're on the safest ground if it's mostly around nonessential features of the job—for example, assistance with scheduling meetings with clients, but not with the core job duty of actually interacting with clients. Examples could include modified work schedules, physical changes to the workplace, modification of a workplace policy, adjusting supervisory methods, and job coaches (Latham and Latham, 2002).

If you're going to seek accommodations by invoking the ADA or its state or local equivalents, you'll probably get the best response from your employer if you've proven yourself a capable and desirable employee first—that is, someone they would want to keep and are willing to go out of their way a bit for. The way to get the absolute worst response is to wait until you've dug yourself a giant hole and are half a step toward being fired—it may not be official yet, but your boss has probably made up her mind about you and is now just waiting to document enough to get rid of you. So grab the bull by the horns and start this whole process early, when there's still good will on both your parts.

The Job Accommodations Network website (www.jan.wvu.edu) has a comprehensive list of reasonable and effective accommodations for a variety of disabilities, including ADHD. It would probably be beneficial to review the list of possible accommodations before even talking to your employer, to create a short list of requests. The more specific you can be, the less your boss will worry that you're going to ask for everything under the sun. You may also want to share this website with your boss, so she can see examples of common accommodations.

Documenting a Disability

In order to get accommodations, you need to first prove that you need them. This involves an evaluation and report by an appropriate professional. You may have had psychological testing as a student, but that report probably won't quite suffice for a job-related case. A letter from one of your current treatment providers will almost certainly not be enough either. It's really important to get an evaluation that meets the requirements *exactly* so that your employer's lawyer can't get the report thrown out. You will want to work with an evaluator who has experience doing specifically ADA employment evaluations. Your lawyer may be able to give you some names of locals who do a good job.

These evaluations are probably fairly expensive (up to several thousand dollars), since they need to be thorough and that means quite a bit of time by a trained professional. This will come out of your pocket, so you need to make a judgment call as to whether it is a worthwhile investment.

One risk of applying for accommodations is that it opens up your full medical record to your employer and its lawyers. They will want to know the full extent of your disability and have the right to see if there is anything else in there to justify their not offering accommodations. Although you may not feel that the rest of your medical history is relevant, your employer will seek full access so that it can make its own legal case. Therefore, you will need to convince the judge that certain parts of your record are not relevant.

The bottom line is this—I'm clearly not a fan of getting lawyers involved to solve these sorts of disputes. Sometimes it's your best option, in which case I wish you the best of luck. However, I hope that you go into this fully informed of what to expect, including both the best-case scenario of how it could work out as well as what your risks are. Things may not always work out the way that we want, but I don't think anyone can fault you if you made a reasonable decision based on complete information.

Sometimes It's Better to Just Find a New Job

Whether you fell into a job that used to be OK but not great or you sought a job that used to be rewarding but now isn't, you may find yourself wanting something more. Unfortunately, some people are determined to keep their job, even when it isn't a good fit for their strengths, weaknesses, and interests. I admire their tenacity in many ways, but would also wish something better for them. Persistence is admirable, but stubbornness isn't. The trick is knowing where one ends and the other begins. So let's talk about some of the many reasons why you might feel compelled to stay with a job that isn't working out well and what you can do about it.

- *A sense of loyalty.* I admire those who feel loyal to their employer, coworkers, and customers. There are times, though, that this commitment can prevent someone from making a change for the better. So don't forget your commitment to yourself and your own happiness.
- *A need to prove someone wrong.* Some people are unwilling to give up because that would be perceived as failure or an admission of not being able to handle the job. The target of this pride could be a boss, coworker, or someone outside of work. I certainly have my own share of stubbornness, so I can relate to this, but it's really just not a good enough reason to stay in a job. Moving to a job that is a better fit is a sign of wisdom, which I think trumps admitting that this current job isn't the best for you. It's far wiser to admit it and move on to something better than to continue to suffer just to prevent someone from saying "I told you so."

- *Perceived lack of other options.* Those who spent most of their lives undiagnosed may be pessimistic about their abilities and believe that they couldn't get hired anywhere else, so there's no point even looking. If you truly do a thorough job search and find nothing available at that time, then so be it, but until you really take a look, I'm hesitant to give up hope.
- *Sense of hopelessness of finding a job that's any better.* Related to the last point, some adults with ADHD may feel as if there's no reason to look for a better job because all of their jobs have been bad, so there's no reason to expect any better on the next one. I would counter that the combination of a well-informed job search and getting their ADHD treated can change their odds of finding a job that they can enjoy more.
- *Lack of time to look for anything better.* Many people can't afford to be without a job while looking for another one, yet don't feel that they have any time to look while they're still employed. This is quite a catch-22. This is also a great incentive to really work on your time management skills and find ways to be more efficient, so that you have more time each week to job hunt. Getting on top of your ADHD should help with this. You may also need to look at your schedule for the coming months and forgo some activities so that you can invest that time into your job search.

Should You Work for Yourself?

Working for yourself can be a great option for some people. In fact, adults with ADHD are three times more likely to be self-employed owners of small businesses than people without ADHD (Young, 2000). Should you start your own business? It depends on what your goals are and how you think you would handle the freedom and responsibility. As much as working for yourself can bring some fantastic opportunities, it also requires more skills and diligence than working for someone else. This is because you need to not only be good at whatever your trade is (business consulting, plumbing, computer repair, psychology, whatever) but also capable of managing the details of running a business (or be smart and lucky enough to hire someone who can do it for you). You also need to be a self-starter since there's no boss to get on your case for showing up late and not getting anything done.

There are many reasons why someone with ADHD might start his own business, including

- desire for independence,
- desire for greater income (and tolerance for greater risk),
- seeing a golden opportunity,
- being tired of working for someone else,
- feeling impatient with the slow process of climbing up the ranks, and
- feeling limited by not having certain academic credentials.

If a number of these apply to you, you may want to consider it. However, keep in mind that it usually takes a lot of work up front to get a business going and that your income will probably take time to grow. Therefore, you have to have both the time and willingness to put in those hours, as well as another source of money to pay the bills until the business turns a profit. So you may want to keep your day job and do as much as possible during nights and weekends before taking the plunge.

The Small Business Administration is federally funded and offers tons and tons of resources for those starting or running a small business. They have a lot of good information on their website, www.sba.gov, as well as local offices, where you can speak with their staff in person. They also offer grants and low-interest loans. If you're considering starting a business, spending some time with the SBA can help you decide whether you should proceed and also help you prevent a lot of common problems. It's an investment that's well worth your time—especially since all of their services are free.

Epilogue: The Suffering of ADHD

I'm tired of people crying in my office—young kids, full-grown adults. I'm tired of hearing about the lifetime of pain and suffering that these people have endured before finally being diagnosed with ADHD. My heart goes out to them each and every time. And each and every time I ask myself why it had to get this bad. Why are there still so many people suffering, when there is so much that we can do to improve their functioning and improve their lives?

As much as many people still think of ADHD as a kid thing, it's the adults who have suffered the most, especially the ones who were born before 1975. They're the ones who went through school before most people really knew about ADHD. Instead their troubles were explained away with labels like lazy, unmotivated, bad attitude, and troublemaker. It's hard to feel good about any of those. Ironically, some of the kids who wanted to do well but had trouble doing so gradually started buying into those explanations. They just squeaked by or maybe gave up completely. So eventually those explanations actually became accurate. But without ADHD as an explanation for these difficulties, the explanations you're left with all eat away at motivation to do better. So life creeps along, from one potential disaster to the next.

Most of the time, when I tell someone that she has ADHD, she and her family members are incredibly relieved. Finally they have an answer for her struggles that doesn't come across as judgmental or inherently critical. Much of the therapy that I do with newly diagnosed ADHD folks involves educating them about ADHD and dispelling some of the ideas about themselves that they had gotten before they knew about ADHD-in other words, rewriting the lessons learned from a life of excessive struggle.

This is why I wrote this book and why I present on ADHD—to try to share information that is both scientifically accurate and also completely practical. I try to educate members of the public and also the professionals who treat them. I make time in my jam-packed schedule because I know that for every person crying in my office, there are a hundred who aren't crying in anyone's office.

Whether you found out about your ADHD at age eight or eighty, you have the ability to make a good life for yourself. The ball's in your court. Run with it.

APPENDIX: RESOURCES

More and more good information is available these days on ADHD in adults. This appendix is by no means a definitive list—new items come and old items go—but it's a good start. I don't want to overwhelm you with too many things that you will then feel compelled to check out (and feel guilty if you don't). So I've limited this to some of the best.

Nonprofit Organizations

There are a number of nonprofit ADHD information and advocacy organizations, with ADDA and CHADD being the biggest. I encourage you to join them both. You'll get your money's worth in valuable information and opportunities, as well as supporting their efforts to provide awareness and advocacy.

ADDA

ADDA stands for the Attention Deficit Disorder Association. ADDA is focused exclusively on adults with ADHD. The organization puts out a monthly email newsletter, offers teleclasses on various ADHD-related topics, and has a national conference. You can find more information at www.add.org.

CHADD

CHADD stands for Children and Adults with Attention Deficit/Hyperactivity Disorder, so it covers the full age range. CHADD has approximately two hundred local chapters that hold monthly meetings, offer a local provider directory, and may have other services as well. CHADD puts on a large annual conference, publishes the bimonthly magazine *Attention*, and offers other services to individuals and families with ADHD. You can find more information at at www.chadd.org.

ADD Resources

ADD Resources is a smaller organization than ADDA or CHADD, but still does good work, including teleclasses on various ADHD-related topics. You can find more information at www.addresources.org.

Websites

There are lots of websites out there about ADHD. Some are great, whereas others are just plain ridiculous, so use your judgment if something sounds too good to be true or if it seems to be trying to scare you into something. Here's my short list of favorite sites for information and products for adults with ADHD.

- **www.add.org** ADDA's website has lots of information, especially for members.

- **www.chadd.org** CHADD's website has lots of information, especially for members.
- **www.addresources.org** Lots of good information, especially for members.
- **www.additudemag.com** ADDitude Magazine also has an extensive website.
- **www.addwarehouse.com** Provides an extensive list of books on ADHD and related disorders, plus some other items. If it's relevant to ADHD, you'll find it here.
- **www.myadhd.com** Offers a free monthly teleclass and biweekly email newsletter.
- **www.addvance.com** Initially focused solely on the otherwise under-represented women and girls with ADHD, this site has expanded to both genders.
- **www.addconsults.com** Offers a wide range of resources, including articles, online chats, monthly email newsletter, and books and other ADHD-related items for purchase.
- **www.addclasses.com** Offers teleclasses on a variety of ADHD-related topics, the ADD Book Club, and coaching programs.
- **www.addforums.com** An online community where you can post questions and comments.

Professional Directories to Find Qualified Clinicians

It can be a real challenge to find a professional in your area who really understands ADHD in adults. I regularly receive emails from people desperate enough to take a chance that I might know someone in their area, a thousand miles away from where I am. I refer them to the professional directories on the following websites. There's no guarantee that the people listed are any good, but at least you know that they say they have some skill in working with ADHD adults. So you will need to feel them out, but at least you have somewhere to start.

- www.add.org
- www.chadd.org
- www.addresources.org
- www.addconsults.com
- www.psychologytoday.com

Publications

In addition to the growing number of books and websites on adult ADHD, there are other publications that you and your family members may find useful.

Magazines

ADDitude is devoted to living well with ADHD and learning disabilities and offers practical articles with coping strategies and new information. More information is available at www.additudemag.com.

Email Newsletters

Lots of websites offer free email newsletters that are full of useful strategies and good information. You may want to limit how many you sign up for at a time, just so you don't get flooded with more emails than you have time to read. Here are some of the better ones:

- www.add.org
- www.myadhd.com
- www.helpforadd.com (Attention Research Update)
- www.additudemag.com
- www.addconsults.com
- www.addvance.com

Teleclasses and Webinars

Teleclasses are a great way to learn about ADHD and hear presenters from around the country who you probably would never see in person. It's basically a presentation done as a conference call. Everybody calls a certain phone number at the designated time and listens as the presenter(s) talks. Depending on the size of the group, there may be discussion and questions. Many of these teleclasses are moving online, often called webinars (i.e., web seminars). This way you can watch as the presenter clicks through the slides. Because there is no travel involved, it can be much more convenient. Many of these are free. Recordings are often available afterward, sometimes for a small fee or for members. Here is a sampling of the best teleclass providers:

- www.add.org
- www.addclasses.com
- www.addvisor.com
- www.addresources.org
- www.adhdconference.com

You may also find it helpful to subscribe to my free weekly podcast at: www.adultADHDbook.com to reinforce your reading.

References

Barkley, R.A. (2006a). Etiologies. In R.A. Barkley (Ed.). *Attention-deficit hyperactivity disorder, 3rd ed.* (pp. 219-247). New York: Guilford Press.

Barkley, R.A. (2006b). Comorbid disorders, social and family adjustment, and subtyping. In R.A. Barkley (Ed). *Attention-deficit hyperactivity disorder, 3rd ed.* (pp. 184-218). New York: Guilford Press.

Barkley, R.A. (2006c). ADHD in adults: Developmental course and outcome of children with ADHD, and ADHD in clinic-referred adults. In R.A. Barkley (Ed). *Attention-deficit hyperactivity disorder, 3rd ed.* (pp. 248-296). New York: Guilford Press.

Barkley, R.A., Fischer, M., Smallish, L, & Fletcher, K. (2003). Does the treatment of attention-deficit/hyperactivity disorder with stimulants contribute to drug use/abuse? A 13-year prospective study. *Pediatrics, 111*, 97-109.

Barkley, R. A. & Gordon, M. (2002). Research on comorbidity, adaptive functioning, and cognitive impairments in adults with ADHD: Implications for a clinical practice. In S. Goldstein & A.T. Ellison (Eds.), *Clinician's guide to adult ADHD: Assessment and intervention* (pp. 43-69). San Diego: Academic Press.

Barkley, R.A., Murphy, K. & Fischer, M. (2007) *ADHD in adults: What the science says*. New York: Guilford Press.

Biederman, J., Spencer, T.J., Wilens, T.E., Prince, J.B., & Faraone, S.V. (2006). Treatment of ADHD with stimulant medications: Response to Nissen perspective in The New England Journal of Medicine. *Journal of the American Academy of Child & Adolescent Psychiatry, 45* (10), 1-4.

Brown, T.E. (1995). Differential diagnosis of ADD versus ADHD in adults. In K. Nadeau (Ed.). *A comprehensive guide to attention deficit disorder in adults* (pp. 93-108). New York: Bruner Mazel.

Brown, T.E. (2005). *Attention deficit disorder: The unfocused mind in children and adults*. New Haven, CT: Yale University Press.

Connor, D.F. (2006). Stimulants. In R.A. Barkley (Ed). *Attention-deficit hyperactivity disorder, 3rd ed.* (pp. 608-647). New York: Guilford Press.

Crawford, R. & Crawford, V. (2002). Career impact: Finding the key issues facing adults with ADHD. In S. Goldstein & A.T. Ellison (Eds.), *Clinician's guide to adult ADHD: Assessment and intervention* (pp. 187-204s). San Diego: Academic Press.

Ellison, A.T. (2002). An overview of childhood and adolescent ADHD: Understanding the complexities of development into the adult years. In S. Goldstein & A.T. Ellison (Eds.), *Clinician's guide to adult ADHD: Assessment and intervention* (pp. 1-23). San Diego: Academic Press.

Goldstein, S. (2002). Continuity of ADHD in adulthood: Hypothesis and theory meet reality. In S. Goldstein & A.T. Ellison (Eds.), *Clinician's guide to adult ADHD: Assessment and intervention* (pp. 25-42). San Diego: Academic Press.

Goldstein, S. (2006, October). Advanced interventions for AD/HD. Seminar at 18th annual CHADD International Conference, Chicago.

Ingersoll, B. (2006, October). Complementary treatments. Seminar at 18th annual CHADD International Conference, Chicago.

Latham, P.S. & Latham, P.H. (2002). What clinicians need to know about legal issues relevant to ADHD. In S. Goldstein & A.T. Ellison (Eds.), *Clinician's guide to adult ADHD: Assessment and intervention* (pp. 205-218). San Diego: Academic Press.

Nadeau, K.G. (1995). Life management skills for the adult with ADD. In K. Nadeau (Ed.). *A comprehensive guide to attention deficit disorder in adults* (pp.191-217). New York: Bruner Mazel.

Nadeau, K.G. (2002). The clinician's role in the treatment of ADHD. In S. Goldstein & A.T. Ellison (Eds.), *Clinician's guide to adult ADHD: Assessment and intervention* (pp. 107-127). San Diego: Academic Press.

Prince, J.B., Wilens, T.E., Spencer, T.J., & Biederman, J. (2006). Pharmacotherapy of ADHD in adults. In R.A. Barkley (Ed.), *Attention-deficit hyperactivity disorder, 3rd ed.* (pp. 3-75). New York: Guilford Press.

Ramsay, J.R. & Rostain, A.L. (2007). Psychosocial treatments for ADHD in adults: Current evidence and future directions. *Professional Psychology: Research and Practice, 38*, 338-346.

Rostain, A.L. & Ramsay, J.R. (2006). Adult with ADHD? Try medication + psychotherapy. *Current Psychiatry, 5* (2), 13-16, 21-24, 27.

Schnarch, D. (1997). *Passionate marriage: Keeping love & intimacy alive in committed relationships*. New York: Holt.

U.S. Census Bureau. (February 26, 2007). Census 2000, Summary File 1; generated by Ari Tuckman; using American FactFinder; http://factfinder.census.gov.

Wilens, T. (2004). Impact of ADHD and its treatment on substance abuse in adults. *Journal of Clinical Psychiatry, 65*, 38-45.

Wilens, T.E., Zusman, R.M., Hammerness, P.G., Podolski, A., Whitley, J., Spencer, T.J., Gignac, M., & Biederman, J. (2006). An open-label study of the tolerability of mixed amphetamine salts in adults with attention-deficit/hyperactivity disorder and treated primary essential hypertension. *Journal of Clinical Psychiatry, 67*, 696-702.

Young, S. (2000). ADHD children grown up: An empirical review. *Counselling Psychology Quarterly, 13*, 191-200.

Index

A

E

F

M

N

O

P

T

V

W